# Unleash
*Your*
# Vitality™

## 8 SIMPLE STEPS TO
## MAXIMIZE YOUR HEALTH
## WITH NUTRITION

# ROB VAN OVERBRUGGEN PH.D

## AUTHOR OF "HEALING PSYCHE"

## Unleash your Vitality™
## Copyright © 2015 by Rob van Overbruggen
## Version 2015.1

Ordering Information:
This title is available at special quantity discounts for bulk purchases for sales promotions, premiums, fundraising and educational use. Special versions or book excerpts can also be created to fit specific needs.

### For details, contact our office at:
### office@helpforhealth.com

# Word-of-mouth is CRUCIAL
# for any author to succeed.

If you enjoyed this book then please let us know *WHAT you LIKED and WHY* so we can give you more of that. If you didn't please tell us WHO this book is more suited for.

Leave your review at amazon, even if it's only a line or two. Other people will be grateful for your insights too.

Thank you for this, your review is a **huge help** !"

**Click to review:**
**Amazon USA :** http://gnoo.net/uva_us
**Amazon UK :** http://gnoo.net/uva_uk

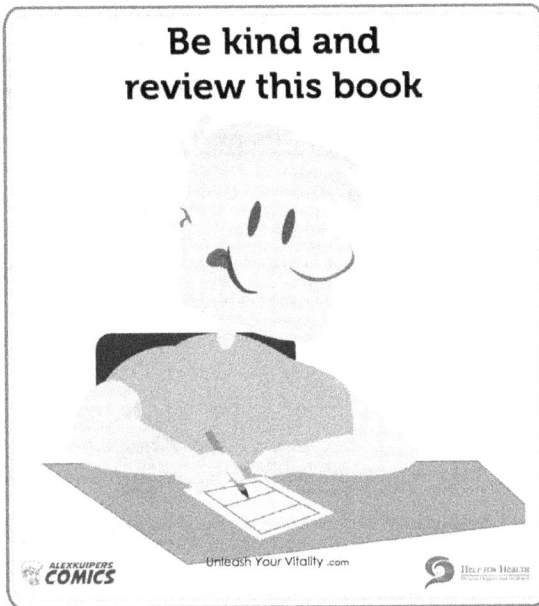

Be kind and
review this book

Download the special resource pack with additional chapters, exercises, checklists, whitepapers and other cool stuff.

Click here to access your resource pack
(http://www.unleashyourvitality.com/resource)

*If reading on e-reader, tablets, phones or computers you need it for the exercises*

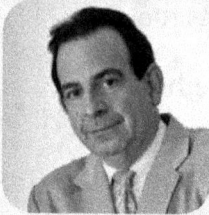

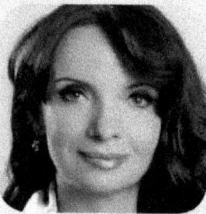

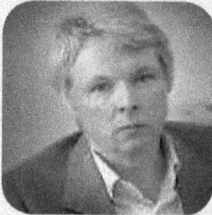

Dinner is destiny, per lifestyle medicine expert David Katz. If you want to **upgrade your destiny**, dive into Dr. van Overbruggen's fabulous book titled the "Unleash Your Vitality™ - 8 Simple Steps to Maximize Your Health (with Nutrition)".

Every cell in the human body needs a complex set of nutrients to perform at its best. This book is an **engaging** and thorough reference and summary of the contribution to nutrients for human thriving.

*Margaret Moore/Coach Meg, MBA*
*Founder & CEO, Wellcoaches Corporation*
*Co-Founder & Co-Director, Institute of Coaching,*
*McLean Hospital, a Harvard Medical School affiliate*

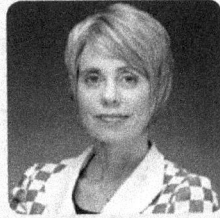

---

I've now read parts of your new book and I can see that I will love the words of wisdom here as much as I did Healing Psyche, the other of your books I read. Your intelligent approach to the facts, told in such simple and yet elegant prose, is sure to bring the audience "to use the book" which you define as an '*action book*'. I applaud you for your work and appreciate your voice being added to this important conversation

*Ann Fonfa*
*founder of Annie Appleseed Project*
*Alternative and natural approaches to cancer*

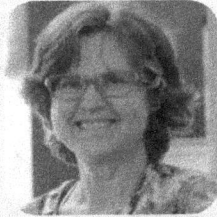

---

Thank you very much. It is **exceptionally good**, especially the tables, flow charts and **assessment** sheets. They were user friendly and scientific. I also like your principle in empowering people to heal themselves. Congratulations

*Hanan Marie, MD*
*Gynecologist, Halifax, United Kingdom*

Unleash Your Vitality™ - 8 Simple Steps to Maximize Your Health (with Nutrition) brilliantly present a new map for **understanding and treating disease** based on principles of functional nutrition. It is an ecological view of the body where all the networks of our system interact in a dynamic process that creates dis-ease when out of balance and promotes health when in balance.

This book accurately frames the transformational awakening in science towards a paradigm shift from medicine by cause to medicine by symptoms. As an integrative and functional medicine practitioner, I feel strongly that we are on a verge of a true transformation in medicine.

Unleash Your Vitality™ contributes to spreading the knowledge of what creates health. It engages the reader in the concepts of what restores balance by getting to the root of the symptoms.

Rather that promoting a pharmaceutical symptomatic intervention, the books illustrates what primarily causes dis-ease and what nutrients are able tore store balance in dose-dependent manner.

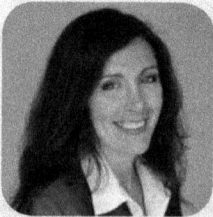

The time is certainly ripe for a radical transformation in health: *Unleash Your Vitality™ clearly offers all the tools for this change to occur.*

**Manuela Boyle PhD ND**
*manuelaboyle.com.au*

Unleash Your Vitality™ *hits the bull's-eye* for all those seeking an answer to good vitality, with inside information that is rare. There are plenty of books out there with information on how to live, but this is a book *I wish I had at my start of my career*, 33 years ago when I was building my interest in orthomolecular medicine. This book is innovative, no-nonsense, packed with up-to-date information and with literature references. It shows that there really are ways to improve your health: *those who want to make effort can reach out and change their lives*.

As an orthomolecular educator for many years, and also a orthomolecular therapist I can recommend this book as a genuine start for those who are interested in orthomolecular medicine and healthy living. It is not only for people with existing diseases, but especially for people who want to prevent disease.

*Go for it! Live to the max! naturally and responsibly.*

### Jan Blaauw
*Director and founder of Ortho Linea,*
*one of the leading institutes in orthomolecular health*
*www.ortholinea.nl / www.praktijkblaauw.nl*

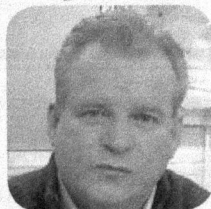

---

A clear and practical book. With lots of information about nutrition, which not only remains information, *but is also directly practically applicable*.

Rob says it is a book about nutrition, but it goes beyond just food. Because knowing a lot about nutrition is one, but what does it do with my body? That's the question. And the answers are in the book, when you work it trough.

'*Optimal nutrition for optimal vitality*' is sure true and to achieve with this book.

### Trudy Vlot, MD
*Integrative Medicine by clinical PNI*

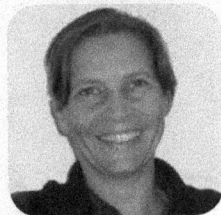

Food and the way we produce and consume it, is the nexus of most of our world's health, environmental, climate, economic and even political crises.

As a doctor, it is my job to figure out the best way to keep my patients healthy. *Food is medicine, the most powerful drug* on the planet with the power to cause or cure most disease.

Rob talked about facts that amazed even me. You'll enjoy your reading journey from the start till the end with *up-to-date, evidenced based information that will transform your life.*

I would like to express my sincere gratitude to Rob van Overbruggen and to take this opportunity to let you know how much I respect and admire you as a dedicated professional.

### Laila Moustafa Kamel MD
*Vice President of the Egyptian Nutrition and Health Coaching Association*

---

I love this book! Being an avid follower of all things health related I was delighted when this gem came my way. Having experienced amazing personal life-changing success for myself, and my family with nutritional healing through diet modification and supplementation, I became joyful and content as a side effect. I would like these feelings to become contagious!

Rob van Overbruggen's idea of making this into a practical workbook particularly appealed to me and also helped kick-start me into raising my game and being even more proactive.

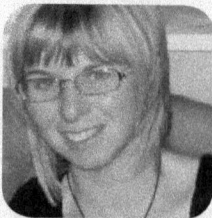

*Don't dig your grave with your knife and fork! Follow Rob van Overbruggen's advice and watch the magic unfold...*

### Jo Trewartha
*(Health and Wellness Facilitator)*
*freeyourmindsolutions.com*

Dear, dear Rob, Believe it or not, only today I could stay and have a look on your great masterpiece!

I can't believe that you have provided such guidance, in my opinion, such a book should take you a lifetime.......but instead, *it is for a lifetime*!

Congratulations, it will take time for me to follow all the steps, and I am sure many of my students and healthcare professionals who interact with, will take advantage of this valuable guide. Actually it's so great to share your incommensurable experience and knowledge.......

I am sure the few words that I have send to you cannot express my "wow" for your expertise and all you have done for all mankind. You are really great!!!!!!!!!

I am really impressed with your last volume, it's amazing...........it's extremely organized and helpful......it's wonderful, I am sure we will translate it for other people, it's a must, thank God for people like you.

I am so grateful,

*Professor Hab. Liliana Foia M.D.*

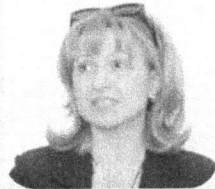

A *comprehensive, cogent guide* and workbook on salutogenesis: a focus on health creation and self-efficacy in a soon-to-be bygone era of disease care.

*Glenn Sabin*
*Author of forthcoming n of 1: How one Man's Triumph over Terminal Cancer is Changing the Medical Establishment*
*Director, FON Consulting*

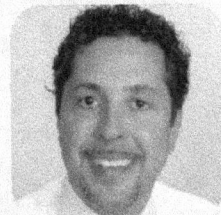

The book came at the perfect moment, when I had already committed to honoring my physical body more, in order that I can live a long and healthy life. Unleash Your Vitality™ - 8 Simple Steps to Maximize Your Health (with Nutrition) *gives me the tools to do just that*, by providing great insight into health and wellness through the medium of diet and supplementation.

As a mind: body: spirit based therapist, using Meta Health, EFT and Matrix Reimprinting, I have worked with the emotional connection between health and disease to great effect, supporting myself and others to release diverse symptoms and to feel better. I began to look for solutions to improve my personal vitality through what I put into my body on an ongoing basis - nutrition - the building blocks of life.

The book explains in simple terms what happened to our food and water, and how to achieve nutritional balance, with the promise of feeling great!

The material is presented in a readable fun way, distilling complex messages into easily digestible bite-size chunks.

I like the tests and supportive (quite firm) guidance to enable you to get from where you are now to your desired health goal.

I was already negotiating the supplement minefield, so the information in *this book has taken the stress out of making healthy choices*.

I decided to use the supplements suggested in the book and I am *already feeling the benefits*. So much so, that I have decided to be a coach, *sharing the information with others*. In this process I will learn even more and support others to achieve their vibrant vitality too.

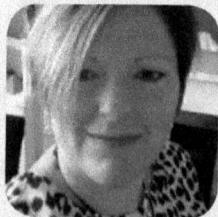

*Feeling great and grateful!*

**Sarah Ridout**
*positivelifezone.com*

# *Table of Contents*

## 8.   CALL TO ACTION - ARE YOU REALLY READY? ..................... 281

## 9.   BECAUSE YOU'RE WORTH IT - HOW TO SELECT THE BEST OF THE BEST..... 289

# 14.  YOUR USEFUL RESOURCE PACK ... 369

# 15.  RECOMMENDED READING ........... 375

# 16.  COMMONLY ASKED QUESTIONS .. 377

# 17.  REFERENCES ..................................... 385

# 18.  SYMTPOM INDEX ........................... 421

# 19.  MEET THE AUTHOR ....................... 431

# Exercises

# Insights and Actions

# *Overview of your actions*

Write down **WHEN** you are going to implement **WHAT** action and **WHY** do you want that. What is your motivation to do that action, what results do you want to achieve.

This will help you complete your mission towards unleashing your vitality

Write down these components while working through this book.

Cross them out once you have completed them.

If you need more room download the sheet from the resourcepack from: http://www.UnleashYourVitality.com/resource

| WHEN | WHAT | WHY |
|---|---|---|
| | | |
| | | |
| | | |
| | | |
| | | |
| | | |
| | | |
| | | |

NOTES

# Glorious Food
## that extra bit more that's all we live for

Until recently I had no knowledge whatsoever about food. For me, food was the stuff that I shoved into my mouth until my stomach was full. Depending on the location or situation I was in, my diet consisted of snacks, vegetables, potatoes, meat, fried foods: almost whatever I liked and got my hands on.

> *"To eat is a necessity, but to eat intelligently is an art."*
> ~ *La Rochefoucauld*

Having spent many years' working professionally and studying health and wellbeing my predominant focus was on emotions, beliefs and their relationship to health. All my trainings and events revolved around the effect of emotions and beliefs on health and how to change that. My first book "Healing Psyche" explains in depth the relationship of emotions, beliefs and the progression or remission of cancer.

When I started researching into food, vitamins and minerals I was amazed how much scientific research was available: research I believe will turn your life around. Many allopathic doctors do not yet recognize the vast amount of research that is available about the effects of food and dietary choices have on diseases.

During my research I became convinced that taking my daily vitamins, minerals and other supplements was a necessity to stay healthy. The next challenge was to find the right ones. This painstaking journey of trial and error took quite some time to complete.

My goal in writing this book is to raise your personal awareness, helping you make more conscious and informed choices about what you decide to put into your own mouth and body; thus offering you opportunity to maximize your health in 8 simple steps. I am sharing my findings so that you can avoid the pitfalls I experienced and make profound changes easily and rapidly.

## 1.1    Zest ! Sparkle!, Zing!, Oomph ! Vigor and Vivacity! The Vitality Model

This book is about nutrition and health. One thing we all know is that nutrition and stress influence your health levels. For me this has always been difficult to understand. I studied beliefs, emotions and health for many years and I have seen the transformational changes in people's health when working on their stress levels. On the other hand I saw people change their nutritional patterns and they too had transformational changes in their health. How is that possible?

I struggled with these apparently conflicting elements how could both stress and nutrition influence health. How is it possible that someone who has tremendous levels of stress does not get sick? How is it possible that someone with a very poor nutritional diet does not get sick?

On the other hand, I have seen people with low stress levels get sick and I have seen people with an apparently healthy diet get sick. I knew both stress and nutrition has an effect on health, but I could not explain the interaction between stress and nutrition. I was looking for a kind of "theory of everything" related to health.

These questions have been running around in my mind for some time now.

I tried out many different models and explanations and none of them really were hitting the mark, until I was explaining to someone the value of nutrition and there was suddenly an epiphany of a new vitality model. This model explains very easily how health, vitality, stress, nutrition and many other elements work together.

**Searching The Theory of Everything**

Instead of focusing on disease, on what caused it and how to prevent it, I am now looking at it differently. I started looking into what causes health.

When you think of it, health and vitality are normal states of being. Look at a child, in most cases they are born in perfect health and not with diseases that need to be fixed. This vitality, (also referred to as life force, life energy, qi) is omnipresent in the baby and child. However as we grow older, the more this vitality tends to disappear. Why does it disappear and how can we get it back? What is vitality and how does stress and nutrition play a role?

### Vitality Levels

When your vitality is high you have plenty of energy, you feel great and you are not limited by your physical body. You spend your day in excitement and joy. You have enough vitality in your 'vitality pool'.

When your vitality drops a little, you might start to feel some minor discomfort, like lack of energy, fatigue, sometimes a little headache, some minor discomforts, but nothing really serious. At the end of the day you may feel tired and exhausted. You have just enough vitality in your 'vitality pool' for the day.

Should your vitality levels drop even further, more obvious physical symptoms develop. Maybe a skin issue, ongoing fatigue, digestive problems, elevated blood pressure or maybe high cholesterol levels or even a light anxiety or increased worries may develop. You find yourself becoming more susceptible to stressors and small frustrations. Your 'vitality pool' is below acceptable levels.

**Low levels in your Vitality Pool leads to disease**

If your vitality drops plummets from this point, diseases will develop. This might be a chronic disease like irritable bowel disorder, heart disease, or even cancer. You are easily stressed and maybe have some emotional outbursts. Your 'vitality pool' is at a dramatic low, action is needed immediately.

By this point if nothing is done to remedy the situation and vitality drops continues to drop even further, your 'vitality pool' will be empty and then all the life force will go and life will end

### Vitality points

Everything we eat, do or think has vitality points. Some things have very high points, others have lower points, others even have small or large negative points. All these points influence your vitality. Positive points raise your vitality; negative points reduce your vitality.

Eating, doing, thinking something that has negative points is not good or bad; it depends on your total vitality levels.

When you eat fast food (which gives negative vitality points), your total vitality will drop a little because the fast food drains vitality out your system. This is not bad in and of itself. If you eat fast food every day, there will be lots of vitality draining from your system. If you are highly stressed, the stress drains out from your vitality pool. If you are worried a lot, vitality is draining out. If you live in a toxic environment, vitality is draining out. None of these have to be a problem, as long as there is not too much draining and enough vitality is refilled.

Getting a good night's sleep will increase your vitality, having proper food will increase your vitality. Relaxation increases your vitality. Drinking clean water increases your vitality.

Your main concern should be to keep your vitality levels as high as possible. When you have a high vitality level, and you eat fried foods, nothing will happen to damage your health. However, when your entire vitality is low, and you eat the same foods, your stomach might be upset or symptoms or diseases might develop.

If your vitality level is high and you experience a major stressor, you can cope with it easily. However, if your vitality level is low, and you experience the same stressor, then you develop symptoms or diseases.

In order to unleash your vitality potential, you only need to follow 3 simple steps:

1. *Remove existing vitality drains*

2. *Prevent new vitality drains*

3. *Add more vitality boosters*

It is imperative to work with all three simultaneously every day to gain and keep optimal health.

Just removing the existing drains will not be sufficient if new drains arrive. Just adding vitality boosters does not work if there are many drains.

So it is not a bad thing if you eat, do or think something that reduces your vitality, as long as you know what you can do to prevent further damage.

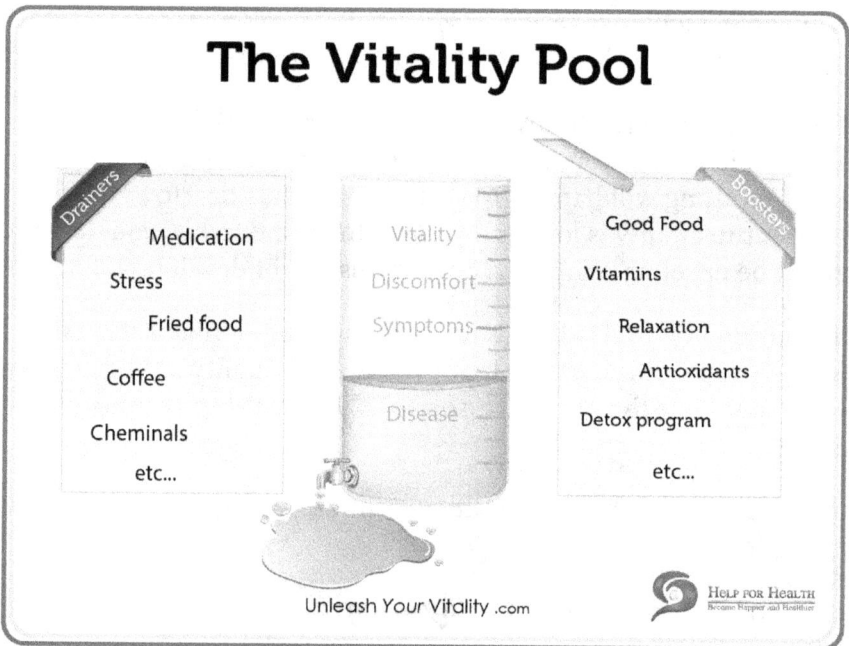

# The Vitality Pool

Drainers

Medication
Stress
Fried food
Coffee
Cheminals
etc...

Vitality
Discomfort
Symptoms
Disease

Boosters

Good Food
Vitamins
Relaxation
Antioxidants
Detox program
etc...

Unleash *Your* Vitality .com

HELP FOR HEALTH

*Health is like a bank account. During your life you should deposit enough so you can enjoy it when you grow older. If you make too many withdrawals without deposits you will suffer in the end.*

## 1.2 A warm welcome handshake!

Nutrition is the base of all life. Every living organism on the face of the planet eats. Microscopic bacteria, plants, fish, animals and humans alike, eat in order to survive. Food is on our mind from the moment we are born, and we spend a significant part of our lives eating. A person can go without food only for so long until the vital organs stop working efficiently.

✓ *Are you afraid that the modern lifestyle might affect your health in a way that will endanger your future?*

✓ *Have you ever considered what the constant exposure to pollutants and stress will do to you?*

✓ *Do you notice that people tend to get sick very often, and you are afraid that you might be next?*

✓ *Are you looking for means to protect yourself and those you love, in order to live a healthy and disease free life?*

If so, you might want to know that there are simple ways to do this, all of which relate to a notion everyone is familiar with: nutrition.

The quality of our nutrients is even more important than the quantity, and this has been debated over and over in the media, by scientists and nutritionists, in magazines and online, and it's on everybody's minds and lips. Eating is not just about filling the stomach, eating is about feeding and hydrating every cell in your body, food is the spark that ignites the engine of life.

---

*What you eat and drink today – walks and talks tomorrow!*
*~ Dr Ishan Abdeen*

---

In the past few centuries, the industrial revolution has completely changed the way we view and produce food, and more importantly, the way our body responds to it.

For thousands of years, humans as a species had access to a wide variety of, what we call today, organic food. We gathered fruits, worked the land, raised our own animals and we didn't use any chemicals or genetically modified organisms (GMO). The soil was still rich in nutrients, and it was able to sustain the growth of plants. This provided us with a perfect balance of nutrients, which ensured the survival and the evolution of humankind.

This evolution made us thinkers, we became focused on intellectual growth and rapid development. We, no longer had the time and the resources to eat the right things, and, sadly the right and clean foods became increasingly hard to obtain.

With our development, we changed the balance of nature. We changed food and how it affects us.

An apple is no longer just an apple. The molecules that compose it have changed, and the nutrients inside are drastically reduced. It has a different taste, a different texture and it is filled with chemical and hormonal substances that make it grow faster. It is so deprived of vitamins and minerals that we can hardly call it an "apple" anymore. In order to get an appropriate amount of vitamins, we would have to eat much more than a single piece of fruit. To fully to obtain the same amount of nutrients as your grandmother did when she ate one (real) apple as a youngster. Nowadays you need to eat multiple "apples" to keep the doctor away.

> **An apple is no longer an apple**

This changes completely the meaning of the saying into a more appropriate: "10 apples a day keeps the doctor away."

Thankfully, modern life has its advantages. We developed science, and with its help, we can now improve the quality of our life, by choosing what to give our body, so that it becomes healthier and more efficient.

We all know that we are what we eat, but what does that really mean, and how can we nourish ourselves, when real food is so scarce?

Modern society made us dependent on doctors, and we trust them to fix us when we become sick, even though it would be much more efficient to not become sick in the first place. Not only that, we've become accustomed to the idea that it is normal to become ill, but we've also silently accepted the fact that chronic disease is a threat even for young people.

---

*People have given their health to their doctor,*
*Their money to their banker,*
*Their soul to the preacher,*
*Their children to the school system,*
*and in doing so...*


*Have lost the power to control their lives !*
*~ Rolling Thunder*

---

Given the actual circumstances, by the year 2020, half of the population will be suffering from diabetes[1].

## Which half will you belong to?

This is not the worst part. Due to the constant decay of nutrients in our food, and the lack of interest in prevention, trends show that for the very first time in the history of humankind, parents will outlive their children on a massive scale![2]

We tend to invest in trying to prevent objects from breaking. We take our car for a tune-up, we have protection for our Smartphones, and we even use firewalls for our computer. Therefore, why not work at preventing atrophy in our own bodies? Makes sense doesn't it?

✓ *What do you do to tune-up your health engine?*

✓ *What is your health "firewall"?*

The intention of this book is to shed some light on this difficult matter. It is not a book about food, or about what is right or wrong to eat. There are already many great books that discuss diets in detail.

Instead this book is about the most essential aspect of our eating habits and vital nutrients. It will take you on a journey to the

**Parents outliving their children ?**

molecular level, but I promise it is easy to understand. I will take you to the place where everything is taking place. It is a book about nutrients and how to choose them. It is a book that gives you the secrets to unleash your vitality. Ultimately, it is a book about life, because learning to feed your body will give you more time and energy to experience the joy of living.

Today, we know that 90% of all diseases can be prevented, so inside this book, you will find the means to do exactly that, along with information that will take your vitality status to a much higher level.

However, the information alone is not enough; you have to implement this information into your life to actually experience it.

Ask yourself:

✓ *Are you really willing and ready to embark on this journey?*

✓ *Are you ready to take the steps to ultimate vitality?*

✓ *Do you really want to get healthy?*

If not, then please give this book to someone who really wants to or needs to change their life.

### 1.2.1   Do you have the latest release?

This book is updated regularly with new sections, questions and research. Our specialists are constantly on the lookout for new information and the latest in research.

Make sure you have obtained this book from a reliable source. That can be either a physical copy or an electronic copy from one of the main booksellers or straight from our website. When you have obtained this book through any other means, just send us an email so we can send you the latest version.

Also make sure you download the resource pack from: http://www.UnleashYourVitality.com to do the exercises and get more background information. This will also allow us to send you updates and new sections when we have finished them.

### 1.2.2   How to use this book

Please read the title again… did it say "how to read this book"?… Nope… This is an action book. This is one of those books that you will want to come back to. From it, you will learn a lot of important information. At times this information might seem overwhelming so, remember to re-read certain parts of this book and even take notes. Fill in the exercises, mark the

> **To DO or NOT to DO.**
> **That is the question**

symptoms you recognize and write down your insights and actions that you commit to do.

### *Make this work play and play with fun!*

The first and foremost thing is to read and work through this book/ resource with pleasure. Congratulate yourself on the fact that you made the decision to engage in an activity that will improve your health, wellness and life in general in the long run. You are already so far ahead of many people who procrastinate and promise themselves that they will make changes yet never take life enhancing actions.

How do you go about driving to another place? Do you know where the traffic signs are along the route already?

☐ I wait until all the traffic lights are green
☐ I start driving and get closer to my destination, navigating signs as I approach them

I guess you start driving, right?

That is the way that I would like you to approach working with this book. Start applying it now. Right away! You will get closer to your goal, only when you implement the suggestions we give you!

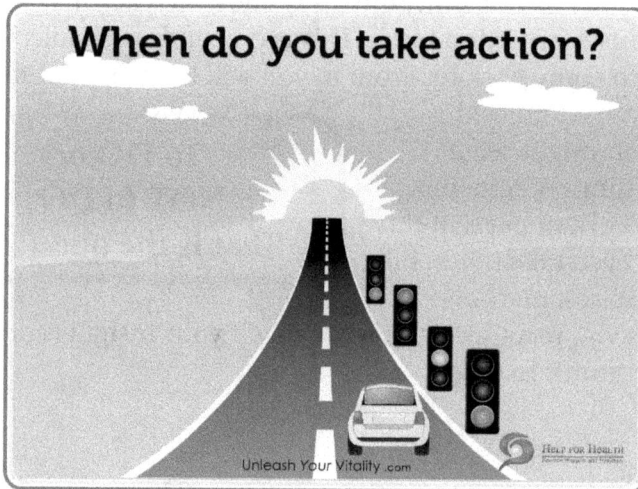

# Well done for getting this far!

### Makes notes

When you go over this book make notes again in the borders: notes of important sections for you, notes of reminders, actions to take, sections to re-read. Make it a WORK-Book, and not a read-book.

### Exercises that change your life

To re-iterate, this book is designed not to be read but to be done. At certain points, you will encounter exercises. Doing these will give you a deeper level of awareness regarding very important matters. Do all of the exercises, as they come, and be as honest as possible. Fill in the exercises right inside this book. This will allow you to better digest and implement the information. It also makes it easier to come back and adjust your insights and actions.

Add your own comments and thoughts inside the book. Many people also find it useful to share the new information with friends. This helps them learn in a faster and more enjoyable way. So go ahead and share your insights with friends and online.

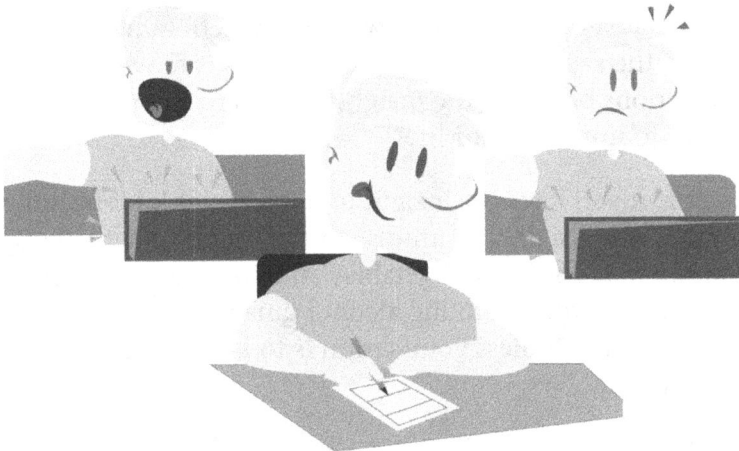

### Mark your symptoms

Whenever you find a symptom or a description in this book that resonates with your life, then mark it, by a checkmark or highlight it. This will allow you to easily recognize what you can do to start changing it. We will come back to these items during your Personal Nutritional Plan, so mark all the symptoms that you recognize.

### If you want to skim this book

If you don't have time right now, and you just want to read the bare minimum, you should at least read the chapter on soil depletion and the one that teaches you how to choose a good supplement. However, this book is designed to work through cover-to-cover to ensure optimal results.

### Your insights and personal actions

While working through this book you will gain rich plentiful insights. Write these down. Each chapter includes an insights and actions section. By writing down your main insights you commit them to memory and you will find them easier to remember.

An insight is just nice, an insight without an action, however, is just a dream. So the second part of those exercises is to write down your personal actions based on the insights. How are you going to use that insight to improve your life?

For example if you have the insight to buy vegetables for dinner tonight, that is just a dream, unless your action is to actually go to the supermarket, select the vegetables and purchase them. If you have an insight to quit drinking alcohol during the week, then that is just a dream, unless your action is to keep the bottle closed during the week.

Get my drift?

It is the insight that sparks your interest and the action is to implement it into your life. Write down both and they help you to change your life and reach your vitality goals.

### *Use our coaches !*

Worldwide we have several coaches to help you. In your action plan you will learn how to access them for FREE. They will help and assist you in your process and how to get the most out of this program. Use them, they are there to help.

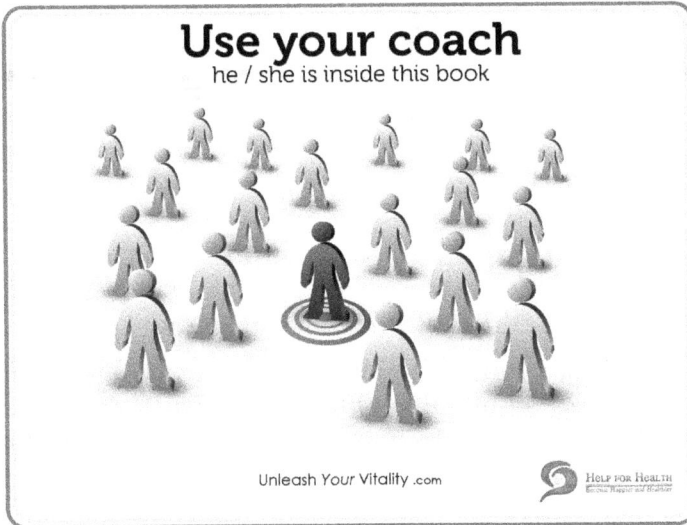

## Use your coach
he / she is inside this book

Unleash Your Vitality .com

Help for Health

### *Re-read sections*

Use colored post-it for the pages you will want to return to. The amount of information is high, and this technique will really come in handy when you want to find something in a hurry.

### *Additional Resource Pack*

There is an accompanying resource pack available for free. It contains the exercises from this book so you can do and repeat them. Especially if you are reading this on an e-reader, then you need this resource pack to complete the exercises. The resource pack also contains additional materials that I could not include within this book. So get your resource pack now.

## Download it from:
http://www.UnleashYourVitality.com/resource/

# Congratulations on taking this step to unleash your vitality ! !

*"Do the best you can until you know better. Then do better."*
*~ Maya Angelou*

### 1.2.3    Important note

With this book we provide scientific information on the health aspects of dietary factors and supplements, foods, and beverages for the general public. The information is made available with the understanding that the author and publisher are not providing medical, psychological, or nutritional counseling services on this site. The information should not be used in place of a consultation with a competent health care or nutrition professional.

The information on dietary factors and supplements, foods, and beverages contained on this book does not cover all possible uses, actions, precautions, side effects, and interactions. It is not intended as nutritional or medical advice for individual problems. Liability for individual actions or omissions based upon the contents of this site is expressly disclaimed.

**Let us help you**

We promote healthy life through a balanced diet, exercise and emotional support. None of the information in this book is intended to diagnose, treat, cure, or prevent any disease. We will not diagnose or prescribe any supplement. Read entire labels and recommendations before use. We recommend you consult a qualified physician before starting any diet plan and/or taking supplements. We are not responsible for individual use of this product. These statements have not been evaluated by the Food and Drug Administration.

Whatever your ultimate decision or decisions may be, the authors disclaim any and all responsibility for that choice. You are the one responsible for your own health and for the health of your family.

Take this responsibility for your health seriously.

> *"Take responsibility for your own health or give me your wallet and pray I spend it wisely."*
> *~ Rob van Overbruggen*

*Warning*

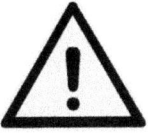

When you start living healthy and implement the changes from this book and the associated resources from Unleash Your Vitality™ website, you will see a **significant improvement in your health**.

This will result in **positive changes** for example, to blood values and blood sugar levels. If you are taking prescribed medication of any kind you must be checked regularly.

**Implement and feel health improvements**

Contact your physician immediately so that he or she can readjust your medication when needed. This is especially important in the case of insulin, cholesterol and blood pressure medication.

NOTES

# Food ain't what it...
## Your Granny wouldn't Like It, Food ain't what it used to be

Before you continue reading any further, take a moment and think about your past and the time that you were most vibrant and healthy.

> *"Today, more than 95% of all chronic disease is caused by food choice, toxic food ingredients, nutritional deficiencies and lack of physical exercise."*
> *~ Mike Adams*

## 2.1    Your Zippy, Smart and Speedy Survey

When you think about your health status, now and in the past, how is that different? Below, you will find a series of questions; answer them honestly, to get a better understanding of your health. You will be able to notice the differences that have emerged in your health in more recent times.

Do this exercise now.

# Exercise: 1 – The Healthy You

This is a two step exercise. In the add-on pack (http://www.unleashyourvitality.com/addon/) you will find a way to get a downloadable visualization that can help you with this exercise.

This exercise consists of two parts whereby you answer the same question twice. Once for a time in the past, once for your current situation in life.

## Step One:

Take a moment and think back to the most vibrant and healthy time in your life. Maybe it is only recently, maybe it was when you were a child. Really step into that moment in time and re-experience your life as it was back then. While staying in that memory, answer the following questions as if you were there at that moment in time. So if your most healthy vibrant time was when you were 6, then you answer as if you were aged 6.

Fill in your answers in the PAST column only, leave column NOW empty

## Step Two:

Excellent, you've now made a first quick assessment of your health and vitality from the past. This exercise will help you later on in developing an action plan. So make sure that you have completed this exercise before you continue !

Now look at your present life, and answer the questions again today at your current biological age. Assess your vitality with the same questions based on your current situation in life.

Fill in your answers in the NEW column.

**1. How old are you?**

| PAST AGE | PRESENT AGE |
|---|---|
|  |  |

## 2. What are you doing at this moment?

| PAST AGE | PRESENT AGE |
|---|---|
|  |  |

## 3. How did/do you rate your general health status?

| PAST AGE | PRESENT AGE | |
|---|---|---|
| ☐ | ☐ | Amazing |
| ☐ | ☐ | Very good |
| ☐ | ☐ | Ok |
| ☐ | ☐ | Poor |
| ☐ | ☐ | Very poor |

## 4. How did/do you feel in general?

| PAST AGE | PRESENT AGE | |
|---|---|---|
| ☐ | ☐ | Happy |
| ☐ | ☐ | Good |
| ☐ | ☐ | On top of the world |
| ☐ | ☐ | Sad |
| ☐ | ☐ | In pain |
| ☐ | ☐ | Weak |
| ☐ | ☐ | Tired |

## 5. How was/is your vitality?

| PAST AGE | PRESENT AGE | |
|---|---|---|
| ☐ | ☐ | Amazing |
| ☐ | ☐ | Very good |
| ☐ | ☐ | Ok |
| ☐ | ☐ | Poor |
| ☐ | ☐ | Very poor |

## 6. Did/do you experience any pain?

| PAST AGE | PRESENT AGE | |
|---|---|---|
| ☐ | ☐ | Bone pain |
| ☐ | ☐ | Joint pain |
| ☐ | ☐ | Muscle pain |
| ☐ | ☐ | Head-ache |
| ☐ | ☐ | Pain in other areas |
| ☐ | ☐ | No pain at all |

## 7. What was/is your energy level?

| PAST AGE | PRESENT AGE | |
|---|---|---|
| ☐ | ☐ | Amazing |
| ☐ | ☐ | Great |
| ☐ | ☐ | Good |
| ☐ | ☐ | Decent |
| ☐ | ☐ | Low |
| ☐ | ☐ | Awful |

## 8. How often did/have you feel/felt unwell during the year?

| PAST AGE | PRESENT AGE | |
|---|---|---|
| ☐ | ☐ | Never/Rarely |
| ☐ | ☐ | Occasionally |
| ☐ | ☐ | Often |
| ☐ | ☐ | I was sick all the time |

## 9. How restful was/is your sleep?

| PAST AGE | PRESENT AGE | |
|---|---|---|
| ☐ | ☐ | I sleep amazingly well |
| ☐ | ☐ | Great restful sleep |
| ☐ | ☐ | Decent, guess it is ok |
| ☐ | ☐ | Low energy when I wake up |
| ☐ | ☐ | Awful, I wake up not refreshed at all |

Now that you have completed the exercise you can compare both sets of answers. How did it change over time? Are you feeling better or worse? How have your results changed over time?

Think back to how you felt on the best day of your life, e.g. when you were a happy, energetic child or adult. This is exactly the way you should feel now. The energy doesn't just fade away, it is chased away by events that squeeze it out, but it can be recaptured by giving your body and brain what they need to rebuild what has been damaged.

If there is no difference between the best day in your life and now, or if your health and vitality has increased – Congratulations! You have done an amazing job to maintain your vitality, not many people are able to do so. Continue reading on to discover how you can keep this vibrant health for many years and raise it even higher still.

If you are not feeling as good as you did back then, thank you for your honesty. This means that you don't have proper nutrients to help your cells to be healthy. Statistics show that if you do not change your nutritional intake, your energy and health will decline even further over time, and illnesses and symptoms will appear and become more serious.

If nothing changes and your lifestyle stays the same consider how will your quality of life be when you grow older, when you will be sick? If you think that you can take the pain and suffering, and bear them with pride, think about how boring it will be to be forced to live in a hospital or indoors.

I am sure you will agree that it is better to take action now. It is easier to make minor modifications now than to live with regrets later when it will be harder to make changes.

### 2.1.1    Current Symptoms

At the end of this book we will develop a Personal Nutritional Plan together to increase your health and vitality. One of the pointers to start working on is the symptoms that you are currently experiencing. Those can be symptoms as in severe diseases but think also in terms of small frequent recurring symptoms like a cold, ongoing small aches, small discomforts etc.

Go to your "Your Action Plan Workbook" (chapter 12) and fill in the symptoms only. The rest of that exercise will be discussed later on in this book.

Go to the section and do that exercise now.

The result of that exercise will be used later to create your Personal Nutritional Plan towards vibrant vitality.

## 2.2    Boom! We are in a Mega crisis!

We are facing an international crisis, and that crisis is illness, disease and decrease in vitality. Healthcare and health technology are increasing, but this does not show in the disease statistics. Many scientists are working to understand disease, yet chronic diseases and other serious illnesses are still on the rise.

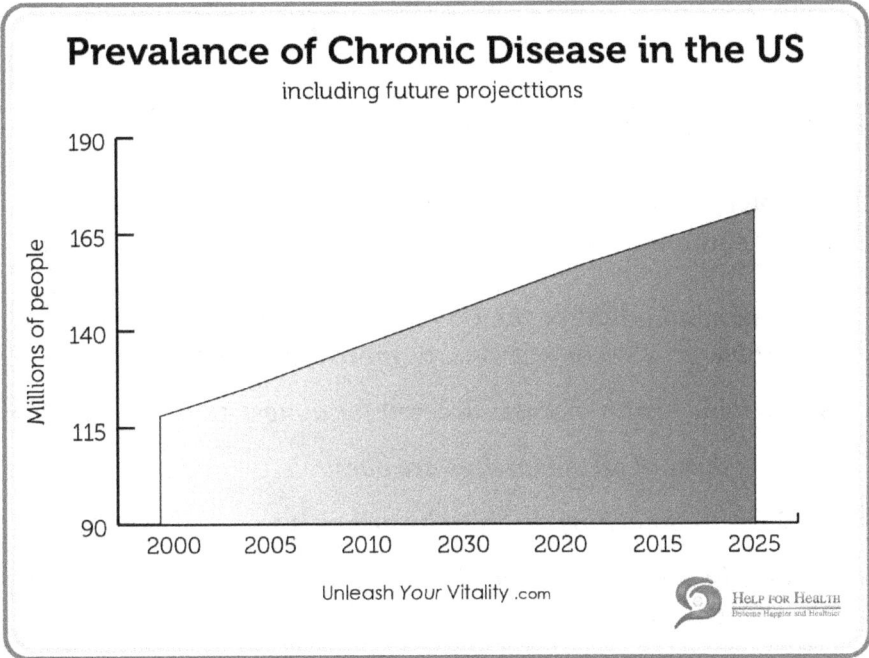

**Prevalance of Chronic Disease in the US**
including future projecttions

Unleash *Your* Vitality .com

Source:[3],[4]

Take diabetes and obesity for example. Diabetes incidence has quadrupled in the last 30 years and obesity is considered a worldwide epidemic, not in the sense that it is contagious, but it is spreading and increasing like wildfire.

*"Chronic disease is the great epidemic of our times"*
*~ British Medical Journal*[5]

When we look at a more detailed view we see staggering increases in some diseases.

| DISEASE | 1980 | 1994 | % INCREASE |
|---|---|---|---|
| Heart condition | 75.4 | 89.4 | 19% |
| Chronic Bronchitis | 36.1 | 56.3 | 56% |
| Asthma | 31.2 | 58.5 | 87% |
| Tinnitus | 22.6 | 28.2 | 25% |
| Bone issues | 84.9 | 124.7 | 47% |

Per 100,000 people of the US population.[6]

The Center of Disease Control describes these chronic diseases as the most common, costly and preventable of all health problems.

> ✓ *Half of all adults in the US have one or more chronic health problems. 25% have even 2 or more chronic health problems*[7]
>
> ✓ *Chronic health diseases account for almost 48% of all deaths*[8]
>
> ✓ *One third of all Americans are obese*[9]
>
> ✓ *23% are somehow disabled by arthritis*[10,11]
>
> ✓ *One in every three over 50 will break their bones because of osteoporosis*[12,13,14]

So what is going on? Why are the statistics not improving? But even more important is the question what can you do about it? What can you do to fall outside of these statistics? If you already have one of those illnesses, what can you do to start reversing it?

In this book we are going to look at one of the possible – and easily preventable causes of the rise in diseases: Food and nutrition.

Although we will touch on the mind and emotional wellbeing a little bit in this book we will not go into much depth on how this influences health. For that topic you need to take a look at my other book "Healing Psyche". That describes in depth how your mental and emotional state influences diseases processes.

Ok, let's jump in. Our food has a direct impact on the cause of many diseases, so it can also help in reversing it. But why are there more people getting sick instead of less?

Did our food change over the years? Do we eat different things now to that which our grandparents did? Or is something else going on?

## 2.3    Widespread Malnutrition

*"The food you eat can be either the safest and most powerful form of medicine or the slowest form of poison."*
*~ Ann Wigmore*

We are educated to consider feeding directly related to eating, food simply isn't what it used to be, and it doesn't `feed` us any more, at least it doesn't do a very good job of it.

This is why scientific studies focused on researching malnutrition, as a form of disease that we are not familiar with: Malnutrition without weight-loss.

Did you ever consider the possibility that an obese person can suffer from malnutrition? These two terms seem to be in perfect opposition, don't they?

We tend to view people who suffer from malnutrition as thin and weak, when the fact is that malnutrition doesn't refer to one's weight, but to the nutritional status.

**Obese people suffering from malnutrition ?**

Anyone can suffer from different forms of this affliction, and anyone can be exposed to it.

Malnutrition is a disease that develops when a person doesn't get enough nutrients from their diet, it can be caused by lack of a certain vitamin or minerals or by not having the right combination of nutrients in the diet. We are encouraged to think that a malnourished person will be pale and skinny, but in reality a person suffering from such a condition can even be obese. One of the early signs of malnourishment is just being tired.

Lack of micronutrients will influence the evolution of one's health to the point where other serious disease develops, related only to the nutritional status.

A study led in 2010 in the U.S. by the Universities of Tennessee and Pennsylvania, along with hospitals from other regions of the country, showed that "Malnutrition is common among hospitalized patients in the United States, and its coded prevalence is increasing.[15]" The study researched older and newer data, and showed that even if the quality of life, in general, has improved, the level of malnutrition is similar to the one found in the 1970's. Moreover, it has found that, on an average, 40% of the patients hospitalized, suffer from malnutrition[16,17,18].

> **Malnutrition common in hospitals**

The interesting fact is that they weren't hospitalized for their nutritional status, but for other diseases, and being malnourished affected the outcome of their diseases, by slowing the healing rate, increasing the risk of infection and complications, and finally, increasing the risk of mortality[19,20].

> **When depleted of micronutrients you cannot heal yourself**

So, the fact that they didn't have enough nutrients prevented them from healing properly.

Due to this malnutrition, administered treatments in the hospital are less effective or produce many more side effects and increase existing symptoms. Some hospitals even provide proper nutrients to counteract this malnutrition before they start the actual treatment.

Lack of nutrients might be one of the main (but preventable) reasons why people have to go the hospital at all. Besides that, it is one of the reasons we see so many deaths in our hospitals. Many people just lack the vitality to survive a serious treatment.

The reverse is also true; people who took care of themselves and made sure their nutritional status was at a good level when they had to go to the hospital were in a far better position. Healthy patients left the hospital much faster and their entire recovery was significantly faster, almost twice as fast[21].

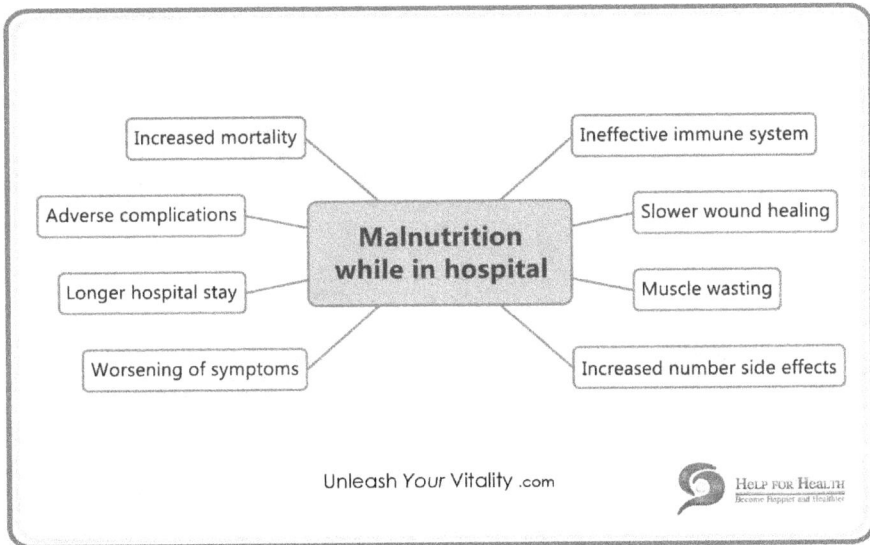

Increased mortality

Adverse complications

Longer hospital stay

Worsening of symptoms

**Malnutrition while in hospital**

Ineffective immune system

Slower wound healing

Muscle wasting

Increased number side effects

Unleash *Your* Vitality .com

Help for Health

Malnourished patients were re-admitted over and over again, where properly nourished patients we not re-admitted at all[22,23]. Well-nourished people tend to recover faster than physicians expect.

This stands as an uncontestable proof to the fact that an organism that is depleted of micro and macro nutrients becomes unable to heal itself. It tries, but it is just missing the right building blocks.

Are you wondering how can some people suffer from malnutrition and obesity at the same time?

Let's try to understand how this happens.

### Why malnutrition can lead to obesity?

Our body can feel hungry when it is missing certain nutrients, and it emits signals that tell our brain to eat. This is not the same feeling as hunger, it is different because hunger occurs when the digestive tract has been empty for too long. This feeling is weird, and we interpret it as cravings for certain foods. It is a defense mechanism against malnutrition, and it is due to our evolution.

In the past foods were much richer in nutrients, but now they contain only 30%, maybe, if you are lucky, 40% of what they used to[24,25]. We will go into this more in depth in Chapter 4.5 - But where did our food go?

# *Your Amazing Insights and Actions*

Date: __ / __ / _____

## What are your insights and learnings from this section?

Now we have come to the conclusion of this chapter. Write down your main insights about what you learned and about yourself.

## What are you going to do differently starting today?

Insights alone will not unleash your vitality. You need to take actions. What are the actions you are going to do in order to implement these insights in your life?

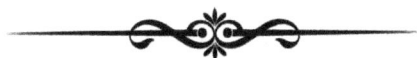

## 2.4    But where did our food go?

We learned to eat to satisfy the body's hunger for nutrients and obtain them from our food. This is an inherited behavior, designed to help us survive.

Nowadays, it isn't exactly straight forward, since what we eat cannot provide us with enough of what we need. An obese person who suffers from malnutrition will feel the need to eat even if the stomach is full, because the body wants to obtain nutrients. Obesity itself can even be a symptom of malnutrition[26].

It is a vicious circle, which can only be broken with adequate nutrition, but before we discuss how to break the circle, let's learn a bit more about this obesity "syndrome".

> *"A deficiency of a vitamin or mineral will cause a body part to malfunction and eventually break down - and, like dominos, other body parts will follow."*
> *~ James F. Balch, M.D.*

*Malnutrition is an everyday problem in every country.*

This is a common health problem, and it doesn't just happen in third world countries, where hunger is an everyday problem. It is encountered all over the world, and most of the time it is found right in front of us. Anyone can be affected. You might even have friends or family who suffer from this condition, which could easily be called "the hidden killer".

**Malnutrition is The Real Hidden Killer**

We've already learned that the body burns calories in order to keep moving, and that these calories come from carbohydrates, protein and fat. Most people get enough of these nutrients from their daily diet, which means that they keep burning energy, while also depositing fat.

The human body is wired to build reserves, and the most abundant nutrient it deposits, is fat. However, fat is used only for its energy releasing proprieties, which means that it cannot give your cells the nutrition they long for.

Did you notice how fast, after a big fatty meal, you feel the need for more food? Did you realize that if you eat a lot before going to bed, you feel hungry the next morning?

### Feeling hungry is the bodies cry for nutrients, not stomach fillers!

This doesn't happen because you need more food, but because you need more nutrients. A nutrient deficiency is also called a "hidden hunger", because we define hunger as a feeling that we perceive and can pinpoint, and also as a deficient intake of calories. However, a

**Nutrient deficiency ... "The Hidden Hunger"**

nutrient deficiency cannot be easily noticed, unless it starts showing symptoms like fatigue, upset stomach, acne, gas or other small discomforts.

Malnutrition should be taken seriously, and every person who wants to be healthy, must take into consideration the fact that they might suffer from it.

Answer the following questions to get an indication of whether you have symptoms of nutrient deficiencies or not.

# Exercise: 2 – Malnutrition Indicator Scale

We've already established that malnutrition should be taken seriously, and is more commonplace than you previously may have imagined. Every person who wants to be healthy should take into consideration the fact that they might be affected by it.

Do you want to know if you are malnourished? Then go over a few questions. Answer the following:

| | NO | YES |
|---|---|---|
| Do I take a long time to recover from infections? (If a common cold doesn't completely go away in a week, it's taking too long.) | ☐ | ☐ |
| Am I feeling tired all the time? | ☐ | ☐ |
| Am I finding it hard to keep warm? | ☐ | ☐ |
| Do I have difficulties concentrating? | ☐ | ☐ |
| Is my skin dry? | ☐ | ☐ |
| Is my hair falling out? | ☐ | ☐ |
| Are my nails frail? | ☐ | ☐ |
| Is my appetite too high? | ☐ | ☐ |
| Is my appetite too low? | ☐ | ☐ |
| Do my gums bleed? | ☐ | ☐ |
| Do I have more than five infections per year? | ☐ | ☐ |
| Do I occasionally experience dizziness? | ☐ | ☐ |
| Do I experience depression? | ☐ | ☐ |
| Do I have trouble concentrating? | ☐ | ☐ |
| **Total 'YES' responses** | | |

# Results:

Count how many yeses you have, and fill that in at the bottom of the questionnaire.

Make a mark on the scale below with the number of yes responses.

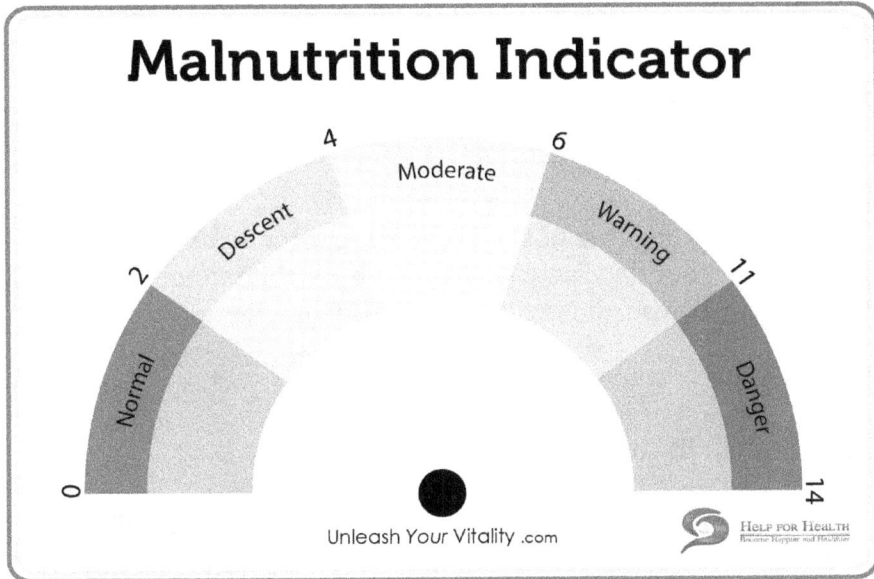

## Malnutrition Indicator

4    6

Moderate

Descent    Warning

2    11

Normal    Danger

0    14

Unleash Your Vitality .com

HELP FOR HEALTH

Place an X on the scale. If you have 5 yeses, draw the x in the yellow box. If you scored 9 yeses, draw an X in the orange box. Now draw a line from the center black point to your X. This is your malnutrition gauge.

## Score 1-2 – Very Low – Dark Green

Place an X in the dark green box

You are doing superbly, you do not show signs of malnutrition. This is an amazing accomplishment. Keep up the good work.

## Score 3-4 – Mild – Light Green

Place an X in the light green box

You are doing well yet are likely to be experiencing a very mild case of malnutrition. Look at your diet and what you consume. You might want add some supplementation to maintain and boost your health.

## Score 5 – Moderate – Yellow

Place an X in the yellow box

Your score is not good, not bad. There are some signs of malnutrition but they are probably not too debilitating. Start supplementing your diet with high quality nutrients.

## Score 6-11 – Warning – Orange

Place an X in the orange box

Your score indicates a warning level. You are suffering from a moderate case of malnutrition. If you want to keep your health you need to look into supplementing your diet.

## Score 11-14 –High – RED

Place an X in the red box

You are experiencing a serious case of malnutrition, and you probably have been suffering for quite a while. You are in a bad shape, and you are seriously lacking in nutrients. Thankfully, with an adequate diet, and proper supplementation the condition is reversible, but you must act now, because if the condition worsens it can affect your day-to-day life if it is not already doing so.

In order to reverse this process and become healthier and more energetic, you must do something about it now. The sooner you are healthy, the sooner you will be able to forget about being tired or worrying about disease. Reducing the nutrient deficiencies and completing your body with all the missing nutrients takes a bit of time. It took some years to get depleted.

If you noticed the fact that you suffer from malnutrition, no matter how mild, you must do something about it now. The complications can be life-threatening, and it is not complicated at all to restore the natural balance, at least not in the early stages. The sooner you take action, the sooner you will be rewarded with positive results which will be well worth your efforts.

In order to stay healthy, for as long as possible, the human body needs the very nutrients that it is composed from. We, as owners of the body, need to provide these, if we expect to be spared from pain and suffering.

Are you curious to see, how many people suffer from this condition? Do you have any other questions about your nutritional status?

Don't just keep this idea in the back of your head!

Do something about it, be proactive and act now, rather than later. There is something you can do to prevent these symptoms. You will learn about this in the next chapters.

*There is something you can do to prevent these symptoms*

2.4.1    <u>Your Key Points to Remember</u>

# Exercises

✓ *Did you complete Exercise: 2 – Malnutrition Indicator Scale*

# Main points to remember: Nutrients

✓ *Your vitality now should be as energized as during your best days*

✓ *Realizing the problem is the first step to fixing it*

✓ *Chronic diseases are still increasing every year, and there is no indication that this will stop*

✓ *Malnutrition is a serious matter that affects millions world-wide*

✓ *You can't see if you are malnourished, it doesn't always show clear visible signs*

✓ *Even obese people can suffer from malnutrition*

✓ *Many people who end up in the hospital with diseases are malnourished, although that was not why they were admitted*

✓ *Lots of people in developed and rich countries are malnourished too*

✓ *One of the first symptoms of malnutrition is feeling tired*

✓ *If left untreated, malnutrition can lead to extremely dangerous complications*

✓ *Malnutrition is one of the main reasons for which people don't heal efficiently*

✓ *If addressed correctly, malnutrition can be cured with the use of proper nutrition and supplements*

✓ *The hunger feeling is more the need for nutrients than the need for food*

## 2.5    Drugs – Devastating Effects

*He who takes medicine and neglects to diet*
*wastes the skill of his doctors.*
*~ Chinese Proverb*

Besides the fact that most people do not get the proper nutrients and are malnourished, there is another problem. The problem of medication decreasing your nutrient levels, and preventing your body from actually absorbing the nutrients you do consume.

You're probably aware of the fact that medication has some side effects. What doctors usually don't tell you is that drugs can also influence the way you absorb and process nutrients. Medication can actually be a cause of malnutrition.

> **Medication can cause malnutrition**

Many prescribed and over the counter drugs deplete your vitamin and mineral levels, and in some cases this happens quickly. This is one of the main reasons for the actual side effects of those medications. So in essence it is not a side effect of the medication, but the result of nutritional deprivation while taking the medication.

Imagine that for some situation you take medication X, that medication happens to prevent your body from using the vitamin C from your foods.

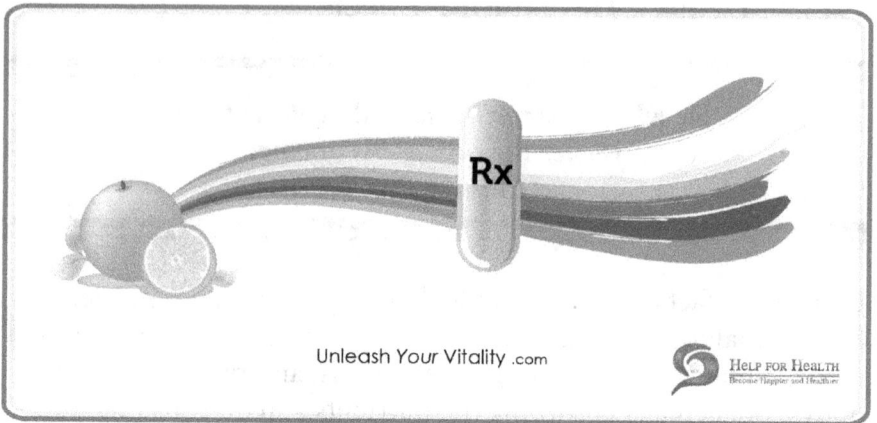

Unleash Your Vitality .com

HELP FOR HEALTH
Become Happier and Healthier

Eventually you would develop symptoms because of your lack of usable vitamin C, for example scurvy1. Eventually when this medication X becomes widespread everybody will get Scurvy. Scurvy becomes one of the listed side effects on the labels. However, this is not totally true, yes it is a side effect, but a preventable one when you supplement vitamin C.

Some of the medications do this so slowly that you only start to notice it over time, and then there is no clear connection anymore to starting on the medication.

Most antibiotics interfere with the intestinal flora, making it difficult for your body to absorb nutrients. Besides the fact that food no longer contains all the vital nutrients, the medication worsens the situation by preventing the absorption of the little nutrients that are present.

---

1        Scurvy characterizes itself by poor wound healing, loosing of teeth and jaundice. In the beginning it shows itself by feelings of lethargy and malaise. It is generally accepted that scurvy is a disease that results from a vitamin c deficiency. Although it does not occur that much anymore, it still can be found with children and elderly. Originally it was a long distance sailors disease, whereby people spend months on the oceans

Actually, all drugs change the way your body is able to absorb nutrients. This is why people that take any kind of medication, should always choose a good supplement to counterbalance that effect.

### 2.5.1   Mechanisms

There are three mechanisms in place explaining how medication can create nutrient depletion:

✓ *Lack of absorption*

✓ *Disturbed metabolism*

✓ *Increased excretion*

#### 2.5.1.1   Lack of absorption

Medication changes the total environment of the body and therefore can prevent nutrients from being absorbed. For example calcium requires an acidic environment in the stomach. Stomach acid suppressors (antacids) do exactly what their name implies. They make the stomach less acidic, whereby calcium is no longer absorbed. When calcium is no longer absorbed you will develop bone decalcification and osteoporosis over time, which is one of the known side effects of antacids. Do you see the connection?

#### *Stomach Acid Reducers (Antacids)*

Let's dive into this a bit more.

Antacids (stomach acid reducers) are used to relieve heartburn or indigestion due high levels of stomach acid. Their main goal is their main problem at the same time. These medications reduce the acidity of the stomach, so they reduce the ability of the stomach to function.

It is like putting a speed limiter on a racing car. The function of the racing car is to go fast, but now with the speed limiter it no longer can perform its duties.

By reducing the acidity in the stomach, the stomach cannot perform its duties optimally. The body is deprived of nutrients like vitamin A,B,C and many minerals. Especially the deprivation of B12[27,28,29] and calcium[30, 31] can lead to problems if not supplemented.

In the case of magnesium, reports show a direct relation between low levels of magnesium and using these medications[32,3334,35,36]. The FDA actually issued a warning for people using these drugs that their magnesium might be dangerously low[37]. This can lead to several problems.

In chapter 6.2.2 - Magnificent Magnesium I explain this further including the possible symptoms related to those deficiencies.

### Cholesterol Drugs/ Statins

Take statins (Lipitor, Crestor, Zocor etc.) for example. They prevent cells from using Coenzyme Q10. Depending on the type and dose this can be as large as 52% reduction of CoQ10[38,39] uptake. Deficiency of CoQ10 is often associated with muscle aches and pains. One of the much known side effects of these drugs is pain in the joints and muscles.

See the connection?

More statins equals less CoQ10. Less CoQ10, more muscle pain.

When supplementing with CoQ10, patients reported a significant decrease in pain[40]. Supplementing extra CoQ10 will then be very beneficial.

### 2.5.1.2    Metabolism

In other cases, the medication changes how the body uses nutrients. When the body has absorbed, nutrients, it then needs to process them for further use. Medications can interfere with this processing and prevent the body from actually using the nutrients.

Imagine taking a candy that is wrapped in plastic; you need to unwrap the candy before you can indulge in the taste, right? Putting a wrapped candy in your mouth is not that enjoyable, you cannot experience the taste.

You can see medication as preventing the body from un-wrapping the nutrients for further use. So you take the nutrients, your body absorbs them. Then, because the medication prevents the unwrapping, your body cannot use the nutrients and excretes them again.

### Antibiotics

Antibiotics are used to treat bacterial infections. They disrupt how the stomach and intestines work, by killing the good bacteria that support digestion. These good bacteria can no longer process the food properly, which results in deficiencies in vitamin B's and K's[41,42,43,44].

Look at the common listed side effects of antibiotics and compare them with the vitamin B deficiency symptoms (more in the chapter on vitamin B).

Do you see the connection?

| ANTIBIOTICS SIDE EFFECTS | VITAMIN B DEFICIENCY |
|---|---|
| Diarrhea or Constipation | Diarrhea or Constipation |
| Nausea | Nausea |
| Headaches | Migraines |
| Rash | Eczema |

### 2.5.1.3    Increased excretion

Diuretics or water pills are commonly used to treat symptoms such as high blood pressure. They reduce the blood pressure by assisting the body to urinate more to reduce blood volume and therefore blood pressure. More urinating also eliminates more sodium, potassium and water. This results in lower potassium levels.

Look at the table below. On the left you see the side effects of using this type of medication. Then look at the right to the general effects of low potassium levels (also referred to as hypokalemia).

Do you see the connection?

| DIURETICS SIDE EFFECTS[45] | LOW POTASSIUM SIDE EFFECTS[46] |
|---|---|
| Extreme tiredness | Fatigue |
| Dizziness | Weakness |
| Muscle cramps | Muscle Cramps |
| Heart rhythm problems | Heart rhythm problems |

Apparently, using diuretics will give you the same side effects as when you have low potassium levels. The body excretes more potassium due to the medication and the low potassium levels lead to symptoms. The symptoms are not caused by the medication directly, but the reduction in potassium uptake creates the symptoms. Supplementing potassium in these cases might be beneficial to reduce the side effects.

### More Examples

This list of examples with specific medications can go on and on. In the resource pack there is a more extensive list of the interactions of different medications on nutritional status and what to do about it.

If you are using any medication it is wise to study this list.

## Download your resource pack at:
http://www.UnleashYourVitality.com/resource/

### 2.5.2    Your Key Points to Remember

*Medications*

✓ *Drugs have a tremendous impact on your nutritional status*

✓ *Many side effects of drugs are actually caused by a lack of vitamins/ minerals*

✓ *Drugs reduce vitamin/mineral absorption and the way the body can use the vitamins/minerals*

✓ *Side effects may be reduced by taking additional vitamins and minerals*

## 2.6  It sure ain't pretty - Toxic Build up

Modern life has exposed us to just about anything you can imagine. Everything we encounter has some sort of chemicals either inside it, around it, or on its surface. Even air has something in it, and it's not something pretty.

We are exposed to toxins from:

- ✓ *The air that we breathe*
- ✓ *The food that we eat (but also medication and other stuff we put into our mouth)*
- ✓ *The water that we drink*
- ✓ *Personal hygiene and grooming products that we put on our skin (creams, deodorants, shampoos, cosmetics etc.)*

Toxins from processed food, from polluted air, from water polluted with fluoride and bacteria and from drugs, tend to build up inside the body and inside its cells.

When this happens, we can't function properly, we can't absorb nutrients efficiently, and we feel tired all the time.

Symptoms of too much toxicity could be weight gain, loss of energy, more frequent colds, low immunity, but the list is much longer than that.

# Effects of Toxins

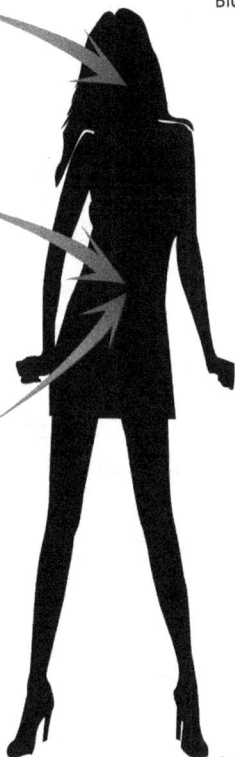

### Air
**Toxic**

### Food
**Toxic**

### Water
**Toxic**

### Topical
**Toxic**

Headaches

Memory loss

Blurred vision

Nausea

Cancer

Birth defects

Allergies

Acid Reflux

Joint stiffness

Kidney failure

Skin rashes

Asthma / bronchitis

Cough/ThroBirth defects

Back pain

Weight gain

Liver damage

Low testosterone in men

Irritable Bowel

Joint inflammation

Fatigue

Depression

Heart disease

Anxiety

Food intollerance

Unleash Your Vitality .com

HELP FOR HEALTH

### Symptoms of toxicity:

- ☐ Loss of energy
- ☐ Depression
- ☐ Heart disease
- ☐ Cancer
- ☐ Anxiety
- ☐ Mental fog
- ☐ Poor nutrient absorption (leads to many other diseases)
- ☐ Nausea
- ☐ Allergies
- ☐ Food intolerance
- ☐ Headaches
- ☐ Muscle stiffness
- ☐ Unable to lose weight

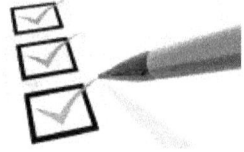

*When you recognize any of these symptoms, mark, and check or highlight them and complete the action plan.

Toxicity is also one of the reasons why the immune system fails to do its job, why we retain water and fat, and why we develop diseases like cancer.

# 2.7 Adam's Ale! Water– The liquid behind it all

*"Water is the driving force of all nature"*
*~ Leonardo da Vinci*

Why are we discussing something as basic as water? Well, because it is basic, and this means it is of utmost importance, and people often neglect it. Water is vital for your health, without water you will starve to death.

Your body is made of water, it is composed of other things too, but over 70% of its composition is water, simple H2O. It is found in the blood, tissues of all sorts, in the brain, inside each and every cell. The heart and brain are for example, 73% water, your skin is for 76% water even your lungs are 83% composed of water. Even the densest part of your body, your bones, are very watery (31%)[47]

*"Water, air and cleanliness are the chief articles*
*in my pharmacopeia."*
*~ Napoleon 1*

If the water levels start to drop, you will begin to feel horrible. However, the quality of the water you drink is even more important than the quantity. Before we start talking about that, we should see what water does for us.

# The benefits of water

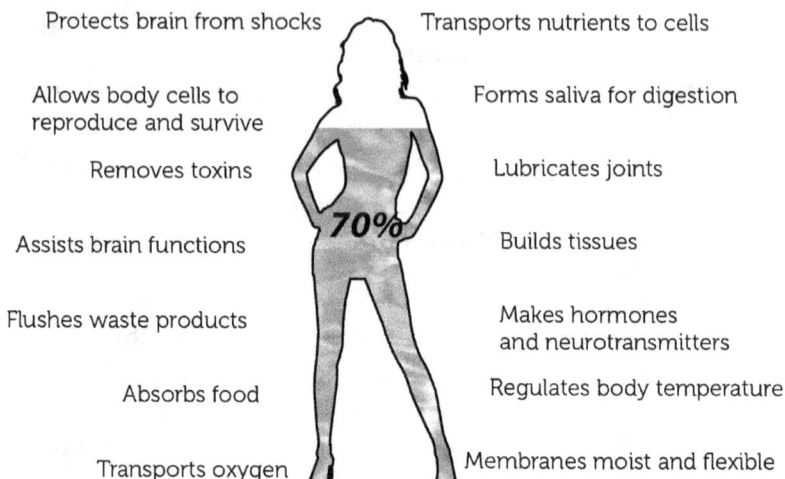

Protects brain from shocks

Transports nutrients to cells

Allows body cells to
reproduce and survive

Forms saliva for digestion

Removes toxins

Lubricates joints

Assists brain functions

**70%**

Builds tissues

Flushes waste products

Makes hormones
and neurotransmitters

Absorbs food

Regulates body temperature

Transports oxygen

Membranes moist and flexible

Unleash *Your* Vitality .com

HELP FOR HEALTH
Become Happier and Healthier

Let's start at the molecular level. In order for a cell to function
properly, it needs water; even our DNA uses it.

Moreover, water is nature's lubricant. It is used for digestion, for
your joints, for the eyes, for the blood that transports nutrients and
oxygen, even for your ears.

This lubricant quality is what keeps the bones in your knee from
rubbing against each other until destruction. Water liquefies food,
in order to be absorbed. Water allows the cilia in your inner ear to
move in order for you to maintain balance.

Did you ever ask yourself why drunken people lose their sense of
equilibrium?

Well, the answer rests in a combination of factors. Your body is
in perfect balance because the brain interprets signals from your
eyes, sense of touch, and from the balance mechanism inside your
inner ear. Alcohol interferes with the neurotransmitters, but it does
something even more interesting.

It dehydrates the body, and by doing that the liquid inside the inner ear becomes thicker and it doesn't allow the cilia to move properly. This is also why dehydration, by all other means, has the same effects as drunkenness.

Not only does water keep the entire mechanism that is the human body moving, but it also keeps it from getting sick.

Water is the main ingredient for the mucus in your nose and throat, and it keeps your skin and eyes moist. These are defense mechanisms, because the water transports white blood cells, which keep the microbes away. This is why, if you keep forgetting to drink water, you will become exposed to all the germs that are spread around and, unlike nutrients, there are plenty of germs in nature, for everybody.

Did you know that you can prevent headaches just by drinking plenty of clean water? Sometimes, when you take an aspirin, the water that you take it with, will have more to do with the easing of pain, than the aspirin itself.

Another important aspect of hydration is the fact that water regulates your body's temperature. It might not seem like a big deal to you now, but just you wait for the torrid summer days, or for the cold winter. As you are exposed to the elements, the body uses its water to keep you at a comfortable temperature, in order to survive. When

> **Toxicity shuts down the immune system and causes cancer**

you are exposed to the cold, the skin sends the blood to the inside, leaving just enough to survive at the exterior. When you are exposed to heat, your brain sends the water to the cells that are dehydrating, and additional water to your skin, in the form of perspiration. This could be an annoying feature, because most people hate sweating, but otherwise you would overheat and die.

If you are not convinced, imagine the Cheetah, it is the fastest animal on the planet, it's so fast that a Ferrari would be jealous of its acceleration, but it can only run for 30 to 45 seconds, after that it has to stop or it will die. This happens because it is unable to sweat, so it can't cool down. You on the other hand, can run for miles, if you are hydrated enough, of course.

What else can water do? Well it can clean you up, and not only on the outside, but also deep inside. Water transports the toxins you are exposed to away and it cleans your organs. If you don't drink enough water, or if the water itself is contaminated, you will build up toxins inside your cells. This toxin buildup in the tissues, manifests through headaches, rashes and other, not so pleasant symptoms.

**Clean water prevents diseases**

You can tell that you are not hydrated properly when you are tired most of the time, you become somewhat slow, your bowel movements are not regular, and your skin isn't as clear as it used to be.

Water is probably the most important substance you put in your system every day, so you must make sure that it is of the best quality possible. But what makes water good, and what could possibly be bad about it?

### 2.7.1    Chemicals in water

Nutrition is an important aspect of everyday life, and the quest to stay healthy doesn't stop just at replenishing depleted nutrients. A very important part of nutrition itself is the avoidance of toxins.

It is essential to:

✓ *Increase the nutrients*

✓ *Remove ALL the toxins*

There are always elements that could harm you, and before you embark on feeding your body, you must first learn what to eliminate in order to stay on the safe side.

This is also in the case of 'plain' tap water, because 'plain' water might be not as plain as you would expect it to be. The problems start appearing when the water is contaminated with different substances, sometimes organic, sometimes chemical and often dangerous.

### Water: H2Oh !!

During my chemistry lessons in high school I learned that water was H2O. However, when you look at the research water used for consumption contains much more than that.

Medications like painkillers, contraceptives, antibiotics, mood stabilizers, blood pressure and many more end up in the water supply. During a test researchers found these drugs in 24 major metropolitan areas in the USA. Apparently drinking water cleansing systems were not efficient in removing these pharmaceuticals. However, you expect your tap water to be safe, right?

This is a major problem to such an extent that fish in the Potomac River are now found to have both male and female characteristics due to the levels of pharmaceutical estrogens in the water. The male fish are being drugged and develop female characteristics.

Now you may think… but I use bottled water, which is safe, right? I pay much more for my bottled water so it must be safe, right?

Wrong, sorry about that. There is no scientific reason to assume that bottled water is any safer than tap water. Both tap water and bottled water have their own problems.

The only thing you can be sure is that both are sold as drinkable water and bottled water is much more expensive.

Let's take a look at both tap water and bottled water.

### 2.7.1.1    Tap water

Tap water often contains many ingredients, including harmful substances.

Can you remember the definition of water that you've learned in school?

Water is supposed to be a transparent, odorless, tasteless liquid. Most of the time, tap water doesn't meet this principle, theoretically it isn't water; Definitely not H2O alone.

- Fluoride
- Parasites
- Iodine
- Chlorine
- Bacteria
- Viruses
- Cocaine (and other drugs)
- Anti-conception
- Hormones
- Heavy metals (lead, arsenic, mercury)
- Other pharmaceuticals

*Tap water pollutants nationwide 2004-2009*

518 Chemicals

187 Above health limits

Unleash Your Vitality .com

HELP FOR HEALTH

Source[48]

In 2010 a study was published whereby they tested the US major cities tap water. The conclusion was devastating; in 89% of the tested cities they found the cancer causing chemical chromium-6[49]. This means that people in those cities drank that chemical for years without knowing. Long-term effects for these people are not looking good. Sutton, the lead researcher, reported:

> *"Getting a water filter is a great way to protect yourself and your family"*
> *"Bottled water is not necessarily any safer than tap water"* [50]

2.7.1.2    Bottled water?

One of the major arguments for people to buy expensive bottled water is that they think and hope it is of better quality. Unfortunately this is not the case. Bottled water is never tested to be any cleaner than tap water. The only thing you know for sure is that you pay a very high price for it.

Bottled water has to state its source and ingredients, if it doesn't it probably is plain tap water (see the problems of tap water above). Of all brands available about 25% is just tap water, sold in a fancy bottle.

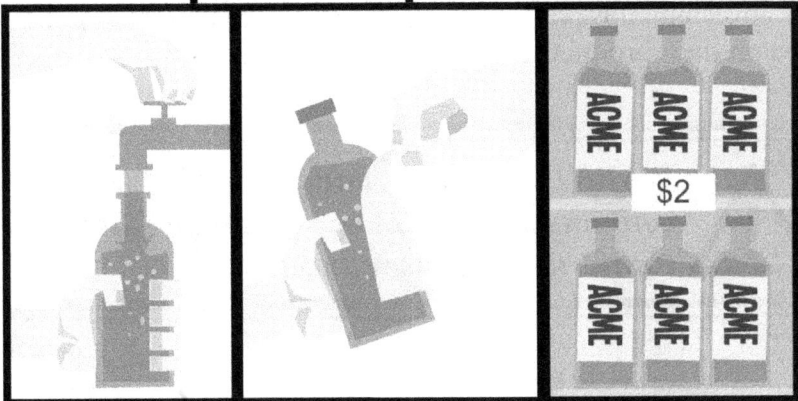

# 25% of bottled water is just plain tap water

ALEXKUIPERS COMICS          Unleash Your Vitality .com          Help for Health

### *The Water inside the bottle*

The company aims to sell us its product with beautiful pristine pictures of mountains, forest and glaciers to make us think that the water is pure. Unfortunately evidence suggests otherwise.

Not all bottled water comes from these pristine pictured water sources. Most of the water companies use the cheapest source of water (plain regular tap water) or they bottle water from surface sources. This water has to be filtered and cleansed, therefore you are also drinking chlorine and other disinfectant agents.

Natural Resources Defense Council tested 103 brands[51] of water and found that a stunning 33% of these contained pollutants like chemicals, bacteria and some even carcinogens[52]. Some brands even exceeded maximum safety levels and were dangerous to drink. Although this is a report from 1999, no subsequent studies have been performed, and the standards or regulations have not been changed. So the risk is still there.

The Environmental Working Group[53] found that 90% of the bottles they tested contained many chemical pollutants; some even contained cancer-causing agents and exceeded legal safety standards. That is just a complex way of saying that it is dangerous for your health to drink those brands.

The government is now requiring those manufacturers to put a label on their product:

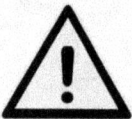

> **WARNING: This product – bottled water – contains a chemical known to the State of California to cause cancer.**

# 'Pristine' bottled water

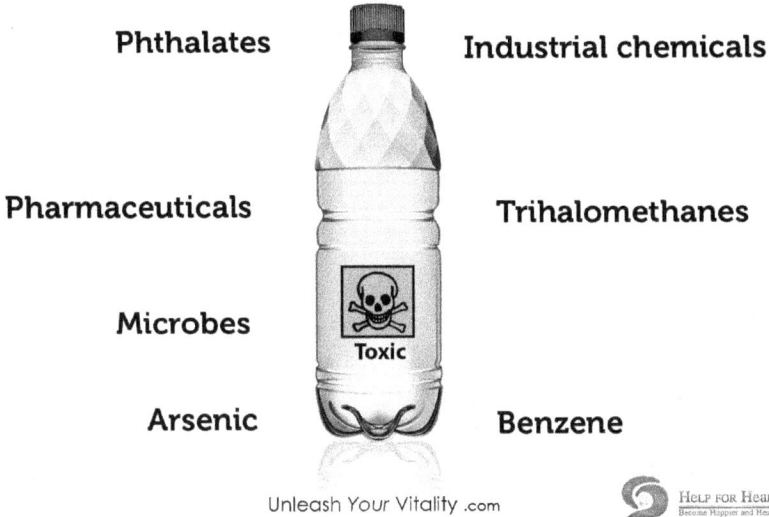

Phthalates

Industrial chemicals

Pharmaceuticals

Trihalomethanes

Microbes

Arsenic

Benzene

*Unleash Your Vitality* .com

HELP FOR HEALTH

Bottled water still contains chemicals and pollutants like phthalates, mold, microbes, benzene, pharmaceuticals, trihalomethanes, and industrial chemicals, even arsenic and sometimes even E. coli (a bacteria that causes food poisoning)The University of Missouri[54] even found that one of these bottles increased the size of a breast tumor by 78% within 4 days. And you thought bottled water is better than tap water?

*"Bottled water is not better regulated, not better protected and not safer than tap"*
*~ Eric Goldstein, co-director NRDC*

Bottled water is regulated for safety, but that is just a fluke. The FDA overlooks bottled water in the USA, which is correct. However, if the bottled water never leaves the state it was bottled in, then the FDA approves it without looking at it. About 70% of the bottled water never leaves the state, so that water is also never tested and is free of FDA interference. Out of 188 bottles tested only 3 provided the basic labeling as to where the water was sourced. The rest came from unknown sources, probably tap water, but you still pay a high price for that.

### *The bottle*

Besides the water quality, the bottle itself is a health concern. Several studies were conducted on the effects that plastic bottles and containers have on the health of the consumer. BPA (Bisphenol A) is a chemical found in plastic, and is has been linked to breast cancer and other diseases. This chemical, once inside the body, mimics estrogen hormones.

Therefore, it can cause different types of cells to mutate into what we know as estrogen dependent cancer. In 2004, the CDC (Centers for Disease Control) examined all the urine samples collected that year, and checked for this compound. They have found that 93% of the subjects, aged 6 years and older were carrying this BPA chemical. Due to this toxicity, it is now banned in many countries for the use of baby bottles. However, it is still in use for other bottles.

BPA doesn't stay in the body for more than a few days, and the results of the study show that we are constantly exposed to this chemical. So, basically you are also drinking plastic, along with the expensive water.

### *You are also drinking plastic*

# BPA Dangers
**used in many plastic bottles, not only bably bottles*

Brain Tumors

Polycystic Ovarian Disease

Insulin Resistance

Learning disabilities

Lack of fertility

Miscarriage

Loss of memory

Heart disease

Prostate cancer

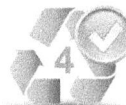

*Only a 4
inside is safe

Increased drug abuse

Hyperactivity

Erectile dysfunction

Breast cancer

Asthma

*Unleash Your Vitality* .com

HELP FOR HEALTH
Become Happier and Healthier

## PET

Most other bottles are made from polyethylene terephthalate, abbreviated as PET or PETE. Although these bottles are generally safe, scientists have now discovered than when it is stored in warm temperatures, or stored for 28 days or more[55,56] (from the time it was bottled) the plastic bottle releases chemicals into the water.

> *"Leaving bottled water in a car changes the chemical equilibrium so that the materials from the plastic go into the water"*
> ~ *Ken Smith, PhD, American Chemical Society*

One of the toxic chemicals that the PET bottle releases into the water is antimony, which causes nausea, vomiting and diarrhea. Others chemicals released into the water are formaldehyde and acetaldehyde which both have cancer-causing properties.

### How to recognize

The type of plastic used in a bottle is easy to recognize. Just look at the recycle logo. If there is no recycle logo, then be aware. When there is a recycle logo, look for the number 4. This is the safe plastic.

# Plastic Selection

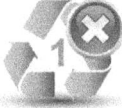 **PET or PETE**
**(polyethylene terephthalate)**

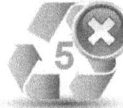 **PP (polypropylene)**

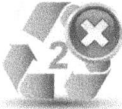 **HDPE**
**(high density polyethylene)**

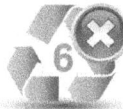 **PS (polystyrene)**

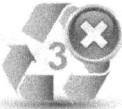 **V (Vinyl) or PVC**

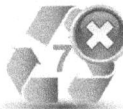 **All Others**

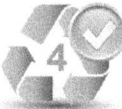 **LDPE (low density polyethylene)**

Unleash Your Vitality .com

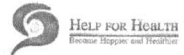

### *Environmental toll of bottles*

Besides the actual health effect of the bottle, just think for a moment about the effects those plastic bottles have on the planet.

- ✓ *That bottle that takes just three minutes to drink can take up to a thousand years to biodegrade*

- ✓ *The energy used each year making the bottles consumed in the United States is equivalent to more than 17 million barrels of oil. That could fuel a million cars for a year*

- ✓ *If bottlers had used 10% recycled materials in 2004, they would have saved enough energy to electrify more than 680,000 homes for a year*

- ✓ *Three million water bottles are trashed every day in California*

- ✓ *As of 2013, the total amount of un-recycled bottles can be used to create a two-lane highway that stretches the entire United States. The amount is still increasing*

- ✓ *The recycling rate in 2004 for all beverage containers was 33.5 percent If it reached 80 percent, the greenhouse gas emissions reduction would be the equivalent of removing 2.4 million cars from the road for an entire year*

- ✓ *Every 27 hours Americans drink enough bottles of water to circle the equator with empty plastic containers*

To support the environment instead of reducing the number of cars, reducing use of the car, or emission from factories, you could reduce the number of bottles you consume[57].

It you still like to buy bottled water, look at least for the NSF (National Sanitation Foundation) certification so that you ensure that it has been tested on some level. The bottle should be labeled as BPA free, and never store your bottled water for a prolonged period or in warm temperatures. But even better is to use a steel bottle and purify your own water.

### 2.7.1.3    Effects of toxic water quality

If you drink water (tap water or bottled water) that isn't purified from all agents, you are being exposed to:

- ☐ Anemia
- ☐ Parasitizes infestation
- ☐ Kidney stones
- ☐ Gastritis
- ☐ Liver problems
- ☐ Nervous system damage (frequent headaches are a symptom)
- ☐ Cancer

### 2.7.2    Water solution

Where can you drink water from, if tap water is contaminated and bottled water has chemicals?

In order to have access to clean, pure water, you need to create your own conditions, to become independent from all the water brands. This way you can ensure that you provide yourself and your family with the best water available.

**Water is essential to maximize your health**

Probably, one of the most convenient ways to do make sure you have clean water is to use a purifier.

A **good purifier** removes all chemicals and toxins and makes the water safe to drink for you and your children.

If you decide to buy such a device, make sure you choose wisely, because it must be able to clean out ALL the impurities: chemical, physical and bacteriological. Once you have one of these, especially if it is an appropriate size, you will be able to carry it with you, and use any water source you have available, including regular tap water to purify your own source of healthy, clean water.

Whatever the source of the water, make sure to keep your body hydrated at all times. No matter how many nutrients your diet has, you will still need water to detoxify your cells and to carry those precious nutrients to where they are needed.

When considering a water purification system, look at the filtration and purification process. The quality of purification is indicated in % of viruses, bacteria, hormones, drug residues, heavy materials and other contaminants it filters out. A very basic filter will already get out more than 90%, the more advanced filters take out 99,9999%. Easy to remember, the more 9's the better.

For example, one of the harmful substances in water is fluoride, removing that from your water is very hard. Most standard water filters on the market will not remove fluoride at all. So you think you drink purified water, you still ingest too much fluoride. When you buy a purification system make sure it is certified for fluoride removal. For more information about the dangers of fluoride see chapter 2.8 - Fluoride.

> **Use your OWN purifier to clean your water**

Also look for the NSF (National Sanitation Foundation) certification. This states that the water system meets certain purity standards.

### Important note

Besides the clean quality of water, one other important aspect should be considered. When you start drinking more water the body also flushes out minerals. These minerals are necessary for your wellbeing. Always take additional mineral supplements when increasing your water intake.

2.7.3    Your Key Points to Remember

# Water

✓  *Water and water quality is vital for your health*

✓  *Tap water contains all sorts of bacteria, viruses, drugs, chemicals and heavy metals*

✓  *Plain tap water is not safe to drink*

✓  *Bottled water is often regular tap water*

✓  *Bottled water still contains chemical and other pollutants and even known carcinogens*

✓  *Some bottled water brands need to carry a warning label*

✓  *Plastic bottles often contain dangerous chemicals*

✓  *Bottled water contains a dangerous substance that is widely considered a carcinogen*

✓  *Look for the number 4 in the recycle logo for safe plastics*

✓  *The safest and cheapest way to stay hydrated, is by creating your own clean water*

✓  *Use a water purification system with more 9's in its percentage of purification*

✓  *Make sure the water purification also removes fluoride*

✓  *The NSF certification gives an indication that the purification system creates really clean water*

## 2.8    Fluoride Jeopardy

You probably already know that fluoride is one of those toxic things you can find in your water. Some countries actually add it to tap water. This is such an extensive topic that I had to create separate chapter for it, because it is not only related to water. It is present in many toothpastes and other dental products. Just take a look at the label.

So, what is fluoride? It is an odorless compound, which is found in many forms in nature. Ironically, the Merriam Webster dictionary defines fluoride as a chemical that is sometimes added to drinking water, toothpaste, mouthwash, floss, to help keep teeth healthy. Besides the use in dental products, air sometimes contains fluoride particles and it is even found in some prepared foods.

You probably already know the fact that our tap water is fluorinated in some countries because it is said to prevent the formation of cavities.

Before we start talking about how fluoride can harm you, let's focus on what it is thought and said to do: that is, prevent caries.

In 1940, fluoride was used for the first time to fight and prevent cavities. The foundation for most studies, which demonstrate the fact that fluoridation helps improve oral hygiene, is related directly to the fact that since water fluoridation was introduced, the number of caries in children and in the general population, dropped. Although this is true, it might have more to do with the fact that quality of life improved, and more people had access to calcium and vitamin D3 supplements, water and a …toothbrush.

The evidence however is quite shaky as they found in a review of all the available studies[58]. That is why in more and more countries water fluoridation is not used or even forbidden. Countries like: Austria, France, Germany, Luxemburg, Norway, Switzerland, and many others, don't add fluoride to their water. Their population has experienced the same improvement in oral health as the rest of the world.

The general consensus nowadays tends to be that excessive fluoride leads to an increase in cavities throughout life (or even worse symptoms can develop), and not so much the decrease of cavities. Besides that effect on cavities, you are still exposed to a chemical compound that is not properly researched and could have serious health implications.

### 2.8.1    Natural

There are countries where the water contains too much fluoride from natural sources, and this affects the population in the long term. So, if it can cause problems, and if it's not a guarantee that you can avoid caries by ingesting it, why would you drink fluorinated water?

**Fluoride and other chemicals pollute your water**

Fluoride is abundant in the earth and the waters of the earth. The levels depend on the type of soil, minerals and location. This is a natural process occurring but it does not mean it is healthy for humans.

Although the World Health Organization[59] promotes the use of fluoride in "optimal" levels to prevent dental caries, the problem in this is that the optimal levels cannot be determined.

There are many sources from which fluoride enters our system. Besides your general fluoride exposure, it also depends on the person's nutritional state. For example a poor diet and lack of calcium will increase the levels of fluoride retention. With the same dose, a person with a poor diet will have more problems with the fluoride than a person with higher calcium and vitamin C levels in their diet[60,61]. This means that you need to prevent fluoride intake as much as possible and have a nutritional diet with enough calcium and vitamin C to prevent the storage of fluoride that you still might ingest.

Why are we discussing it? Because it is found everywhere, but most importantly it is sometimes added to your water, and while you need to stay hydrated, you also need to stay healthy.

Since you are obviously trying to improve your health, and you want to take proactive measures before it's too late, you must be thinking that you should find another water source. Do keep in mind that other sources can be naturally fluorinated, and the exact quantity of fluoride probably isn't stated on the label of bottled water.

The only way to stay safe, and protect your family from the risks that fluoride poses to their health, is to create your own clean water.

Before moving on to the next chapter, take a minute to do an exercise. Get up and go to the bathroom. Once there, read the label on the back of your toothpaste tube. What is on it? Fluoride?

### 2.8.2    Effects of fluoride

A few issues should concern you with regards to the fluoride that you are ingesting. The most obvious ones are also the most researched. Excess fluoride can lead to dental and skeletal fluorosis. Dental fluorosis is a condition that affects the way your teeth look. An excess of fluoride is deposited on the teeth, which will make them appear stained. This esthetical effect is only shown in children, adults will not show these early signs, but they will experience the more severe symptoms.

It doesn't only affect looks. It affects the bones. Since fluoride has to go somewhere, it enters the bones, making them less elastic, therefore prone to fractures.

A study published in the Journal of Toxicology and Environmental Health[62] , showed that in regions with an increased level of fluoride, the fertility rate was lower. Therefore, adding unwanted fluoride to your diet may interfere with a woman's capacity to conceive a baby. Even if you don't plan to have children, there is other striking evidence that should motivate you to rethink what you drink.

**Excess fluoride causes diseases**

Probably one of the most disturbing effects of fluoride is related to the mind. Just a few milligrams can affect the way you think and your decision-making. There used to be a myth that communists used fluoride to make the population more submissive. There is no evidence to sustain that statement, but what we know for a fact is that fluoride decreases the IQ of children.

There were quite a few studies that researched the neurological implications of fluoride, but one in particular, published in 2007, in the Environmental Health Perspectives Journal, found that children's intelligence and growth is affected in a very negative way by high concentrations of fluoride by decreasing the IQ[63] by several points. The IQ drop was even 2 points greater than the IQ drop for heavy marijuana users. So it is safe to say it is smarter to smoke marijuana than to drink fluoride!

In addition, a study led by Harvard scientists[64], published in the same Environmental Health Perspectives Journal, showed that fluoride affects children's intelligence in a dramatic way, and that the neurotoxic effects could be devastating.

*"The children in high fluoride areas had significantly lower IQ than those who lived in low fluoride areas."*
*~ Anna L. Choi*

On a similar topic, research published in Current Science, in May 2010[65], showed that avoiding fluoride during pregnancy decreases the risk of developing anemia, lowers pre-term births, and overall increases the survival rate during pregnancy and childbirth, for both mother and baby.

Early symptoms of flurosis include headaches, pains and stiffness of joints.

When these symptoms are ignored the next phase is where the bones harden and fracture more easily and the muscles and nervous system is damaged.

### *Excessive fluoride could lead to:*

- ☐ Sporadic pains
- ☐ Stiffness of joints
- ☐ Headaches
- ☐ Stomach ache
- ☐ Muscle weakness
- ☐ Reduced fertility
- ☐ Thyroid disease
- ☐ Bone cancer
- ☐ Dementia
- ☐ Arthritis

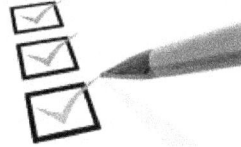

Unfortunately, up until now no effective treatment is known to treat these conditions. The only remedy is prevention by making sure you keep fluoride out of your system and to detox your system.

### 2.8.3  Fluoridation Detox Program

When you have a buildup of fluoride in your system you need to get rid of it. So how can you get it out of your system? There are a few things to remember:

✓ *Prevent ingesting fluoride*

✓ *Prevent storing of fluoride*

✓ *Assist in flushing fluoride out of your body*

### Prevent Ingestion

Remove fluoride from your products and make sure your water is free from fluoride (see Water solution). Use a good NSF certified water purification system that is suitable for fluoride removal.

### Prevent Storing

Increase your nutritional balance. You need additional supplementation of magnesium and calcium and vitamin C. Calcium catches the fluoride and prevents it from settling in the bones and teeth. Magnesium inhibits the absorption of fluoride in your cells and prevents fluoride poisoning.

Additional intake of iodine showed an increase in fluoride in urine, thus promoting excretion of fluoride from the system. However, the use of iodine also increased the excretion of calcium. Therefore, if you use iodine also use extra doses of calcium in addition to the one you are already using during your fluoride detox.

### Fluoride Detox Program

One of the important aspects of removing fluoride out of your system is a cell-detox program. These programs remove the toxins that are stored deep inside your body, inside the individual cells. More information about effectively detoxifying your body you can find in Chapter 11.1.5 - Step 5 – Your Cell based Detox.

### 2.8.4   Your Key Points to Remember

# Fluoride

✓ *Is sometimes added to tap water*

✓ *Damages your teeth*

✓ *Is dangerous for your health*

✓ *Makes your bones weaker*

✓ *Affects fertility.*

✓ *Decreases your IQ, It is smarter to smoke marijuana than to consume fluoride*

✓ *Remove it from your system with the detox program*

When you want to have a more in depth knowledge about your current health status go straight to the action plan and perform Step 1 – Your Extensive Health Check

# *Your Amazing Insights and Actions*

Date: __ / __ / _____

## What are your insights and learnings from this section?

Now we have come to the conclusion of this chapter. Write down your main insights about what you learned and about yourself.

## What are you going to do differently starting today?

Insights alone will not unleash your vitality. You need to take actions. What are the actions you are going to do in order to implement these insights in your life?

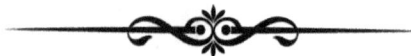

# I Desire to be Healthy

You probably noticed that your health can be improved, maybe just a little, or maybe a lot. Whenever you want to go somewhere, it is good to have a goal. With a goal you know what, where and why you are spending your time and energy.

There are many people in the world, some are rich, some are poor, some of them live long fulfilling lives, and experience every moment. Other people are bound to a hospital bed or stuck in a wheelchair. Life itself is a challenge, but we all experience that challenge.

*"If you aim at nothing, you will hit it every time."*
*~ Zig Ziglar*

Have you witnessed the pain and the emotional torment that disease can bring upon people? Have you seen old grandparents playing with their grandchildren in the park?

How do you want to feel 50 years from now? Do you want to be sad and in pain, or happy, healthy and very much alive?

So, what is your goal health-wise? If you have no goal, think again, why did you pick up this book?

> *"If you don't know where you are going, you will probably end up somewhere else."*
> ~ *Lawrence J. Peter*

Think also how you want your health to be and how you would like to feel when you reach 60, 80, 90 or even 120 years of age. Being old can be fun, if you are healthy. There will be nothing holding you back from going for an entire weekend to Amsterdam and enjoying all of life's pleasures. I know from experience that Amsterdam has quite a variety of them, both for young people and old people young at heart.

A healthy body will allow you to do anything you want and like, you can go dancing, take flying lessons, skydive, and many more activities that only people who care for their health can do at an old age.

Moreover, being healthy is not just about you, it's about your family, your legacy, and the evolution of the entire species. Teach your children to be healthy, because they are our future, and also your biggest accomplishment. Remember that the statistics show that this is the first generation of parents that will witness the death of their children. Many parents will simply outlive their children unless they do something about their health and change it.

**Investing in your health is your best retirement plan ever !**

Having a clear picture in your mind of your desired situation helps you tremendously in actually getting there, finding the ways to continue when it is a bit harder.

We are now going to set personal goals for you. If you tend to have a cold too often, work on improving it within a time frame. If you have allergies, record this, and choose a time frame in which you will resolve this issue. If you want to lose weight, write down how many pounds you intend to lose and during what period of time.

> **Teach your children to be healthy. They are the future**

A goal without a time frame is just wishful thinking. Simply by writing down your problems and goals, you will start realizing how to reach them.

Do you want to know an advanced strategy for accomplishing your goals? Share them with your friends and family. Research showed that more goals are being accomplished when they are communicated to the world.

As I said in the beginning, this is a WORK book… not just a book to be read. Continue filling in this information as you continue through the text and exercises. Refer back to this section often to see if something can be added.

Be realistic when building your goals. For example you can't say that starting tomorrow, I won't get sick anymore. Nothing, not even nutrition is a quick fix. It can take up to six months to rebuild a broken system. For some people, nutritional deprivation lasted for years and their body is so far depleted that it will take a while to replenish. Even then, it is likely to take a bit more time to reach optimal levels. So stick with it.

## *Goal Setting*

A healthy goal must be Inspiring, Timed, Enforced and Measurable. They must be I.T.E.M.

# Your Health Goals

- ➤- **Inspiring**
- ➤- **Timed**
- ➤- **Enforced**
- ➤- **Measurable**

Unleash *Your* Vitality .com

HELP FOR HEALTH
Become Happier and Healthier

### *Inspiring:*

The goal must be something you really want. Or even better, something you must reach no matter what. The more inspiration and motivation you have, the easier it is to reach your goal.

### *Timed:*

There must be a time connected to your goal. This allows you to plan and measure progression.

# *E*nforced:

People who reach most of their goals have other people to help them achieve them. Sometimes this is a friendly supporting help, or sometimes a kick in the butt to keep working at it. Have someone that can help you with your process. This can be a friend that keeps you on track and

**Share your goals and they become easier**

keeps you accountable. Another really powerful way is to use social media for help with this. When you post your goal online, other people will know, which will help you to stay on target and accountable.

# *M*easurable:

The only way you know if you reach your goal is to have a way to measure it. At the end of the book there is a measuring tool that you can use as an additional way of seeing if you have fully met your targets. When formulating your goal, include ways of how you can actually see that you have reached your goal.

One way of finding more information about what your vitality goals might be is to complete the health-check. Just go to: http://www.UnleashYourVitality.com/healthcheck. When you have finished these questions you will see a drawing showing your stronger and weaker areas.

## Now let's continue formulating YOUR goals.

# *Exercise: 3 – Your Ultimate Health*

Where do you want to go health wise? What do you want to have changed?

Let's start creating a health goal together. Let's make sure it is really inspiring. Describe what you will do, how you will feel once you've achieved your goal and how you can measure it. Note when you will have accomplished this by, and who can keep you accountable and how.

In order to help you with this we created a visualization for you. This will help you answering the questions below. Get it from the add-on pack at:

http://www.UnleashYourVitality.com/addon

Date: __ / __ / _____

## <u>What does having maximized health mean to you?</u>

| | 😖 | 😐 | 🙂 | 😄 | 😁 |
|---|---|---|---|---|---|
| How is your energy? | ☐ | ☐ | ☐ | ☐ | ☐ |
| How refreshed do you wake up? | ☐ | ☐ | ☐ | ☐ | ☐ |
| How strong are you? | ☐ | ☐ | ☐ | ☐ | ☐ |
| Are all the aches gone? | ☐ | ☐ | ☐ | ☐ | ☐ |

## Describe your life when you have this vibrant vitality:

## When you have reached your goal, what evidence will you have that you reached this new level:

1. *What you see happening in your life differently?*

2. *What people may say about the 'new' vibrant you or what your own self-talk might be about reaching this target?*

3. *How you feel inside about achieving this goal?*

You can even use the downloadable version from: http://www.UnleashYourVitality.com/resource , print it out and put it on a visible place. This will help you to complete the exercise and gain the insights you need.

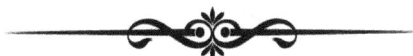

### *Share your goals*

To help you reach your goal and to gain encouragement and support it is good to share your goals. Tell as many people as possible. Tell your family and ask them to support you. Tell your friends, and let them know about what you have learned and what you are going to do about it. Post your target on Facebook and ask your friends and family to help support you towards your goal. Post updates to show yourself and others how far you have progressed.

Share your goals on our page so we can help you:
http://www.UnleashYourVitality.com/results

This is a very efficient way to stick to your plan and achieve your desired results because people want to help you.

Now that we have a goal, let's take a look at what you can do to obtain it: what to look out for, what actions to take, and what additional information you might need. The first step we are going to take now is to look into nutrition.

# Are you ready?

# The Truth...
## Swallow this, Nutrition – the unpalatable truth!

We all know that nutrition is important and that it's the center of our existence, whether we like it or not. But what is it, and how does our body extract nutrients from food?

You never gave it much thought, did you? We all learn in school the basics of it all, but when we take a bite from a pizza slice we don't exactly stop and think how much energy we will get from it.

## 4.1 Nutrition 101

The human body is an incredible mechanism. No matter what condition we are in, it does its best to function properly. Every day our organs work, in order for us to live the way we want.

---

*"The doctor of the future will no longer treat the human frame with drugs,*
*but rather will cure and prevent disease with nutrition."*
*~ Thomas Edison.*

---

A human heart has the longest life expectancy, which separates us from all other primates. It beats 3.5 billion times in a lifetime. It pumps blood at an amazing rate. All the blood circulates around your entire body three times every minute. This happens 24 hours a day, seven days a week, 365 days a year, for as long as you live.

The lungs breathe an average of 28,800 times a day, oxygenating your blood and organs, while keeping your mind clear…most of the time.

Every single cell in your body has the ultimate purpose of keeping you alive. To function properly, every

**Every cell needs nutrition**

cell needs food; specific cell nutrients. Therefore, as with every organism on this planet, the better it is nourished, the better it will perform, and the more happy and healthy you will feel.

All this hard work requires energy, and that is provided by eating and drinking. To keep up with all the movement needed for surviving, the body burns calories.

When we eat, the digestive system transforms food into simple nutrients like carbohydrates, proteins and fats. These are the basic ingredients that are burned down into energy, or deposited to suit our needs at a later time.

Our food is mostly composed of carbon, hydrogen, oxygen and nitrogen. Carbohydrates (or 'carbs') and fats are the main energy source for muscular cells and are found in most foods of plant origin, and a smaller proportion is found in foods of animal origin.

Carbohydrates are converted to glucose and transported to tissues. These carbs are also converted into glycogen and stored in muscles and the liver for later use.

Fats release a high amount of energy during effort. This is why the body prefers to deposit glucose in the form of fat, instead of simply eliminating the excess.

Proteins can also be used to create energy, after being transformed into glucose, but it's a strain on the body to do it, so it prefers other resources. They are also used as a base for creating cells and tissues, so it is always important to have a good source of protein in your diet.

Until now we've talked about energy sources, but the body needs much more than simple fuel to burn.

Every day we "use" cells. Did you notice how much hair you lose? Or how your skin tends to exfoliate on its own, from time to time? These are events that you are able to see, but on the inside too, every cell, that has reached its life expectancy, dies and it is replaced by a new one.

The human body is an amazing machine, it functions like a Swiss watch, every part is tightly interconnected with every other part. But the human body is even more amazing. Constantly, it recreates and replaces old parts. The fact that we are able to regenerate, gives us incredible powers.

Our skeleton is fully replaced with new cells every trimester. We have an entirely new liver every six weeks. Our skin regenerates entirely every 35 days, a new stomach lining is produced every 4 days and some parts of your stomach are replaced every 5 minutes. One of the most interesting features of the body is the

**Nutrition builds life**

fact that it is able to change its brain cells entirely, while still keeping memories from years ago. This is evolution's gift to us, but everything comes at a price.

For the process of creating new cells, the body needs much more than simple elements that are converted into glucose.

It needs micro and macro nutrients, which could be considered building blocks for the new cells, for the healing of tissues, and for the prevention of diseases.

These nutrients have many shapes and forms, they are vitamins, hormones, minerals and trace elements, and they are the foundation of our entire system. We start processing these nutrients, long before we are born, and they help our cells multiply from the moment we are a single-cell organism inside the womb of our mothers.

Nutrients act in the most interesting of ways, and a simple deficiency can turn into a fast-developing disease within a small amount of time, if not addressed correctly.

Did you notice the fact that with every year that passes, people around you seem to get sick more often? Society, even doctors, tend to blame this on something as simple as ageing. The truth is that ageing has very little to do with disease. As a matter of fact, the major thing about ageing is prolonged deprivation of nutrition to such an extent that the body cannot cope with it anymore and becomes very susceptible to diseases; something that would not have affected the body a couple of years ago could now become a problem.

*Remember that there are not "symptoms" of growing old, as people are inclined to say.*
*However, there are symptoms of your body's nutrient reserves being depleted.*

Cells are replaced every day, and the way our body does that is pretty simple. It copies information from its own DNA, and uses nutrients to build new cells, based on that information. When the information is right but it doesn't have the right building blocks, or the building blocks are faulty, errors appear in the result, which lead to disease.

Think about a game of LEGO®. When you want to build a house, if you don't place the brick correctly or you have missing pieces, the final result will either collapse or, it will look really weird. You need all the right LEGO® pieces to form a beautiful, steady construction.

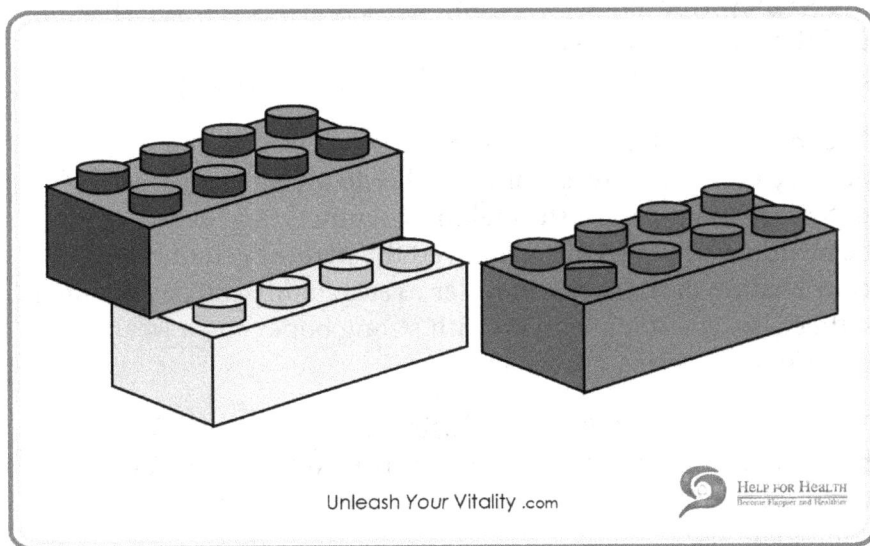

Unleash Your Vitality .com

HELP FOR HEALTH

Your body needs all the nutrients to form healthy cells. When you want to build a house, but you are missing the roof tiles, your house will leak. Or if you want to build a car, but you are missing the wheels, the car won't move. You need all the pieces to have the right result. Remember this analogy as we return to it several times. You need all of the right building blocks to form a proper house.

The most common disease, caused by cells being cloned improperly, is cancer, which affects a huge amount of people worldwide.

This is not a pretty picture, and it definitely isn't something to look forward to.

What does nutrition have to do with cancer? Everything.

But this is a story for another chapter.

In order to prevent diseases, to live a long and healthy life, without worrying about how disabled you will be during your senior years, it is important to understand what you need. Learning a few simple details about your nutrition will help you improve your life expectancy, your fitness level, and more importantly, your health and the future of your children. Supplementing your daily diet may not merely improve quality of life, but it could actually save lives.

The important idea here is not to focus on just one nutrient, because these molecules work together to create the perfect outcome. You can't just start taking vitamin C, and expect to be healthy your entire life, you need the perfectly equilibrated combination of nutrients, in order to sustain life and development. Otherwise, you might end up with strong bones and a weak heart, or clean kidneys but a weak liver.

You cannot build a LEGO® tree, using just blue bricks. You need brown and green blocks. The same is true for your body; it needs all the right nutrients in the right shapes, amounts, forms and combinations.

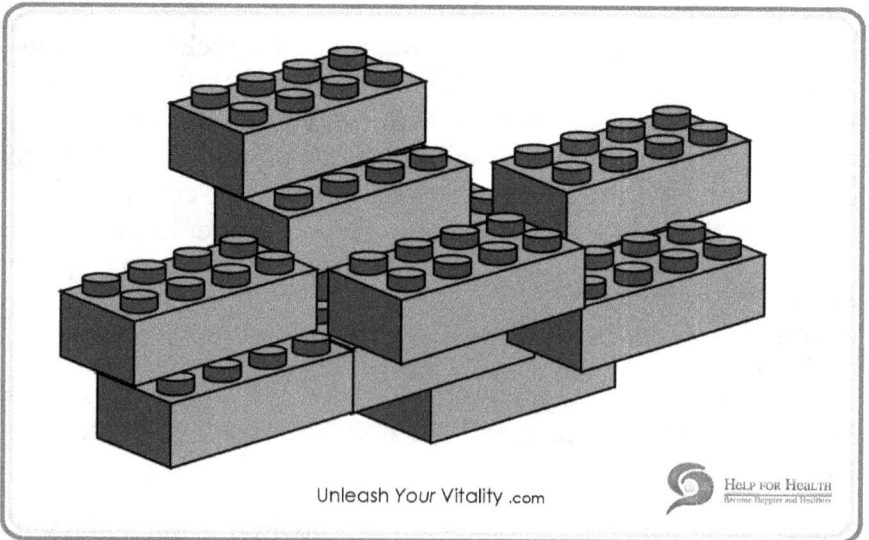

Unleash Your Vitality .com

HELP FOR HEALTH

Think about it like this: you are a car. A car doesn't just run on gas, it needs oil for the engine and the gear box, water for the radiator, additives for the gas, and other consumables that will make it run smoothly.

The human body is the same. It isn't exposed to the same wear and tear of a car, but it has its own tricks and quirks, and it needs more than simple food. It needs something to sustain it and maintain it. The sad part is that you can buy a new car, but you can definitely not buy a new body (currently!), not even if you had all the money in the world.

The best thing you can do to protect your body, is to care for it and provide the best materials available, the building blocks it needs to rebuild every broken cell. This way you can stay disease free and strong for a very long time.

Health is the ultimate richness, and once lost it is very difficult to gain it back. Lack of proper nutrition almost always leads to disease, and it is a shame that people neglect such a simple point, because they end up regretting it sooner or later. No one lives forever, but some people might live for many years without worrying about being in poor health and without having to depend on others.

The question you want to ask yourself is: How do I want to live my life? Do I want to be an active person, full of energy? Or do I want to be tired all the time and hardly make it through the day?"

If you want to live a long life, without fearing the pain of disease, you will need to give your body all the nutrients required for optimal functioning, maintenance and repair. This wasn't always an easy task, but now, with all the advancements in science, proper nutrition is at your fingertips, you just have to learn what you really need, and how to get it.

> **Maximizing your health requires optimal nutrition**

This is exactly what we are going to teach you in the following chapters.

What is your opinion on this? If you are reading this book now, you must be interested in your health and what you are feeding your body. Don't be afraid to express your opinions and concerns, about the effects bad nutrition has on you and your family. The fact that you are interested in having a better life is the first step that one must take, in order to change for the better. Call it evolution if you want, the kind of evolution that is supported by science and information, gathered over decades.

In the next chapters, you will learn what nutrients are, what they do, and how they can help you. We will travel inside microelements, and see how they act, and how they influence the growth and development of cells. You will begin to understand how to prevent disease, how to stay fit, and how to live a long and healthy life, by simply giving your body the essential elements that it consists of.

We will discuss nutrients, and where to get them, how to use them, and how to choose them. After you finish reading this book, you will be able to decide for yourself if you need nutritional supplements or not, you will understand the importance each nutrient has, and you will be able to control what happens with your body.

You are on the right path, and to stay on track, you need to communicate, learn and understand. You can buy books, read studies and watch documentaries, but the truth is that modern society has brought us an amazing tool, which brings all the information and all the people together: The Internet. So, next time you have questions, or you feel the need to share your opinions with others, turn on your computer and write on a forum, it is simple and it will help you, and others like you.

## Join our community and learn from each other.
## http://www.UnleashYourVitality.com

### 4.1.1   Your Key Points to Remember

✓ *Ageing is less about passing of years. Ageing is all about nutrition*

✓ *The human body uses carbohydrates, proteins and lipids only as fuel*

✓ *Nutrients are the building blocks of every cell, including those inside the DNA*

✓ *The quality of nutrients is more important than the amount*

✓ *Nutrients are needed constantly, the body replaces used cells every day*

✓ *You need all different types of nutrients to support your entire body*

# *Your Amazing Insights and Actions*

Date: __ / __ / _____

## What are your insights and learnings from this section?

Now we have come to the conclusion of this chapter. Write down your main insights about what you learned and about yourself.

## What are you going to do differently starting today?

Insights alone will not unleash your vitality. You need to take actions. What are the actions you are going to do in order to implement these insights in your life?

## 4.2    Free-Radicals, stress and antioxidants

Okay, So It Sounds Boring and Technical, But it's of Upmost Importance to you !

---

*"It's not stress that kills us, it is our reaction to it."*
*~ Hans Selye*

---

Stress is a social notion that seems to be everywhere, and affect everyone. Therapists have developed methods of fighting stress, through exercise, meditation, psychotherapy and other means. In my book "Healing Psyche" I explain more about mental-emotional stress and its effects on cancer.

Besides mental-emotional stress there is biochemical stress. Individual cells in our body are exposed to stress just as much as you are as a whole, but it's a different kind of stress.

Mental-emotional stress is influenced by work, duty, society, frustrations, careers, or any other socio-psychological factor. A little stress can be good, it makes you become aware and do what you need to do to improve the situation. However, too much stress is harmful and could lead to diseases (see "Healing Psyche").

Biochemical stress is caused by living. Breathing, eating, digestion and the production of energy from food creates free radicals in the process. Just as with mental-emotional stress, this is a good and healthy process, however it can become a problem when there is too much biochemical stress; then there are too many free radicals and that leads to disease.

You probably heard this notion before, it is all over the media, and antioxidants are advertised because of their qualities of fighting free radicals.

Do you know what they really are? How do you imagine this invisible threat?

Let's explain the concept, because you need to be able to relate to the idea. It is always important to know what is going on inside your body, because this is what will guide your future actions and your ability to work proactively on your health.

The human body is made from cells, which are tightly united. There are, on an average, 100 trillion cells, alive, in your body, as we speak.

Each cell uses oxygen to create energy. In this process free radicals are formed. Having too many of these free radicals is called oxidative stress.

### How Antioxidants "eat" free radicals for breakfast

Imagine this process as a wood fire. While burning the wood, sparks will be formed; this is inevitable. Depending on the type of wood (type of food) you will have more or less sparks, but sparks will always be there. The sparks are not a problem, as long as there are not too many.

When there are too many of these sparks (free radicals) they start attacking your cells. Left unchecked, the free radical will damage everything surrounding it, including the DNA.

So, what helps us get rid of the excess sparks? The answer is simple, and you probably already know it: antioxidants. They act in a very simple way: they make the free radical inactive. They neutralize the sparks.

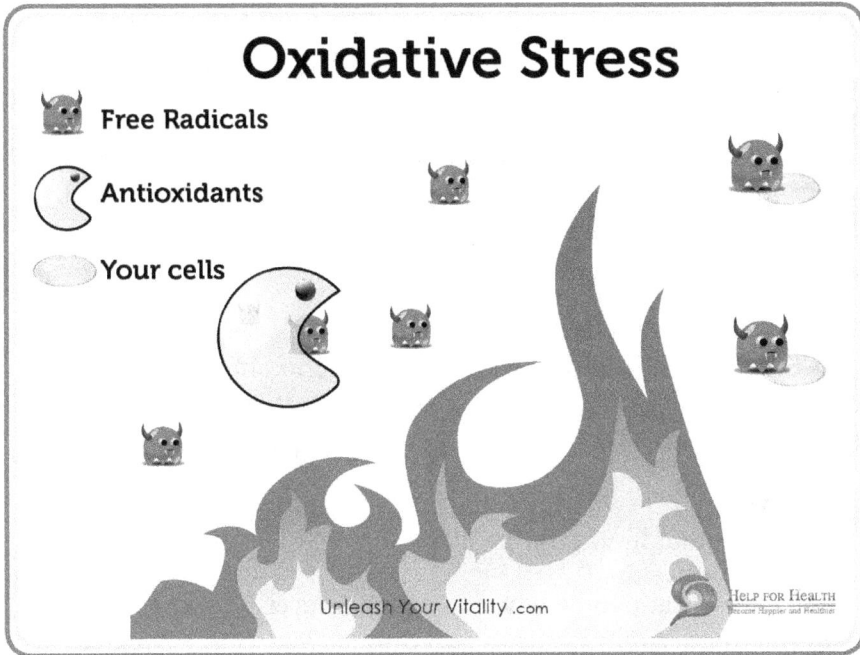

**Oxidative Stress**

Free Radicals

Antioxidants

Your cells

Unleash Your Vitality .com

HELP FOR HEALTH

Antioxidants prevent free radicals from harming our cells. They neutralize the free radical, preventing damage and protecting cells.

There are hundreds of different types of antioxidants, all with their own unique neutralizing properties. There is no single antioxidant that does it all, you need a large variety of them to assist you in your health and neutralize the different types of free radicals.

Did you notice that if you cut an apple and leave it on the table, it turns brown? The process is called oxidation. The apple is in contact with the air and forms free radicals. When enough free radicals are formed the discoloring will be visible. It's the same thing that happens inside your cells, when you are exposed to free radicals.

Did you know that, if you pour lemon juice on that piece of apple, it will no longer turn brown? The free radicals are still formed, there is no difference there, however the antioxidants in the lemon will neutralize the free radicals and that is why the apple keeps looking nice.

Sadly, we can't just drink lemon juice, because in order to get enough antioxidants from it, we would have to drink gallons of it, and it would destroy our stomach lining, causing other serious problems.

What we can do, is to use another antioxidant source, that is concentrated, effective and, most importantly, safe, like carefully controlled supplements. You will learn more about this in subsequent chapters.

Oxidative stress (too many free radicals) was proven to be one of the most important factors in the development of disease and premature ageing. It is caused by so many factors that we simply can't avoid them.

Extensive studies researched the involvement of oxidative stress in the diseases that haunt our century.

It was found that people who have higher levels of free radicals in their blood are suffering from conditions like:

- ☐ Cancer
- ☐ Diabetes
- ☐ Asthma
- ☐ Heart failure
- ☐ High blood pressure
- ☐ Depression
- ☐ Alzheimer's
- ☐ Parkinson's
- ☐ And many other diseases

---

***Oxidative stress is the root cause of all diseases,***
***Eliminating that stress is the root of all cures.***

---

If you want to improve a condition that you already have, or if you want to prevent developing such illnesses, you need to make sure that you are getting enough antioxidants to cope with the increasing exposure to free radicals.

Regardless of this fact, the medical community still focuses on addressing these diseases after they have settled. A better option would be to teach the population how to prevent the onset of these illnesses by using proper nutrition.

If doctors were paid only to keep a patient healthy, and if that payment would stop when those in his/her care got sick, prevention through nutrition would become the number one concern of the medical community. Until that is the case, you need to take matters into your own hands. So, what are you willing to do, to prevent illness from happening to you?

**Doctors are not paid to keep you healthy**

*The only 'real' life insurance is investment in nutrition*

*"Health is like money,*
*we never have a true idea of its value until we lose it."*
*~Josh Billings*

If there was an insurance policy that would almost guarantee that you would stay healthy forever, what would that insurance be worth to you? Really contemplate this question and come up with a monthly amount.

| MY PERSONAL HEALTH INSURANCE POLICY | |
|---|---|
| **Monthly fees** | ............... |

### *Free radical exposure*

Most of our food is processed or treated with chemicals, which facilitates the creation of free radicals. We live in a polluted environment. We are exposed to ozone depletion, air pollutants, radiation and chemicals every day. There is no place to hide from these factors, and even if we could move and live our lives on a mountaintop, we would still have to cope with the side-effects of modern life.

Causations of extra free radicals:

- ✓ *Radiation from the sun*
- ✓ *Electrical radiation*
- ✓ *Medication*
- ✓ *Chemicals in the air*
- ✓ *Chemicals in the water*
- ✓ *Fast food*
- ✓ *Smoking*
- ✓ *Mental-Emotional stress*

# How exposed are you?

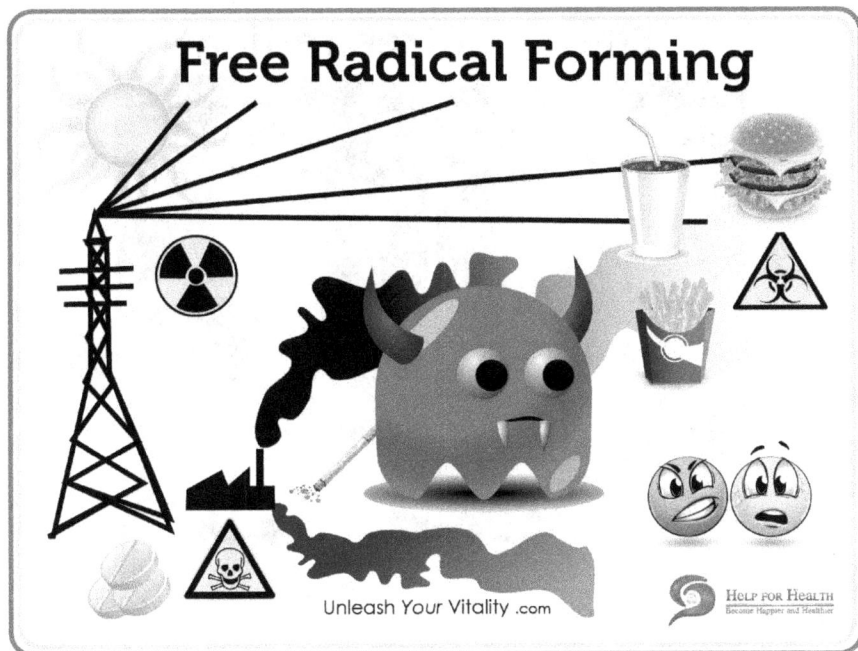

Free Radical Forming

*Unleash Your Vitality* .com

Did you know that even medication itself can cause oxidative stress?

They do this by interfering with the way the cells act. Even if medication is needed in certain conditions, it still creates more free radicals. This then increases the potential damage of oxidative stress.

This is one of those side-effects that you won't find on the label. It is for this reason that, when you take any kind of medication you really should help your body cope with the side-effects by supplementing your antioxidant intake.

If you want to visualize better how oxidative stress affects an individual, take a look at smokers. If you are lucky enough to meet a pair of middle-aged twins, and only one of them is a smoker, you will be amazed at the differences. We found such a case, and you can see for yourself what smoking does to you over the years[66].

# Effects of free radicals

Unleash Your Vitality .com

HELP FOR HEALTH

Look at these images. They represent a pair of twins, who were exposed to different levels of free radicals. The twin on the left never smoked, while the twin on the right smoked for 29 years. You can notice the fact that the smoker shows more signs of premature ageing and lack of vitality.

- ✓ *Look at the loose skin under the eyes*
- ✓ *Lines on her forehead*
- ✓ *Eyelids*
- ✓ *Vitality in the eyes*

Smoking does that by adding more free radicals to your system. This information isn't aimed at encouraging you to stop smoking, even if that would be an excellent idea. The purpose is to illustrate the way free radicals act.

What smoking visibly does to the outer layers of your body, free radicals do to the inside of your body. In the case of these twins, smoking just helps in painting a picture.

Free radicals change cells and the entire DNA, making you age faster than you should. Most of the time you are not even aware of what is happening inside your body, because the effects aren't always noticeable at first. However, with increased free radicals and without the antioxidants to neutralize them you are exposing yourself to disease development.

If you happen to be a smoker, you will have many more free radicals inside your body, so you should know that you also need many more antioxidants than a nonsmoker. One of the best things you could do to get your health on track would be to stop smoking. The next step would be to heal your body by taking antioxidants. But if you do not intend to quit or you cannot quit, then at least take triple the amount of antioxidants. You will learn later in this book where to get those antioxidants from.

Our only chance is to do what evolution has thought us, and adapt to the present conditions; that is reducing the number of free radicals as much as possible and taking plenty of antioxidants to prevent us from getting sick.

Each day, you encounter different agents that could be a danger to your health. The amount of free radicals produced by your body can vary from one day to another. This process depends on many factors, including psychological and physical stress, disease, chemicals and nutrition.

If you want to be constantly protected from the threat of free radicals, you need to supply your body with the right antioxidants, in a balanced manner, so that every time a free radical is produced, there will be something to neutralize it with.

**Antioxidants protect your health**

Nevertheless, antioxidants aren't as simple as they seem, you need to choose them wisely, to make sure that they are perfectly adapted to suit your needs, and that their source is natural.

Think about them as an umbrella that you can carry around to protect you from the rain. To make a comparison with our modern environment, rain could fall every day so, an umbrella is an excellent idea. Antioxidants are your umbrella.

It took science decades to discover the root of most problems, and several years to develop means of neutralizing those problems, but finally it came through, and we can benefit from its advancement.

> ✓ *Are you concerned that your free radical level might be too high, and that your health can be endangered?*

> ✓ *Have you noticed changes in your body that are letting you know that you must take action?*

> ✓ *Are you trying to find ways of protecting your children from this invisible threat?*

Then act now, and stay away from disease by supplementing your diet with powerful antioxidants. Do continue reading this book, as there are some important pitfalls to avoid.

## Let's do an exercise to get an indication how many free radicals you form in your daily life.

# Exercise: 4 – Free Radical Exposure Scale

Answer the following questions to give you an indication of how much you are exposed to free radicals, and how many antioxidants you should take in.

### 1. Where do you live?

| | | |
|---|---|---|
| A | ☐ | Big city |
| B | ☐ | Small city |
| C | ☐ | Country-side |
| D | ☐ | Mountains |

### 2. Do you smoke?

| | | |
|---|---|---|
| A | ☐ | Yes, daily |
| B | ☐ | Yes, occasionally |
| C | ☐ | No, but I am exposed to second hand smoke |
| D | ☐ | No, I never smoke and I am not exposed to second hand smoke |

### 3. Do you drink alcohol?

| | | |
|---|---|---|
| A | ☐ | Yes, more than once a week |
| B | ☐ | Yes, but less than 3 times a month |
| C | ☐ | No, not really, maybe one every other month |
| D | ☐ | No, never. |

## 4. Do you use medications (prescribed or over the counter)?

| A | ☐ | More than once a month |
|---|---|---|
| B | ☐ | Every month |
| C | ☐ | Only one or two times per year |
| D | ☐ | No, almost never |

## 5. Would you say that the place where you live and work is polluted?

| A | ☐ | Yes, very polluted |
|---|---|---|
| B | ☐ | Yes, moderately polluted |
| C | ☐ | Not really polluted |
| D | ☐ | No, not at all |

## 6. Do you eat lots of fatty foods, fast-food, processed foods and foods with additives?

| A | ☐ | Yes, more than twice a week |
|---|---|---|
| B | ☐ | Yes, once a week or less |
| C | ☐ | Sometimes |
| D | ☐ | Never |

## 7. Is your skin exposed to sunlight?

| A | ☐ | Yes, very often |
|---|---|---|
| B | ☐ | Yes, occasionally |
| C | ☐ | Sometimes |
| D | ☐ | Rarely |

## 8. Do you get sick? (even common colds count)

| A | ☐ | Yes, quite often |
|---|---|---|
| B | ☐ | Yes, once a year |
| C | ☐ | Rarely |
| D | ☐ | Almost never |

## 9. Is your house cleaned with chemical cleaning agents?

| | | |
|---|---|---|
| A | ☐ | Yes, very often |
| B | ☐ | Yes, but not excessively |
| C | ☐ | Rarely |
| D | ☐ | Almost never |

## 10. Do you eat organic, unsprayed vegetables and fruits?

| | | |
|---|---|---|
| A | ☐ | Almost never |
| B | ☐ | Rarely |
| C | ☐ | A few times a month |
| D | ☐ | Yes, multiple times a week |

## 11. Do you have emotional stress in your life?

| | | |
|---|---|---|
| A | ☐ | Yes, daily |
| B | ☐ | Yes, often |
| C | ☐ | Rarely |
| D | ☐ | Never |

## 12. Do you drink enough purified water daily?

| | | |
|---|---|---|
| A | ☐ | I drink coffee or tea instead of water |
| B | ☐ | I drink less than 2 liters water |
| C | ☐ | I drink 2 or more liters tap water or bottled water |
| D | ☐ | I drink 2 or more liters purified water |

## Calculate your score

1. *Count the number of A's and write the number in the column below*

2. *Count the number of B,C,D's and write them in the columns below*

3. *Calculate the totals by multiplying the count*

4. *Calculate the overall score by adding all 4 totals*

|  | Count | Total |
|---|---|---|
| A | X 4 | = ...... |
| B | X 3 | = ...... |
| C | X 2 | = ...... |
| D | X 1 | = ...... |
| **Overall Score** |  | = •••••• |

## Score 36-48

You are extremely exposed to free radicals, and your body is in desperate need of antioxidants to cope with this issue. Take action immediately.

You are exposed to free radicals on a daily basis, and you probably notice their influence over your body. Supplementing with antioxidants would be of great benefit to your health.

## Score 24-36

You are moderately exposed to free radicals, and, even if your health seems to be untouched for now, constant exposure will influence your long-term wellbeing. Supplementing your diet with antioxidants would be beneficial.

## Score 12-24

Congratulations, you have successfully managed to avoid constant exposure to antioxidants. Nevertheless, antioxidants would help you prevent disease, and since you have a healthy lifestyle, with proper nutrition you could live a very long and healthy life.

———◈———

The next chapter will show you what diseases derive from prolonged exposure to oxidative stress. These effects shouldn't scare you, instead you should learn from them, and you should motivate yourself to take control over your life.

***Don't allow yourself to get sick before you take action.***

### 4.2.1   Your Key Points to Remember

## Exercise

✓ *Did you complete Exercise: 4 – Free Radical Exposure Scale ?*

## Key points to remember

✓ *Biochemical stress creates free radicals*

✓ *Free radicals damage cells*

✓ *Antioxidants neutralize free radicals and thus protect and repair cells*

✓ *There are hundreds of different antioxidants. You need them all to neutralize the different types of free radicals*

✓ *Smokers need more antioxidants than non-smokers*

✓ *The damage produced by free radicals leads to diseases like premature ageing, disease, slowed immune response, and cancer*

✓ *Supplements with high antioxidant levels prevent and reverse cell damage and diseases*

✓ *Different sources of antioxidants are needed to protect you against all free radicals and to obtain or maintain vibrant vitality.*

# *Your Amazing Insights and Actions*

Date: __ / __ / _____

## What are your insights and learnings from this section?

Now we have come to the conclusion of this chapter. Write down your main insights about what you learned and about yourself.

## What are you going to do differently starting today?

Insights alone will not unleash your vitality. You need to take actions. What are the actions you are going to do in order to implement these insights in your life?

## 4.3 The Extraordinary Awesome and All Mighty Immune System

Do you know why you are able to sit and read this book today?

Because you didn't get sick and die every time you encountered a life-threatening germ. And this is due to… yes the answer is found in the title of this chapter, the immune system.

We tend to overlook and underestimate this beautiful mechanism that nature gave us. Without it, we wouldn't even survive being born, and still we don't give it enough credit.

There are millions of cells running through our blood to keep us safe from outside invaders. During our life, we come into contact with viruses, bacteria and other microbes. Our immune system is there to protect us from getting symptoms.

> *"Regaining health is more difficult than becoming ill.*
> *Becoming ill is a random act of ignorance*
> *and regaining health is an intentional effort in frustration"*
> *~ Richard Diaz*

We all want a strong immune system that can prevent every disease always. That isn't possible, but what we could build is an immune system that can prevent most disease. An immune system that is able to fight cancer cells, bacterial- fungal and viral infections, and all kinds of bugs.

Poor immunity has been linked to a series of factors, and you are going to learn which these are, because it is important to avoid them as much as possible. That is, if you want a strong and effective immune system.

One of the circumstances that can cause your immune reaction to slow down is stress. Often this isn't avoidable, but you can at least try to minimize reactions to stress and create supporting strategies to deal with it.

Stress influences an incredible amount of processes in our body, ranging from how we act, to how we eat and process nutrients. It lends a hand in the creation of free radicals, it forces your adrenal glands to produce more adrenaline, it makes you irritable, it doesn't let you fall asleep and it has a series of other unwanted effects.

*"Insufficient vitamin intake is a cause of chronic disease... it appears prudent for all adults to take vitamin supplements."*
*~ Journal of American Medical Association, June 2002*

What is stress? You've definitely heard about it, and you've most definitely felt it, but really, what is it?

Stress is the fight and flight mechanism of your body. When we evolved, danger was all around us, and we hadn't yet developed the "getting mad" feeling. When you are stressed, the brain perceives it as constant danger, and makes adjustments to the body, to be able to cope with a dangerous situation.

Stress sends more blood to the muscles, it alerts the senses, releases hormones which will increase your heart rate and respiratory rate. It slows down processes that are considered irrelevant in a dangerous situation. One of these processes involves the immune system.

Stress itself should be useful, because it is a survival mechanism. Problems start emerging when we are constantly stressed, and stress hormones run through our blood continuously and produce havoc all around.

Stress is a big factor in everyday life, and the older we become, the more exposed we are. The fact that illness is closely related to stress is…well, an understatement.

> *"When under stress, cells of the immune system are unable to respond properly and this promote disease"*
> *~ Prof. Cohen - Professor of Psychology*

This book is not intended to go too much into this subject, but if you want to find efficient ways of coping with this disease of the century, you can find answers and methods in my book "Healing Psyche" (http://www.healingpsyche.com).

Another important reason why your immune system is not functioning the way it should, is a buildup of toxins.

A crucial part of the immune system is represented by the lymphatic system. If you are retaining water and toxins, the inflammation that results from this will prevent the lymph from circulating properly and will slow down the immune response, allowing the viruses and bacteria enough time to multiply.

**Lack of nutrients breaks the system**

One of the leading causes of immune system malfunction is nutrient deficiency. One particular study demonstrated that malnutrition doesn't just affect the subject exposed to it, but also weakens the immune system of any children they may have. The researchers gave a pregnant mouse a diet that was deficient in zinc. After it delivered, a normal diet rich in nutrients was introduced for her and the offspring. Nevertheless, the mice and their offspring did not ever develop a strong immune system during the course of their entire life. The same way, if you suffer from a deficiency, it will affect your children for their entire life.

Now that you've come to understand the factors that influence your health status and the way your body faces its attackers, let's see what you can do to restore the normal functions that protect you from disease.

As with all aspects of your health, immunity calls for a proactive approach. You need to understand that waiting to get sick, and then helping your body cope with the problem is not your best option. Every time you suffer from an illness, you expose your cells to more free radicals, disturbing the entire balance and creating opportunities for cells to mutate into cancer.

Your immune system needs constant nutritional support as it renews its cells every day, and those cells call for a large number of nutrients.

> *"If you do not invest in your health*
> *then you do not need a retirement plan"*
> *~ Rob van Overbruggen*

Think of that for a second.

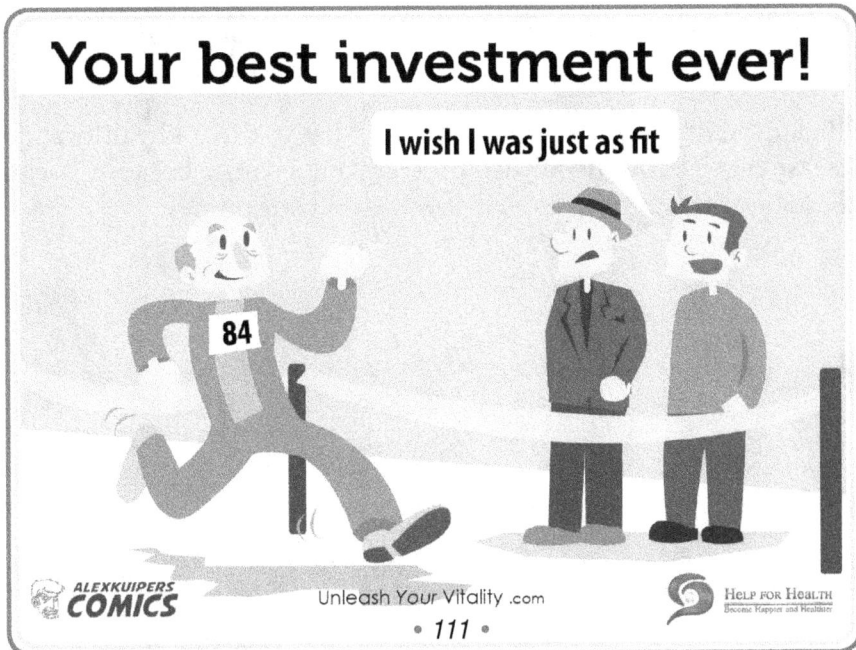

Your best investment ever!

I wish I was just as fit

### What to do?

The first step towards long lasting health is found in your diet. Try to avoid processed, fatty foods, sugar and excess red meats. Furthermore, make sure that what you eat is not filled with chemicals and toxins. You can do that by buying whole grain products, eating organic vegetables, nuts and seeds and cold water fish like salmon.

Make sure you choose a vitamin and a mineral supplement that address the specific needs of your immunity. A good vitamin supplement should be able to provide all vitamins B, a generous amount of vitamins C and D, vitamin E, and if possible grape seed extract, which is famous for its involvement in the immune function.

Don't forget that minerals are a must when you are concerned about your immunity. A supplement containing calcium carbonate and citrate, magnesium, zinc, copper, selenium, cinnamon and natural green tea extract, would be of great help.

Drink plenty of clean purified water to keep your body clean of all the toxins that impair the lymph from circulating properly. Double-check to be certain that you are also getting lots of antioxidants, to prevent cells from going rogue and turning into cancer cells.

A balanced immune system will ensure that you live a healthy and disease free life, but it will also protect your savings, because disease doesn't just waste your time, it also wastes your money.

### 4.3.1  Your Key Points to Remember

✓ *Stress is one of the leading causes of a poor immune response*

✓ *Low immune reactions lead to diseases*

✓ *A diet high in (trans or saturated) fats and a high cholesterol level diminishes the immune response*

✓ *Nutritional deficiencies lower the immune response*

✓ *A child whose mother was malnourished during pregnancy will develop a deficient immune system*

✓ *Vitamins B, C, D and E, interact directly with the immune system, therefore a supplement that contains them will benefit you greatly*

✓ *Zinc, copper and selenium are of great value for the efficiency of the immune response*

## 4.4    Want to be brainy like Einstein? Brain food!

The mind is the invisible force that drives us, it stores our memories, it can be clear or foggy, it dictates our actions, and, it can be fast or slow. We define ourselves through our mind: we are what IT is.

*"The energy of the mind is the essence of life."*
*~ Aristotle*

We take our mind for granted, and we only think about it when we have to learn something new, or when we forget something. It rarely occurs to us that the mind has to eat too.

What does the mind eat?

The philosophical answer would be: ideas. As beautiful and deep as that sounds, before we can nourish our mind with information and ideas, we first have to give it something to sustain it physically.

The brain is the central core of our mind. The brain is the one that dictates our every move, it stores the memory, it controls the heartbeat and it too can become sick if it doesn't receive proper nutrition.

You already know that nutrition can influence your mood, behavior and the way you experience certain events, but did you know that it can affect your brain functions?

Nutrient intake reflects in the brain chemistry, and it can influence the way neurotransmitters act, therefore perturbing or improving your memory, sleeping patterns, mood, emotional status, communication, eyesight and many other brain functions. You will see the effects that proper nutrients have on your mental capabilities in subsequent chapters.

The brain begins to deteriorate when the balance of nutrients drops.

Do you know how much of your energy goes to your brain?

It can use up to 30% of your energy intake, being one of the most demanding organs in your body. If you are stressed, and you need to think about your next move all the time, it takes even more energy. Making decisions and even worrying about issues uses up tremendous amounts of energy.

When it is deprived of essential nutrients it slows down, and when the brain slows down, everything else does too.

Think about how important it is to have good reflexes when you are driving, and how much damage can come from just one second of diminished attention. How debilitating would life be if you could not concentrate or remember your spouse?

Even though the brain controls your entire body it is also entirely dependent on it. This means that if something goes wrong at a different level in the body, it will affect the brain. If you are not getting enough oxygen, brain cells will start dying. If you get an infection, it can pass through the Blood Brain Barrier and infect the brain directly. If you are exposed to a high amount of free radicals, your brain cells will be affected as well. So, having good general health will decrease your chances of having problems with your brain, like dementia, memory loss, poor concentration or lack of focus.

**Your brain needs nutrients to keep functioning**

Take Alzheimer's for example. This is a frightening condition, and most people prefer not to think about it. It completely changes a person, and it is even harder on those around them. Our mind is the only thing we know we can trust, but what happens if it goes away, and we forget who we are, what we like to do and who we love?

The National Institute of Health predicts that by 2050, 100 million people worldwide will be suffering from Alzheimer's.

### What is this terrible disease?

Alzheimer's is a condition that derives from a variety of causes. The exact reasons why it appears aren't yet fully understood, although many medical studies have shown that it could be related directly to faulty nutrition and poor lifestyle choices. It manifests initially through irritability, depression, confusion and latterly, tremendous memory loss. By doing this it changes the people affected, to the point where they would no longer know themselves.

The one thing the medical community has found in all Alzheimer's cases is a high level of Homocysteine[67]. This is the same amino-acid that is related to heart attacks, atherosclerosis and strokes.

What can you do to prevent memory loss and Alzheimer's?

The most important action that you can take is to keep your Homocysteine levels as low as possible, and to do that you will need a good nutritional supplement that will provide you the proper balance of nutrients, and more importantly B vitamins, which were proven to fight against Homocysteine build-ups.

Furthermore, keeping stress at a low level is also important, we've previously discussed its involvement in other conditions, but when it comes to issues of the mind it is of utmost relevance.

### Why?

Professor Robert Sapolsky[68] led research at Stanford University, and showed that under stress, the levels of cortisol raised so much that it actually killed brain cells; in addition to taking B vitamins you need to reduce your stress levels.

Your brain needs more antioxidants than all your other organs. There is so much going on inside it that it needs constant support. The only way that you can make sure that your memory stays fit is to feed your brain, first with the right nutrients, and then with ideas.

**Growing old with a well working mind**

Getting old doesn't mean you have to start losing your mind. There are people in this world, who reach the age of 100, and their mind is sharper than that of a 20 year old. They managed to stay alive and keep their mind active, through nutrition and a balanced diet. On the other hand there are many people who are only as old as 50 who have difficulties remembering where they parked their car.

If you want to grow to be a grandfather who plays chess with his grandchild, while still remembering that you have to fly to Florida for the weekend, you need to start feeding your brain now.

Be proactive; don't wait until you start forgetting what it means to enjoy life.

### 4.4.1    Your Key Points to Remember

✓ *The brain uses up to 30% or more of all your energy*

✓ *High Homocysteine levels in your blood reduces your brain capacity and can lead to mental diseases*

✓ *B vitamins helps you keep Homocysteine levels low*

✓ *Nutrients keep your brain working at optimal levels*

✓ *Without proper nutrients you will have trouble concentrating, trouble with focus, memory and might even develop Alzheimer's*

✓ *Your brain needs high levels of antioxidants*

# *Your Amazing Insights and Actions*

Date: __ / __ / _____

## What are your insights and learnings from this section?

Now we have come to the conclusion of this chapter. Write down your main insights about what you learned and about yourself.

## What are you going to do differently starting today?

Insights alone will not unleash your vitality. You need to take actions. What are the actions you are going to do in order to implement these insights in your life?

## 4.5 But where did our food go?

When speaking about nutrition, the first thing that comes to mind is food, and this is normal, considering the fact that for thousands and thousands of years, we absorbed all the required nutrients exclusively from our food.

---

*"Give a man a fish and you feed him for a day; teach a man to fish and you feed him for a lifetime." ~ Proverb*

---

A balanced diet, with the right amount of fiber, fruits and vegetables, continues to be essential for our wellbeing, but as society has evolved, food itself has changed, and in order to monitor your nutritional uptake, you must be able to understand the changes that "revolutionized" food.

The beginning of the industrial revolution, changed the way we view and produce food, not only at a social level, but also at the molecular level.

The industrial revolution began somewhere in between the late 1700's and the early1800's in Great Britain, and since that moment it has circled the world, turning peasants into people who work from nine to five inside an office. It has brought amazing discoveries in all fields. It is due to this revolution, that today we are able to travel across continents, to have access to medical care and education. It is the reason for which we have information at our finger-tips, and we can communicate with people from all over the world instantly.

It has changed the way we think, act, envision the future, but it has also changed our food, and this is the aspect that interests us the most.

Have you ever wondered how many people there were in the world, in the early 1800's? Today there are a little over seven billion people who live and breathe at the same time you do. So, 200 years ago there might have been fewer people, but the number shouldn't be too dramatic. Right?

Well... it depends on your idea of drama, because in the beginning of the 19th century, there were roughly 1 billion people.

Now, you can probably understand the influence the industrial revolution has had on humankind. Our numbers have increased extremely fast, in a very short amount of time. This is not necessarily a bad thing, since more people usually translates into more gifted minds, and a larger genetic availability, which can only benefit the evolution of the species.

However, there is a downside to this rapid growth, and it's this downside that affects you directly.

In order to have enough food to feed a rapidly growing population, we had to adapt, and make changes in the way we produce and create 'food'.

You can be sure that agriculture has suffered the most in this regard. We had to completely reshape the way we used the land, because what we used to do, simply wasn't enough anymore. With this change, the quality of our nutrients has dropped dramatically.

> **Food is optimized for production, not for nutrients**

Maybe you noticed that some foods don't seem to taste like the original? If you experienced the taste of a nice tomato some years ago then compare that with the current tomato. You may notice that it's almost tasteless nowadays? That even if it is well ripened, it doesn't have that yummy smell anymore?

The food that we eat today has been modified to grow faster because our society needs more than a single crop per year to satisfy the growing demand. Fruits and vegetables are sprayed with chemicals and fertilizers to prevent them from being damaged and to help them grow at a faster pace. No matter how well you wash them, these poisonous chemicals and fertilizers stay on the surface. Some of these poisons even penetrate the shell and sip into the core.

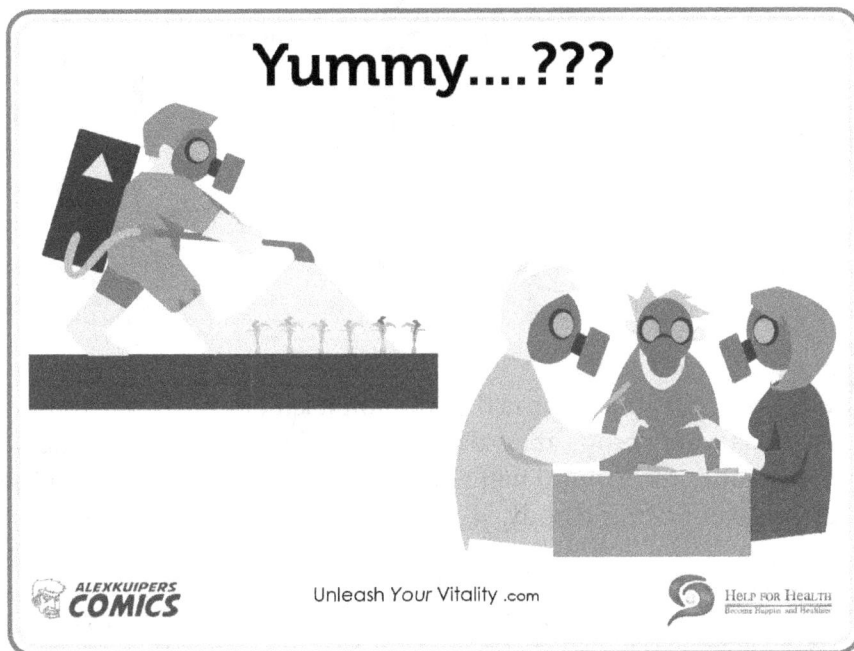

Did you notice that fruits are sometimes bigger than in the past? This is due to genetic tampering. People modified plants to grow bigger and heavier to satisfy demand and financial interests. This doesn't give the plants enough time to extract nutrients from the soil. Most vegetables you can buy are grown on water, rather than soil, this makes them devoid of any vitamins and minerals. The food industry was forced to use this technique due to the scarcity of land, but also due to the low costs that it implies. The plants don't even benefit from sunlight, they are grown indoors with special lamps.

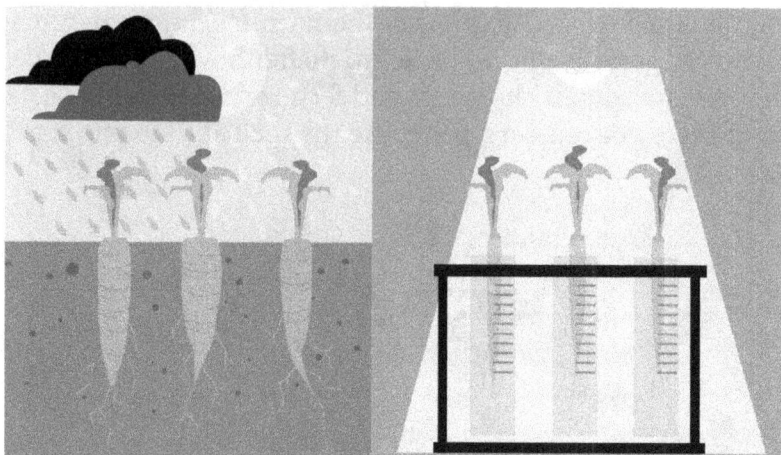

# Growing Carrots

ALEXKUIPERS **COMICS**

Unleash Your Vitality .com

HELP FOR HEALTH

The uglier truth about this is that the soil itself has been affected. Most areas where crops are grown are now depleted of nutrients. What is not in the ground will not be in the plant, what is not in the plant will not be in the body.

Soil is the base of our life. Most of the things we eat grow in it, or feed from what grows in it. Soil has formed after millions of years of evolution, and during its formation, it accumulated the nutrients that today feed our plants. It is the ultimate resource, and even if science can develop alternatives, without soil, the human race, along with all other life on earth will disappear sooner than you can imagine.

Plants, like fruits and vegetables, obtain nutrients from the soil, but if the soil is depleted of these vital elements, plants themselves will not contain nutrients. If plants no longer have a nutritional value, how can you get those precious nutrients to maintain your health?

People who fish might have noticed the fact that angleworms are more and more difficult to find. This is not due to a stroke of bad luck. In fact, they are scarce because the soil is damaged, and not because they are hiding from you.

Soil is home for billions, even trillions of worms, bugs, fungi, bacteria and rodents. Even if you don't like this idea, you must know that all this biodiversity is essential for its health and composition. A single inch of topsoil forms in 500 to 1000 years. This means that for a layer of soil to form around the world, more than five generation of children must be born.

Humans have interfered with this process to the level where soil has been depleted of its nutrients. This happened because we didn't have the time to wait until it formed properly, and we overexploited every piece of land available. Soil degradation is the main cause for which you don't get enough nutrients from your food, and this isn't going to change any time soon.

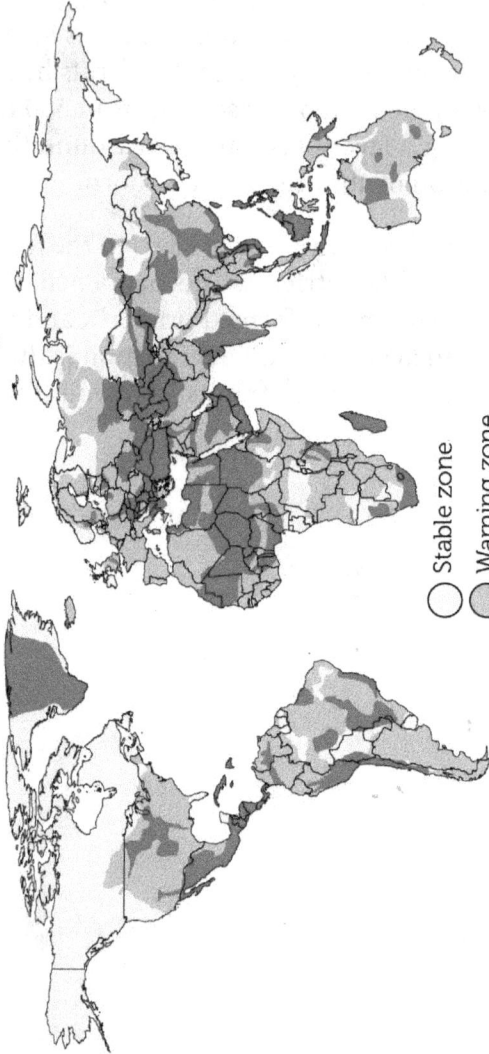

Quality of Soil Worldmap

Stable zone
Warning zone
Danger zone, no vegitation anymore

Unleash Your Vitality .com

HELP FOR HEALTH
Become Happier and Healthier

*Soil degradation over the past 100 years.*

NOTE! This is the status of 1992. There is no indication that it changed for the better.

## Minerals left in the soil

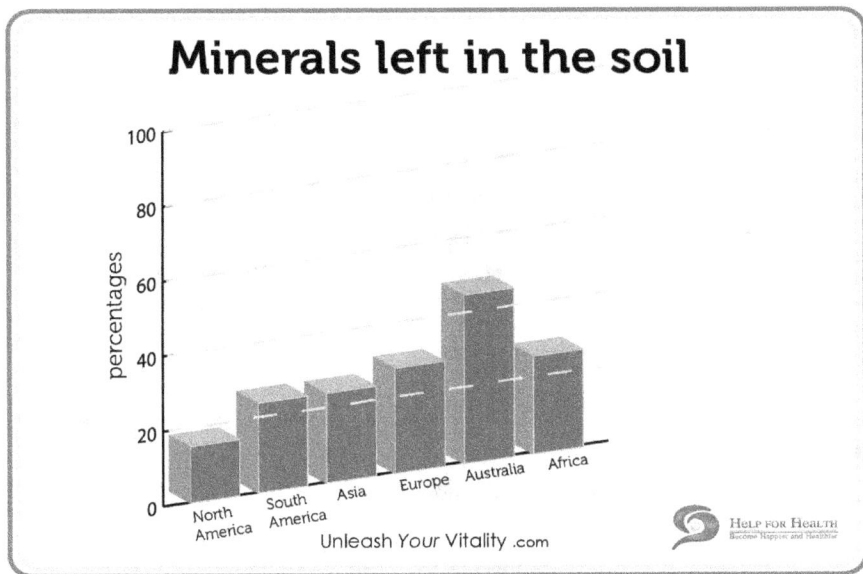

Source:[69]

---

*"There is deep concern over continuing major declines in the mineral values in farm and range soils throughout the world"*
*~ Official Conclusion 1992 Earth Summit*

---

### How does soil become degraded?

The first step in degradation is erosion. This is a natural process that usually happens due to the environment. It is caused by rain and wind and it is a slow process that is normally compensated by the natural formation of new soil. Sadly, mankind is accelerating this process by farming, and by destroying vegetation. On the other hand, if we had the vegetation that we had 200 years ago, and we allowed forests to grow, erosion wouldn't affect the quality of the soil, because it would have the resources needed to regenerate.

The other way humans are influencing the depletion of the soil is by over cultivating. When plants grow, they extract nutrients from the soil, if the same area is cultivated over and over again, it won't have enough time to regenerate. This is why, in ancient times, when there were less people on the planet, farmers never cultivated the same area for two years in a row.

They used to allow the land to lie fallow which means to rest for an entire year, without even letting animals feed from it. The next year they would cultivate it with a different crop than two years before, because different plants require different nutrients. Also, back then the number of trees was much greater, and those trees kept water from over accumulating, therefore from eroding the soil. Trees also helped in the formation of new soil. It was a simple and ingenious system that allowed the soil to regenerate.

**If it is not in the soil, it is not in the food**

Nowadays, we grow two crops in a single year on the same piece of land. We've destroyed most of the forests and we almost never rotate crops.

This practice, combined with the many chemical treatments the soil has undergone to increase production has changed the chemical balance of the soil, and it is no longer able to provide the plants with the right amount of minerals.

This is the reason for which, today's farmers are often forced for profitability reasons to use artificial fertilizers to help plants grow. Even if these manufactured nutrients encourage growth, they cannot supply plants all they need to develop properly, and this is why they smell and taste different, but more importantly, this is why they fail to provide us with what we need nutritionally.

According to the International Soil Reference and Information Centre, "soil is a threatened natural resource", this idea shouldn't be taken lightly, because it influences what we eat, and what we eat influences us.

Did you notice that salad seems to taste like plastic? Well… now you know why that happens.

Nutrition is "sabotaged" by the growth of the population, and as the population grows, food will keep losing its properties, until the point where there will be nothing left for us to assimilate from our food, no vitamins, no minerals and no essential nutrients.

**Food is sabotaged and robbed of its nutritional value**

The food we eat has lost so many nutrients along the path of evolution it often doesn't even resemble the original product anymore. Carrots are still orange and tomatoes are red, but at the molecular level, where every small detail is important, nutrients have become a rarity.

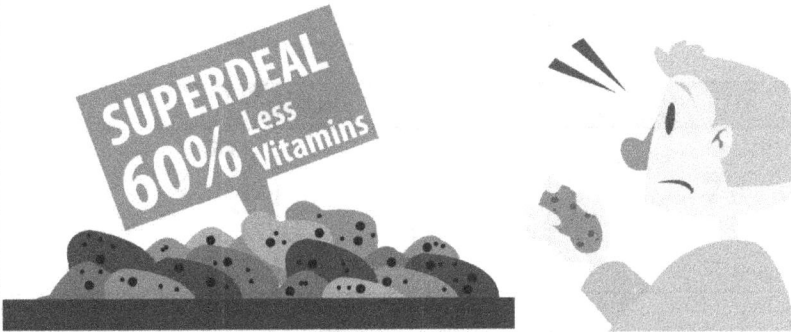

Just take a look at these tables, they show exactly what is happening, and how you are being deprived of what you need.

### *Nutritional loss over the years per 100 grams*

| BROCCOLI | 1985 | 2002 | REDUCTION |
|---|---|---|---|
| Calcium | 103 | 28 | -73% |
| Folic acid | 47 | 18 | -62% |
| Magnesium | 26 | 11 | -58% |
| Iron | | | -46% |
| Cupper | | | -75% |

| POTATOES | 1985 | 2002 | REDUCTION |
|---|---|---|---|
| Calcium | 14 | 3 | 79% |
| Magnesium | 27 | 6 | 78% |
| Iron | | | -45% |
| Cupper | | | -47% |

| CARROTS | 1985 | 2002 | REDUCTION |
|---|---|---|---|
| Calcium | 37 | 28 | -24% |
| Magnesium | 21 | 6 | -71% |

| SPINACH | 1985 | 2002 | REDUCTION |
|---|---|---|---|
| Calcium | 62 | 18 | -71% |
| Vitamin C | 51 | 18 | -65% |
| Magnesium | 62 | 15 | 76% |
| Cupper | | | -96% |

| APPLES | 1985 | 2002 | REDUCTION |
|---|---|---|---|
| Vitamin C | 5 | 2 | -60% |

| BEANS | 1985 | 2002 | REDUCTION |
|-------|------|------|-----------|
| Calcium | 56 | 22 | -61% |
| Folic acid | 39 | 30 | -23% |
| Manganese | 26 | 18 | -31% |
| Vitamin B6 | 140 | 32 | -77% |

| STRAWBERRIES | 1985 | 2002 | REDUCTION |
|--------------|------|------|-----------|
| Calcium | 21 | 12 | -33% |
| Vitamin C | 60 | 8 | -87% |
| Calcium | 21 | 8 | -87% |

| BANANAS | 1985 | 2002 | REDUCTION |
|---------|------|------|-----------|
| Calcium | 8 | 7 | -13% |
| Folium Acid | 23 | 5 | -78% |
| Magnesium | 31 | 24 | -23% |
| Vitamin B6 | 330 | 18 | -95% |

Source: [70,71]

The amount of nutrients contained in food has lowered dramatically, and there are no signs that this continuous decline is stopping. In a few years there will be no nutritional value left.

You would have to eat much more in order to get the same amount of nutrients you would have 20 years ago. Only to satisfy the calcium demand, you would have to eat on average five times the number of vegetables you ate back then, but in doing so, you would be putting your digestive system under a tremendous amount of stress. Can you imagine having to eat 5 times as many vegetables?

If Popeye's loved one Olive were in danger, he would have to eat 5 cans (!) of spinach before he could beat Brutus and save his darling Olive. And that was in 1991. There is no evidence that the decline has stopped since then. Probably he would have to eat 10 or more servings now to get the same amount of nutrients.

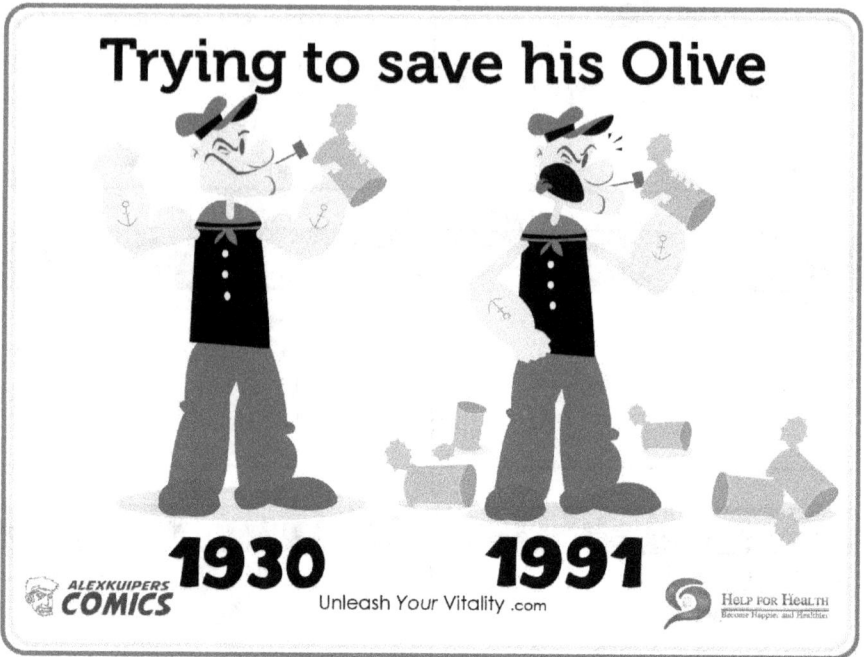

Trying to save his Olive — 1930 — 1991

ALEXKUIPERS COMICS · Unleash Your Vitality .com · HELP FOR HEALTH

## What about the effects of soil depletion on meat?

How do you like your chicken? It is one of the most common meats eaten worldwide. Theoretically, it provides an entire array of nutrients, vitamins B, vitamin D, E, and lots of minerals like calcium, phosphorus and many others. This sounds good, right?

Well this was accurate back when chickens were raised in your grandmother's back yard. The food they received was complete, not genetically modified. The birds weren't stuffed with hormones and antibiotics. In the past, it took a chicken several months to grow in order to be ready to eat. Nowadays, most live in a small cage with artificial light 24/7, and it arrives on your plate having lived only several weeks!

It still looks like chicken, no question there, but how much of it is really useful nutritionally? Will it help you grow new, healthy cells? Or will it just fill your stomach while giving you barely enough nutrients to stay alive?

### Effect of soil depletion

The effect of this soil depletion is easily noticed when you review other research that looked at animals that live off the land and the products that they become. There is a dramatic reduction of the minerals in the final products like beef, turkey and even milk. So, even the animals which live off the land and eat the raw materials are not even receiving enough minerals anymore.

What do you think is happening to your body when you eat similar nutrient deprived meat or vegetables?

|  | MINERAL | 1940 | 2002 | REDUCTION |
|---|---|---|---|---|
| Beef | Sodium | 76 | 62 | -18% |
|  | Iron | 4.7 | 2.9 | -38% |
|  | Copper | 0.25 | 0.04 | -84% |
| Turkey | Sodium | 130 | 90 | -31% |
|  | Calcium | 38.3 | 11 | -79% |
| Cheese | Calcium | 1220 | 362 | -70% |
|  | Iron | 0.37 | 0 | all gone |

Source[72]

### Effect of stolen nutrients

Imagine your body as an older car, one which you need to put leaded petrol in. Everything runs fine and you can just go to the petrol station and get your fuel. Now imagine that you were unaware that the petrol stations removed the lead from petrol. You continue fuelling your car with the now lead-less petrol. Soon your car's engine will break down, because it no longer receives the lead for lubrication. Your beautiful car's engine will be damaged beyond repair.

The general, but false conclusion: Normal wear and tear, it was an old car.

Factual correct conclusion: Engine broke down because it did not get the lead it used to get.

You never changed petrol stations, yet your car is broken down because it did not get the proper 'nutrients'.

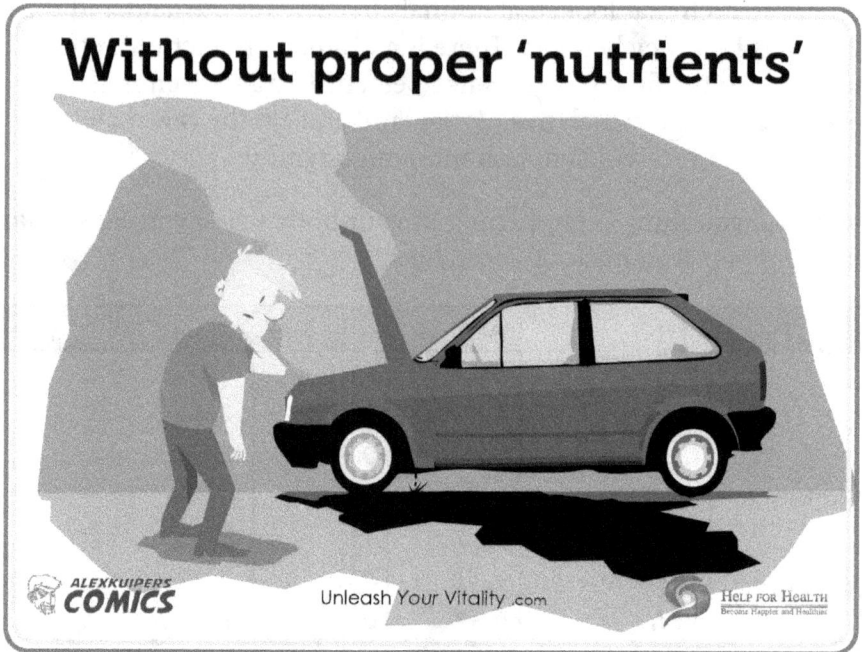

This research data is not new, and you can only imagine that once the trend was set, it would only go downhill. Plants are made to grow faster and faster, and no one will have the time or the money, to stop and consider the implications of malnourished people.

What do you think about the information you've learned in this chapter? Did you know that just eating the right foods is no longer enough? Does this information encourage you to make changes in your life?

### 4.5.1 Your Key Points to Remember

✓ *Food has lost vital nutrients and this reflects in all your cells*

✓ *Nutrient deficiency leads to symptoms*

✓ *Severe deficiency leads to severe symptoms*

✓ *200 years ago the general health status was way higher because of the rich nutrients in food*

✓ *Being old, healthy and happy is possible when you are being proactive and well nourished*

✓ *Food hasn't just lost its taste. The amount of nutrients contained has dropped tremendously*

✓ *Soil itself has lost the nutrients that were needed for growing nutritious plants*

✓ *Most vegetables are grown on water, instead of soil, therefore they completely lack nutritional value*

✓ *Food contains, at most, 20% of the nutrients that it used to have 20 years ago*

✓ *The lack of nutrients in food affects health directly, causing people to suffer from nutritional deficiencies*

## 4.6   The Shocking Truth

Are you afraid that by reading this, you will discover new symptoms? That you might have to admit that you have certain symptoms? Do some members of your family suffer from diabetes or cancer, and you worry that you could be next?

You are reading this book now, and this can only mean one thing: you are determined to stay healthy and reshape your future, in a way that will allow you to take control over your wellbeing. So, use the information we are giving you to do exactly that, and you will know what to do.

You are beginning to know more about how your body works, and the mechanism that drives it. Now, we will take a look behind the mirror glass and see how and why things could go wrong. Knowing what hurts your body will give you the upper hand in prevention.

The scientific community have linked lack of proper nutrition to a wide variety of health and wellbeing conditions affecting the population, and inadequate nutrition can pose a serious threat to life itself.

**Lack of nutrients lead to serious diseases**

Most of these conditions are manageable, but in order to prevent, or treat the underlying problem, we have to take a good look at what causes them. Only by changing the entire scenario that is unfolding underneath our skin, can we change the evolution of disease.

An imbalance in the nutrients received by the body can cause susceptibility to infection, an increase in viral diseases, allergies, other auto-immune conditions, coronary heart disease, diabetes, atherosclerosis, high blood pressure, irritable bowel syndrome, obesity, acne, insomnia, fertility problems, cancer, joint inflammation and erosion, and many others.

In this chapter we will focus on just a few of these conditions in order to shed some light on how to improve your life, and on how to prevent these conditions from affecting you.

### 4.6.1    High Blood Pressure

High blood pressure is a condition that affects millions of people worldwide. High Blood Pressure itself doesn't do much damage, but when it stays elevated for a long period of time, it puts the heart and vascular system under strain and can lead to congestive heart failure, heart attacks, stroke and even kidney failure. It also affects the quality of life due to headaches, altered vision and all the other symptoms that it can bring.

There are a few factors that contribute to this high blood pressure. The consumption of nicotine, caffeine, alcohol, fast foods and stress are important factors.

Some studies revealed that patients suffering from high blood pressure had inadequate amounts of Vitamin C, Calcium and Magnesium in their blood. In 23 scientific studies that were gathered by the Linus Pauling Institute they all showed that a higher calcium intake is related directly to a low, safe blood pressure.

A proper mineral balance (especially the calcium–magnesium ratio: see the respective chapters) with the right Vitamin D, CoQ10 and a reasonable intake of vitamin C can prevent and treat this condition.

### 4.6.2    Diabetes

What is diabetes? Do you have a family member suffering from this disease? Are you afraid that you might be its victim in a few years?

Most people know at least one person suffering from this condition; this idea tells us that there are many people suffering from it. In fact around 24 million people, in the United States alone suffer from diabetes, and this statistic refers only to those people who were diagnosed.

This table illustrates the number of people in the USA diagnosed with diabetes, by year. Sadly, the number is in millions.

| YEAR | NUMBER (IN MILLIONS) |
|------|----------------------|
| 1980 | 5.6 |
| 1990 | 6.6 |
| 2000 | 12.0 |
| 2010 | 20.8 |
| 2011 | 20.9 |

Diabetes is a chronic condition, and once it has settled in, without significant lifestyle changes the prognosis is that you will suffer from it your entire life.

But what is it? What causes it? And most importantly, how can we prevent it?

Your body transforms sugar into glucose, which feeds your cells. In this process insulin is used. Insulin makes your cells permeable, meaning that it allows the cells to use the glucose from your blood.

Without the right balance of insulin, cells won't be able to open their doors, and glucose will be stuck in your blood and cells will starve. Diabetic patients measure how much glucose is stuck in their blood. When cells are starving they cannot perform their duty and symptoms will develop further, for example your skin cannot heal properly from wounds.

Although advancements in medicine have provided those who suffer from diabetes a fighting chance, this is still a common condition, and it is the leading cause of blindness in the U.S. So, even if the disease is manageable, it could impair your life in a very disturbing way.

Type 2 Diabetes, the most common form, can be easily kept at bay with a balanced diet and a proper amount of nutrients.

Many studies have shown that people suffering from diabetes have lower levels of antioxidants than healthy individuals.

Moreover, a study led by endocrinologists Esther Krug at the Sinai Hospital of Baltimore, found that 91% of the diabetic patients had a severe vitamin D3 deficiency. Another study led to the conclusion that a vitamin B12 deficiency is found in the blood of study participants who suffer from diabetes[73]

This information shows us how important nutrition is, and how such a common condition could easily be prevented, just by introducing to the diet a few little, but important nutrients.

Deficiencies are caused by a series of factors like an unbalanced diet, lack of nutrients in foods and an insufficient amount of antioxidants. With only a few simple dietary changes, which add the proper kind of carbohydrates, proteins and fats, along with a proper level of antioxidants, diabetes can disappear.

### 4.6.3    Cancer

This is probably the most hated word in the entire world. There is a good reason for that. Cancer is not just deadly, it is also an awful way to die. Even when it is in remission, psychological damage, and the constant fear of relapse, will haunt a patient for their entire life. If you want to learn more about the psychological aspects of cancer, read my book "Healing Psyche".

Have you noticed the fact that every year the number of cancer patients rises?

All across the media, new information is emerging about things that can cause cancer. The range is so wide that it seems that everything we eat, drink, put on our skin, and even inhale can cause cancer. It is not only what you eat, but even more importantly what do you not eat. Lack of proper nutrients can lead to cancer[74,75,76.]

You probably already know that unprotected sun exposure can cause skin irritation. This happens because the sun's radiation causes a production of high amounts of free radicals, and these free radicals create unstable cells.

This also happens on the inside, when cells are exposed to free radicals without the proper level of antioxidants to protect them. And this is how many cancers emerge[77,78,79,80]. It is a simple notion that many people don't know. Many lives would be saved if only the population were educated in this matter on how to protect themselves against free radicals.

One of the ways cancer develops according to medical research is that free radicals damage the cell[81,82,83,84]. This leads to DNA mutation, and when the mutated cell divides, the mutation will also transfer to the new cell. Therefore, the mutation will lead to more mutated cells. If this development is not stopped in time, it leads to tumors, and if left unchecked, the situation might get much worse.

> **Too many free radicals can lead to cancer**

For a cancer to be seen on a CT or an X-Ray it needs to have a certain size, so it may have been developing for quite some time to reach that size. Doctors then use chemotherapy, radiotherapy and surgery to remove it. These are all invasive procedures that threaten the life of the patient, and physicians cannot promise the cancer won't come back.

As with every disease, the best course of action is to prevent it.

Many scientists have researched how cancer can be prevented with nutrition. One of these researchers is Prof. Dr. Gladys Block, and she brought together 172 studies from all over the world. These studies proved that a high intake of antioxidants decreased the risk of developing cancers, by three times[85,86,87].

Even if nutritional deficiencies are one of the main causes that lead to cancer, research has also demonstrated the fact that emotions and beliefs have a key role in the improvement of the disease. If you are interested in learning how to use your mindset to heal cancer, you can find additional information and research in my book entitled "Healing Psyche".

An adequate intake of antioxidants and nutrients is useful in preventing not just these diseases, but many others. Our mothers and grandmothers never told us to take supplements on a daily basis because they never needed to.

However the world has changed and food no longer provides the nutrients needed. High quality supplements are not drugs; they provide the same ingredients that food would if it wasn't depleted. This is the only option available if we want to stay healthy. Some people refer to these supplements as high doses of vegetables and fruits in a compressed form.

The truth is that if our food were the same way it was 200 years ago, and if we ate the right things and exercised moderately, we wouldn't have to take additional supplements. In reality, things aren't as they should be. Proper food sources to nourish our body are increasingly hard to obtain, so we are forced to take alternative actions.

On the bright side, a good, natural diet plus high quality nutritional supplement, filled with vitamins, minerals and antioxidants won't do us any harm, and will help prevent horrible diseases like cancer.

What do you think? Is proper nutrition worth a try, or do you want to try your chances without it and see where you end up in 5 or 10 years from now?

Now that we've learned what nutrition is, and how it influences our life, let's review the basics and see which its key elements are.

Before we move on to the next chapter, take a moment to consider your nutritional deficiencies. Think about how they have influenced your life so far, and what do you want to improve or prevent.

If you have any other questions, that remain unanswered, or you feel the need to discuss this with others, be proactive, go online and address these concerns now, while you are still enthusiastic about getting your health back on track.

### 4.6.4    Your Key Points to Remember

✓ *Nutrition is directly related your health now and in the future*

✓ *Health doesn't just fade away with time, it is chased away by the lack of nutrients*

✓ *A higher calcium-magnesium intake is related to lower blood pressure*

✓ *A deficiency in vitamin D was found to be related to diabetes*

✓ *A Vitamin B12 deficiency was also related to diabetes*

✓ *A high intake of antioxidants was found to minimize the chances of developing any kind of cancer*

✓ *Free radicals play a major role in the development of cancer*

✓ *Antioxidants like vitamin C, play an important role in overall health*

# *Your Amazing Insights and Actions*

Date: __ / __ / _____

## What are your insights and learnings from this section?

Now we have come to the conclusion of this chapter. Write down your main insights about what you learned and about yourself.

## What are you going to do differently starting today?

Insights alone will not unleash your vitality. You need to take actions. What are the actions you are going to do in order to implement these insights in your life?

**NOTES**

# Do you get enough?
## Key Question: Do you get enough nutrition?

I especially talk about nutrition, not about food. Most people in developed countries do have enough food but lack nutrition. Many people have a full stomach, yet starve on a nutritional level and develop serious illnesses.

## 5.1 RDA keeps you barely alive

What society has taught us, and what we learned from TV commercials, is that we only need a "Recommended Daily Intake" or "Recommended Daily Amount" (RDI or RDA) in order to stay healthy. Sometimes (most of the time), that is not true.

Did you ever wonder how scientists came up with these values? That is a very good question to ask, since every individual is different, and obviously, every person has different needs.

You are probably thinking that the amount of vitamins they tell you that you need has been carefully studied, and it took years to discover the perfect balance that will make your body stay healthy and strong.

Well… that is partially true, but there is more to this story.

History shows the nature of these values. During World War II, the American army established the levels of bare minimum food to be supplied to soldiers so that they could keep protecting the country. Based upon these minimal values, rations were supplied to the soldiers. At least the soldiers were no longer dying due to nutritional deficiencies. That was the only important measurement during a time of war, not the wellness and vitality of the soldiers.

**RDA is the MINIMUM amount you need**

The RDA is debated all over the world, because it is created on the premise of having just enough nutrients not to get really sick.

For example, the RDA for vitamin C is of 75 mg for women and 90 mg for men. If you get less than that you will develop Scurvy.

Another interesting fact is that a guinea pig needs an average of 10 to 30 mg per kg of Vitamin C, in order to stay healthy. Using the same proportion a 70 kg man, would need no less than 2100 mg of vitamin C. Funny right?

These recommendations were created to avoid serious and well-documented disease. The truth is, that in order to function properly the body needs much, much more than the bare minimum. If you were only to take the RDA for a certain vitamin, you will develop symptoms in a very short amount of time that directly relate to deprivation of that particular vitamin.

I am thinking of RDA as Minimal Daily Amount, the bare minimum of what you need not to get too sick. This bare minimum is also based on no physical or mental activity. If you are turning on the remote of your television you already exceed the Minimal Daily Amount and you will need more nutrients.

So my question to you is: do you want to be barely alive or do you want vibrant vitality?

If you opt for the first, then the RDA is sufficient. If you want total health, then the RDA is just the bare minimum.

## 5.2    Is your body starving?

Your body can cope pretty well with a lack of nutrients for a short period of time. However, when it is deprived for a longer time, symptoms will develop. The body needs the essential elements to restore and rebuild what has been damaged. When all the reserves are empty, you will begin to notice some unpleasant symptoms.

If you are a vegetarian or a vegan, you probably are already aware of the need to take good care that you get all the nutrients for a balanced diet, and even the need for supplementation. However, not everybody realizes that yet.

---

*"In order to change we must be sick and tired*
*of being sick and tired"*
*~ Anonymous*

---

The body sends us "telegrams" to let us know that something is wrong. You must learn to interpret the signals that your body is sending you; because this is the only way you can prevent serious illness. It starts showing us that things are going wrong only when it has depleted its reserves. So, simple symptoms like joint pain in the morning or lack of energy can mean that your nutritional status has been low for a while.

Right about now, you probably are considering whether you have deficiencies that impair your life. You might wonder if you can improve your life.

### *What does Unleashed Vitality look like:*

In order to have a better understanding of your overall status, you have to take an honest look at your life. Stop comparing yourself to others, stop finding excuses for your weaknesses and, most importantly, be objective.

- ✓ *A healthy, well-nourished human being should wake up easily, without feeling tired*

- ✓ *When this person wakes up, his joints won't hurt, he will feel relaxed and refreshed*

- ✓ *Such a person would look forward to the challenges of a new day. He would go to work, or do other day-to-day chores, without feeling stressed and overwhelmed, and would complete his job without too much trouble*

- ✓ *He would definitely not pull a muscle while taking out the trash*

- ✓ *He would have the energy to play with his children, or to go out with his friends and have fun*

- ✓ *He would have a healthy appetite, but not to the point where he eats too much*

- ✓ *His weight would be balanced, even if he rarely works out*

- ✓ *He wouldn't be sick and he would only catch colds once every year, even less*

- ✓ *He would go to sleep and fall asleep without staring at the ceiling for a while*

- ✓ *His sleep would be deep, filled with dreams that are not scary or frustrating*

Do you have much in common with that person? If not, maybe you should rethink your nutritional balance. What are you eating and do you get enough nutrients?

Deficiencies can be obscure, and they might not have obvious signs, until it's too late and then you are facing serious symptoms.

This is the trick with our bodies; they are so beautifully engineered that it will give everything it can until it cannot handle it anymore and breaks down. (Remember Zest ! Sparkle!, Zing!, Oomph ! Vigor and Vivacity! The Vitality Model ?) When the vitality pool is drained and the body runs on fumes extreme symptoms will show.

You do not want to wait until you develop serious symptoms. Be alert of even the slightest signs of nutritional deficiency. Being aware and taking action might save your life. That is why it is very important to notice small symptoms and recognize them too as a sign.

In the next chapters we will mention several symptoms. Note them down when you recognize a symptom you experience or have experienced and learn what to do about it

On the other hand, most animals know when they lack certain nutrients. If you are a dog owner, you have probably noticed that from time to time, your dog starts acting like a goat, and eats the weirdest of things. They start eating grass, they lick and chew your walls, they eat dirt, and sometimes they even eat excrement. There are many ideas for why the dog is acting like that, some of them are ridiculous, but the fact is that they eat grass because they extract precious vitamins from it, they eat your walls because they need calcium, eat dirt for minerals and excrement for the good bacteria. This type of behavior could also be a clear sign of iron deficiency. They have an instinct that directs them to eat that particular item because it smells like the nutrient they need.

> **Do not wait until you develop extreme symptoms**

Humans have lost this ability. There are exceptions to this rule: most pregnant women experience cravings for things they never liked before. This is the body's way of asking for its needs to be met. During pregnancy, hormone levels are modified and certain instincts reappear, because humans evolved to protect their children, and by having cravings, a mother is actually trying to provide for her unborn child. Some young children also have this instinct, and this is why you might find them eating all sorts of things. If you'd ask your parents, you will probably be surprised to hear that you did eat dirt and other unpleasant "foods".

### Life expectancy

In the past, people had a very short life expectancy. During the 1800's people died around the age of 40. Science has evolved a lot since then and the average life expectancy today is as high as 80 years. The truth about this data is that it is strictly statistical, and nobody looks deeper into this notion. Humankind is too occupied with bragging about how much medicine has enhanced life span, that it fails to see how addicted we are to drugs.

Why did people die so young, if the food was packed with nutrients?

The answer is pretty simple. Back then people didn't have access to medical care, so almost anything could have killed a person. A simple wound could be fatal because people didn't have the means or the knowledge to properly disinfect it.

Something as basic as pneumonia used to kill thousands, because Penicillin wasn't yet discovered. Appendicitis always led to peritonitis, septicemia and death. Even childbirth often led to death.

Taking all of this into consideration, living to be 40 years old is quite impressive.

Think about your life. How many pills, injections, syrups and ointments have you used? Can you honestly say that you could live safely, just for a year without disinfectant, or without taking a single aspirin? Can you imagine giving birth at home, using only hot water, and nothing else?

Back in the 1800's people could live like that for up to 40 years, and this was due to the nutrients they received from real food. These nutrients provided them with an immune system that would impress any modern doctor. Their bodies were strong, and cancer was extremely rare.

Today's people live for almost 80 years. We receive vaccines from the moment we are born, being immunized against some of the worst plagues, like poliomyelitis and tetanus. We have access to medical care, even if it doesn't seem exactly efficient, it is important, because even fractures can become deadly at any time, if not treated. We are not exposed to the elements while we work as we can wear protective clothes. We take antibiotics, antivirals, analgesics, antipyretics and anti-inflammatories. We have running water to wash our hands with anti-bacterial soap to kill germs with. We even have running hot water to prevent us from losing body heat when washing.

With all these options, and all this science we still have an incredible number of sick people who constantly depend on pills and doctors.

If our ancestors had the medical ability to treat immediate threats, at 80 years of age they would travel across the country, by foot, without even complaining.

Getting old happens to everyone, there is no cure. What everybody wants is to still do things they enjoy, no matter what age they've reached. This is the purpose of nutrition – to ensure a high quality of life.

### Let's try a little experiment.

Find a quiet place inside the house and sit comfortably on the bed or on an armchair. Close your eyes and relax while breathing deeply. After you are completely relaxed, start imagining your life as an elderly person.

How do you picture your 80th birthday?

- ✓ *Do you see yourself as a grumpy, tired person?*
- ✓ *Do you see yourself moving with great difficulty because of joint pain?*
- ✓ *Do you think you will depend on your children for your basic needs?*
- ✓ *Who will blow out the candles, you or the nurse who is taking care of you?*
- ✓ *Will you go biking with your grandchildren or will they push your wheelchair?*

Wouldn't it be better if you could be independent and able to care for yourself and your children and grandchildren if you have them? Don't you want to enjoy the free time of retirement and travel around the world? If you have children, don't you want them to look up to you and follow in your footsteps to a healthy and long life?

You probably like the second option better, and since you took the first step, and you are reading this book, you are on the right track, but you still need to learn more in order to understand how to protect your body from degrading. Also, you need to keep yourself motivated to be able to continue on this path.

Everybody wants to live a long, happy and healthy life, but most people don't.

Many people end up in hospital before they reach the age of 60, and they become dependent on the medical system. Almost all of those who become sick wonder what they've done wrong. Many of them receive elusive answers, which are meant to make them think that is not their fault.

The truth is that if they knew what you now know, they would immediately look at their nutrition and notice that some of the building blocks of a healthy body were missing.

### 5.2.1   <u>Do You suffer from nutrient depletion?</u>

You may think that you are not feeling that bad, and that overall you are in shape and healthy. Nevertheless, if you don't pay attention to the small, seemingly insignificant symptoms, you may wake up one day and realize that you are seriously ill. This is why we are going to finish this chapter with an exercise.

## *So let's do the exercise.*

# *Exercise: 5 – Nutrition Depletion Index*

Decide for yourself if you are malnourished or not.

**1. How would you rate your energy level during the entire day?**

| | | |
|---|---|---|
| A | ☐ | Energy Level 1 – I wake up tired and I stay tired throughout the day, finding daily chores to be energy draining |
| B | ☐ | Energy Level Between 4 and 2 – I wake up with difficulty, and I find it difficult to concentrate and get involved in activities due to the constant tiredness |
| C | ☐ | Energy Level Between 6 and 4 – I wake up refreshed but by noon I become tired |
| D | ☐ | Energy Level Between 9 and 7 – I feel great, but sometimes drowsy |
| E | ☐ | Energy Level 10 – I feel great all day long |

**2. What is your average emotional status?**

| | | |
|---|---|---|
| A | ☐ | I experience depression and sometimes even anxiety attacks |
| B | ☐ | I am anxious and easily irritated |
| C | ☐ | I become irritated easily, and I sometimes feel anxious |
| D | ☐ | I am relaxed and confident, but I do feel irritated sometimes |
| E | ☐ | I am usually relaxed and confident, mostly happy |

**3. How many times a year, would you say you get sick (common cold, the flu, stomach bugs, and other illnesses)?**

| | | |
|---|---|---|
| A | ☐ | Five times or more |
| B | ☐ | Four times a year |
| C | ☐ | Three times a year |
| D | ☐ | Twice a year |
| E | ☐ | Once a year or less |

## 4. How would you categorize your bowel movements?

| A | ☐ | I always have issues in this matter and it affects my everyday life |
|---|---|---|
| B | ☐ | I suffer from Irritable Bowel Syndrome, but it doesn't affect my everyday life |
| C | ☐ | I experience mild diarrhea or mild constipation |
| D | ☐ | I have more than two loose bowel movement each day or I have a bowel movement every other day |
| E | ☐ | I have one solid bowel movement each day, and I experience no difficulty in this matter |

## 5. How fast do you recover completely from an infection (let's use the common cold as an indicator)?

| A | ☐ | Ten days or more |
|---|---|---|
| B | ☐ | A bit over a week |
| C | ☐ | A week |
| D | ☐ | Five to six days |
| E | ☐ | Three or four days |

## 6. How would you describe your skin, hair and nails?

| A | ☐ | My skin is pale and very dry, my hair falls out and has a straw appearance and my nails are frail and break all the time |
|---|---|---|
| B | ☐ | My skin needs constant moisturizer, my hair is lifeless and my nails break easily |
| C | ☐ | My skin easily dries out, my hair falls off moderately and my nails tend to break |
| D | ☐ | My skin is rarely dry, my hair and nails are strong and a bit pale |
| E | ☐ | My skin is moist and radiant and my hair and nails are shiny and strong |

## 7. How would you describe your vision?

| A | ☐ | I can see with my glasses on, if there is light, but at nighttime I'm blind as a bat |
|---|---|---|
| B | ☐ | I have decreased vision in daytime and nighttime, and bright light hurts my eyes |
| C | ☐ | I see relatively well but if the light is to bright or if it's a bit dark, I start experiencing problems |
| D | ☐ | I have excellent vision during daytime but I have a few small issues with nighttime vision |
| E | ☐ | I have excellent vision during daytime and nighttime |

## 8. How much pain do you experience?

| A | ☐ | I experience muscle, joint and bone pain more than once a month |
|---|---|---|
| B | ☐ | I experience muscle, joint and bone pain every month |
| C | ☐ | I have muscle or joint pain when I wake up or go up the stairs |
| D | ☐ | I sometimes have muscle or joint pain when I wake up |
| E | ☐ | I don't experience pain |

## 9. Do you experience food sensitivities?

| A | ☐ | My stomach is upset more than once a month |
|---|---|---|
| B | ☐ | Every month or so I have an experience of an upset stomach |
| C | ☐ | I have occasionally troubles, like a few times per year |
| D | ☐ | I can eat almost anything, very rarely I have troubles with sensitivity |
| E | ☐ | No I can eat everything |

# *Calculate your score*

Now that you've answered these questions let's see how you've done, and how to calculate your score.

1. *Count the number of A's and write the number in the column below*

2. *Count the number of B,C,D,E's and write them in the columns below*

3. *Calculate the totals by multiplying the count*

4. *Calculate the overall score by adding all 5 totals.*

|   | Count | Total |
|---|-------|-------|
| A | X 1 | = ...... |
| B | X 2 | = ...... |
| C | X 3 | = ...... |
| D | X 4 | = ...... |
| E | X 5 | = ...... |
| Overall Score | | = ...... |

## Score 40

If your total score was 40 - congratulations! You can be sure that you don't suffer from malnutrition. If you keep your diet balanced and watch out for any symptoms, you will be fine.

## Score 30-40

If your score is between 30 and 40 points, you are experiencing some symptoms of malnutrition, but nothing too serious. Balancing your diet and supplementing when necessary, will put you back on track.

## Score 20-30

If your score was between 20 and 30 points, you are experiencing moderate malnutrition. Even if the symptoms aren't serious enough to send you running to the doctor, you should still consider the health implications and the fact that, if left unchecked, this condition will develop into something serious in a relatively short amount of time.

## Score 10-20

If your score was between 10 and 20 points, you are suffering from malnutrition. You probably didn't realize it until now, but the lack of nutrients in our food has left its mark on you. Nevertheless, with a balanced nutritional plan, and the proper amount of nutrients, you will rebuild your immune system and your nutrient reserves.

## Score 0-10

If your score was below 20, you are suffering from severe malnutrition. This condition can actually be very dangerous, so you will need to take supplements for at least a year to rebuild your reserves. Even though improvements in your condition will show after just a few weeks, keep in mind the fact that your body was "hungry" for a long period prior to your present condition. This makes it important to continue with your supplementation to keep benefitting from it.

The more you recognize these early symptoms the more your body needs additional nutrients. Your body is starving. If you do not do anything about it, the symptoms will get worse and more serious conditions might develop.

These first signals of your body might not seem too alarming at all, they are often confused with day to day stress or with growing old. Your hair might not look as beautiful and shiny; your nails might become frail and your skin pale. You will catch the flu easier and develop sensitivities that you didn't have before. One of the first signs that you are not getting enough nutrients is being tired when you shouldn't.

---

*Getting older is no reason to get more symptoms,*
*lack of nutrition is the main reason*

---

These small signals are only the beginning, there are many illnesses that are related to deficiencies, and most of them can be prevented, reversed, or improved only by giving a hungry human what he/she really needs. Time is of the essence, if the problem deepens and it isn't addressed in time it might become too late.

## 5.3    Deficiencies lead to illness

Science has proven the fact that a lack of nutrition will lead to disease. Most cancers[88] can be avoided by giving our body what it needs.

> *"Disease or discomfort is nothing more than*
> *a few errors in judgment repeated every day."*
> *~ Adapted from Jim Rohn*

Researchers have focused on the link between nutrition and cancer, and one of the facts that they uncovered is that women with a high level of vitamin D3 had a 50% higher survival rate[89,90,91], than those with lower levels. Vitamin D3 isn't the only "super-nutrient", CoQ10 was also researched, and it too increased the survival rate[92].

Nutrients have an amazing importance in the way the body handles disease. For this reason, there is an entire chapter dedicated to malnutrition, and how it affects people, especially those who have already encountered an illness. It might have surprised you how many people suffer from malnutrition.

**This malnutrition has led to the increase in many different chronic diseases.**

Disease Increase over the years and related minerals

| DISEASE | 1980 | 1994 | INCREASE | RELATED MINERALS |
|---------|------|------|----------|------------------|
| Heart condition | 75.4 | 89.4 | 19% | Copper, Magnesium, Selenium, Chromium, Potassium |
| Chronic Bronchitis | 36.1 | 56.3 | 56% | Copper, Selenium, Magnesium, Iron, Iodine, Zinc |
| Asthma | 31.2 | 58.5 | 87% | Magnesium |
| Tinnitus | 22.6 | 28.2 | 25% | Calcium, Magnesium, Zinc |
| Bone issues | 84.9 | 124.7 | 47% | Calcium, Magnesium, Copper |

Per 100,000 people of the US population[93]

# If you do not take care of your body, where are you going to live?

This is why it is important to learn and understand what we need in order to live a long and healthy life. As the saying goes, "If you don't take care of your body where are you going to live?" Learning a few simple things about your nutrition will help you improve your life expectancy, your fitness level, and more importantly, your health and the future of your children.

Use all the resources available that may help you achieve your goal. You can even post on Facebook your insights, so that your friends can support you, and also learn from you. You will be astounded by the amount of positive empowering remarks that you receive.

Share your results on our community and let people help you, just go to: http://www.UnleashYourVitality.com/results

The fact that you are acknowledging that you need more nutrition than you are getting, and that you want to take control of your health, is the first and most important step towards succeeding in your quest of living a disease free life. This is taking the proactive role, which has been proven[94] to aid your self-healing abilities.

Not many individuals have the motivation needed to succeed, but you are one of the few who do. Keep up the good work and stay committed in unleashing your vitality to maximize your health.

There aren't many people out there that are responsible enough to seek answers that will take them to a better life. The simple act of caring about your future, and reading this book, demonstrates that you are perfectly capable of being an independent and healthy person.

If you might have any questions or you need a bit more motivation, feel free to explore the internet and interact with other people who share your concerns.

## 5.4    Your Key Points to Remember

## Exercises

✓ *Did you complete Exercise: 5 – Nutrition Depletion Index ?*

## Key points

✓ *RDA is the bare minimum you need to stay alive*

✓ *RDA is based on a body that is lying in bed doing nothing*

✓ *If you think or move you already need more than the RDA values of nutrition*

✓ *Nutrient deficiencies shows itself in small symptoms first, change of skin, hair, energy*

✓ *Chronic diseases are on the rise*

✓ *Nutrient deficiencies lead to illnesses*

# *Your Amazing Insights and Actions*

Date: __ / __ / _____

## What are your insights and learnings from this section?

Now we have come to the conclusion of this chapter. Write down your main insights about what you learned and about yourself.

## What are you going to do differently starting today?

Insights alone will not unleash your vitality. You need to take actions. What are the actions you are going to do in order to implement these insights in your life?

# Vitamins and Minerals
## Your Essential Vitality Vitamins and Marvelous Minerals

Vitamins seem to be the new spinach. We no longer see Popeye on TV eating a can of spinach in order to gain extra strength. Now we see mothers being able to cope with daily chores and jobs, at the same time popping a pill. We see old people staying young because they take the right vitamins. Publicity might be excessive, and probably those pills don't do everything they say, but there is a little bit of truth in there.

## 6.1  Vitality Vitamins
Our body has a desperate need for vitamins, especially now that food can't provide them in sufficient amounts. These little, invisible to the naked eye building blocks are the foundation of the entire system that make us who we are.

> *"All those vitamins aren't to keep death at bay,*
> *they're to keep deterioration at bay."*
> *~ Jeanne Moreau*

They literally control the development of our body and our mind, they can make the difference between being smart and the so called… "not gifted".

Did you know that studies have shown that a deficiency of a certain vitamin can even encourage suicide? Or that a massive amount of another vitamin can help cancer patients, in ways no chemotherapy ever did? Surprising, right? Well there is more information about vitamins, that might have never crossed your mind, and we are about to reveal it all.

**Mark symptoms on your action plan**

Before we begin talking about each vitamin, and what benefits they have, let's look at what vitamins are, and how they are defined by the medical society.

The Oxford Dictionary defines the vitamin as being: "Any of a group of organic compounds which are essential for normal growth and nutrition and are required in small quantities in the diet because they cannot be synthesized by the body".

This basically translates into: "An element that you need to eat that is essential for growth and survival". Your body does a lot for you, but providing your body with the right elements is something only you can do.

We are going to review each vitamin, what it does, how it works and most importantly the interconnection with certain illnesses and how to stay healthy for a long period of time.

While reading the next chapter on vitamins and minerals continue working with your "Your Action Plan Workbook" (chapter 12). Mark the symptoms that you recognize in the relevant section and fill in those additional symptoms in the exercise. Complete the column with the vitamins and minerals associated with that symptom or disease.

We will use that information later on when we are working on your Personal Nutritional Plan. When you do the exercises you will have a Personal Nutritional Plan by the end of this book.

### 6.1.1    Astonishing Vitamin A

This is one of those vitamins that many people don't know about.
We learn the importance of certain elements from various sources,
but the truth is that we only know so much about each vitamin, and
in the case of vitamin A, we definitely don't know enough.

Do you remember the old TV commercials that promoted eating
carrots in order to improve night-vision and general eyesight?
The first time it appeared it had another purpose. The radar was
invented, and the military didn't want others to know that, so
they promoted the idea that eating carrots improved their pilot's
eyesight, and that was why they could see enemy planes. Funny
right? This was only possible because there is a measure of truth in
the statement.

Carrots contain beta-carotene, the substance that provides the
orange color, and that is a precursor for vitamin A.

Vitamin A is a fat-soluble, essential vitamin with an entire range
of benefits. It is a very important element in the creation of the
cells of the mucous membranes, and skin, it helps the immune
system develop and it supports the growth of the bones and of bone
marrow.

Are you curious how it does all that?

The human eye is a very interesting mechanism. It has evolved
differently to how you would think. Since all life was born in
water, and then followed the evolution path to earth, our eyes, and
those of all mammals are adapted to see underwater, and this is
why we have a retina, located at the back of the eye. When the eye
encounters light, retinol is converted to retinal, which is sent to the
cells that help you see in the dark. So, without retinol, vision can be
seriously impaired.

If a person has very low levels of vitamin A, they can even go blind.
Now, don't go and eat tons of carrots, they won't help you regain
your lost eyesight, but vitamin A will help in the maintaining of a
good vision, for a very long time. With enough vitamin A there is
no reason for having vision loss when you age[95].

The inside of our stomach, intestines, urinary tract and lungs, is made of cells that can only be built with sufficient amounts of vitamin A. Without this vitamin your linings will not be strong enough and cannot perform properly. This inner layer is our first defense system against viruses, fungus and bacteria. If this layer is not intact, you will be exposed to all those threats.

Retinol – a compound that derives from Vitamin A – is in charge of maintaining the cells, and protecting this first barrier. It doesn't just build an important shield, but it also forms and activates the little soldiers that circulate in our blood to keep us safe – the white blood cells.

All the cells circulating our blood, are developed from the, almost famous, stem cells. What does Vitamin A have to do with this? Well…stem cells are cells that could be turned into anything. Vitamin A comes in and helps them grow into healthy red blood cells; those are the important carriers of food and oxygen.

> **Lack of Vitamin A can lead to cancer**

A few studies showed that supplementation with vitamin A was useful in preventing cancer[96,97] especially in smokers. With enough of this vitamin the body is able to repair the damage created by tobacco, faster and more efficiently. Without this vitamin your body would not be able to do so.

Remember when we talked about how you need to give your body the optimal level of nutrients, in order for the genes from your DNA to be reproduced flawlessly? Vitamin A is responsible for the regulation of gene transcription, meaning it "tells" genes how often to clone themselves. Pretty smart, for the first vitamin of the alphabet, don't you think?

Too little Vitamin A can result in anemia, weakening of the bones, a faulty immune system, dry skin and hair and many other conditions that can become serious.

Nevertheless, too much Vitamin A, can be dangerous, and can make your liver become fatty, give you headaches, and it becomes toxic for the entire body. This is why, if you consider supplementing your vitamin A intake, you should be very knowledgeable regarding the sources of the supplements. To make sure that the supplements are not toxic, check the label to see what sources the manufacturer is using. Natural sources are always safe, because they are built on the same principles as your body. Nevertheless, we will discuss how to choose the right supplement, in another chapter.

### *Deficiencies*

Below, you will find a list of symptoms that are related to a low vitamin A level. If among these, you find ones that you are experiencing, use a pencil to mark them. Remember that this is a WORK-book not a quickly read book.

This will be used later for your Personal Nutritional Plan. By having a have better knowledge of your problems, you will be one step closer to fixing them.

Signs and symptoms of vitamin A deficiency:

☐ Dry skin
☐ Dry hair
☐ Frail nails
☐ Frequent colds
☐ Vision loss
☐ Anemia
☐ Dry eyes (you feel like blinking more often)
☐ Trouble seeing when it's too bright or too dark
☐ Sinusitis
☐ Bladder infections
Sources: 98,99,100

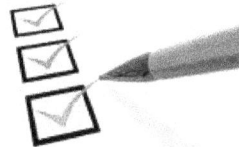

Look at the list above. Did you check everything that you recognize in your life? After you have done so, copy the symptoms to your "Your Action Plan Workbook" (chapter 12). Copy your symptoms and write down Vitamin A in the Nutrients column.

### 6.1.2    Brilliant Vitamins B

Vitamins B are an entire story, there is not just one vitamin B, there are many, which when put together, can help you gain physical and mental health.

The most interesting aspect of the B-group vitamins is that a proper amount can make you feel like you have lots of energy.

We've already talked about the fact that the body uses carbohydrates, protein and fat for fuel. Vitamins B put the burning mechanism to motion, it helps the body burn the fuel more efficiently, and this is only one of the many features of this amazing group of vitamins.

A few things are true for the entire B group of vitamins. They will all help your energy and will make you make you smarter. It increases your mental function[101,102,103,104,105].

One thing you will notice when looking at the vitamin B list is that there are "gaps" in the numbers. The missing B numbers are either not essential for human beings, or they are not real vitamins.

Let's take a look at the most important B vitamins for humans.

### 6.1.3    Vitamin B1 – Terrific Thiamine

Thiamine is a vitamin that is virtually found in all foods. Sadly due to the decline of the quality of food (But where did our food go?), an amazing amount of people suffer from B1 deficiency. Almost 20% of US citizens don't get enough, and the situation is even worse in less developed countries.

Vitamin B1, like all its siblings, plays an important role in transforming fat and carbs into energy. This may not sound like a big deal, but glucose is the main energy source of the brain. This is why Vitamin B deficiency has been linked to Alzheimer's and Parkinson's diseases.

> **Lack of Thiamin leads to non-working immune system**

Thiamine is also called an "anti-stress" vitamin, because like all the other B vitamins, it helps the body strengthen the immune system and it also acts to support important functions, diminishing the impact of stressful conditions.

People who drink high amounts of alcohol, or who suffer from diarrhea, Irritable Bowel disease, and even AIDS, can benefit greatly from an appropriate amount of vitamin B1, especially since diet alone can't provide a sufficient amount of it.

### Deficiencies

Now that you know how important it is for your health, let's see some of the symptoms that derive from B1-Thiamine deficiency. Mark the symptoms that you recognize with a pencil.

Signs and symptoms of B1-Thiamine deficiency:

- ☐ Fatigued
- ☐ Irritable
- ☐ Muscle weakness
- ☐ Anxiety
- ☐ Vague pain and aches
- ☐ Loss of appetite
- ☐ Abdominal bloating
- ☐ Alzheimer's/ Parkinson's
- ☐ Memory loss
- ☐ Attention deficit, lack of concentration

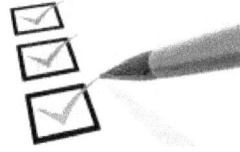

Sources: 106,107,108,109,110,111,,112,113,114,115,116,117,118,119

Look at the list above. Did you check everything that you recognize in your life? After you have done so, copy the symptoms to your "Your Action Plan Workbook" (chapter 12). Copy your symptoms and write down Vitamin B1 in the Nutrients column.

### 6.1.4    Vitamin B2 – Radical Riboflavin

Riboflavin is one of those vitamins that tells you what it is. The "flavius" in the name, means yellow in Latin, they named it like this because, when your diet is rich in vitamin B2, the color of your urine will turn to a bright, distinctive yellow.

It too is valuable in the production of energy, because it helps in the transformation of fat into useful energy.

One of the most known activities of vitamin B2, is its antioxidant role. It is one of the strongest antioxidants in the human body, preventing premature ageing of cells, and promoting health. Remember, antioxidants neutralize the free radicals that damage your body.

> **Lack of Riboflavin leads to anemia and migraines**

A deficiency in vitamin B2 impairs the body's ability to produce red blood cells. This leads to anemia, skin disorders, inflammation of the soft tissue, eye sensitivity to light, and a series of other conditions.

Several studies suggest that people who get migraines may reduce their frequency and severity by taking riboflavin[120,121,122, 123]

Many foods contain vitamin B2, so it should be easy to reach optimal levels. There is a downside, B2 It is light sensitive, and so most foods have already lost their nutritional proprieties once they've arrived on your plate. This could have been prevented if they were transported, processed and packaged in complete darkness, but that never happens for practical reasons.

Light is to B2 as is kryptonite to Superman. It removes all the power from it.

### Deficiencies

Look at the signs of B2-Riboflavin deficiency. Do you recognize any of them? If so mark them with a pencil.

Signs and symptoms of B2-Riboflavin deficiency:

- ☐ Cracks at the corners of the mouth
- ☐ Swollen or sore throat
- ☐ Loss of appetite
- ☐ Nervousness
- ☐ Blood shot eyes
- ☐ Anemia
- ☐ Migraines
- ☐ Weakness/ fatigue
- ☐ Sensitivity to bright light
- ☐ Skin disorders

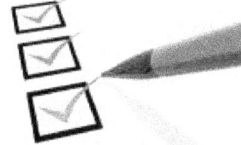

Sources: 124,125,126,127,128,129,130

Now look at the list above, did you check everything that you recognize in your life? Copy the symptoms to your "Your Action Plan Workbook" (chapter 12) and write down Vitamin B2 in the Nutrients column.

### 6.1.5   Vitamin B3 – Nice Niacin

Did you hear about the disease called Pellagra? You probably didn't. Pellagra was a disease that wreaked havoc in the early 20th century. This disease was associated with poverty, and it was considered to be an infectious disease, due to poor hygiene. Its symptoms were called the three "D's" from: Dermatitis, Diarrhea and Dementia. Morbidly enough, these three D's were followed by a forth one: Death.

It was eventually found that Pellagra could be cured with vitamin B3-Niacin. There was no connection to infections or poor hygiene, just that the people contracting pellagra were in the same life circumstances and ate similar foods.

Thankfully, times have changed and science has evolved, and the use of B3-Niacin has been known to be efficient in reversing a series of other conditions, but most importantly for its antioxidant functions.

It has been used to help cancer patients, especially those who have been through bone marrow transplant. Also, it is commonly used to improve the condition of patients suffering from diabetes, because Vitamin B3 is very efficient in helping the body replace tissues, and in this case, pancreatic tissue.

One of the most obvious effects of Niacin is that of vasodilatation (widening of blood vessels). It is obvious because after high doses, the face of the patient becomes flushed.

> **Lack of Niacin could lead to depression and suicides**

No, this doesn't mean that you have high levels of Vitamin B3, just because you blush easily.

This particular property is extremely useful in treating patients with coronary diseases and hypertension. Niacin is also used by the body to make a variety of hormones, including sex hormones. This is why it is useful for those suffering from hormonal imbalances.

Many studies proved that adequate nutritional supplementation with niacin reduced: irritability, aggression suicidal tendencies and especially depression and anxiety. This is due to the fact that vitamin B3 is used for the production of serotonin, a hormone that regulates mood and feelings.

### *Deficiencies*

Now that you know how important it is for your health, let's see some of the symptoms that derive from B3-Niacin deficiency. Mark those symptoms that you recognize with a pencil.

Signs and symptoms of B3-Niacin deficiency:

☐ Increased cholesterol levels
☐ Vomiting
☐ Coronary disease
☐ Hypertension
☐ Aggression
☐ Suicidal tendencies
☐ Diarrhea or abdominal discomfort
☐ Fatigue
☐ Depression
☐ Dry, cracked or scaly skin
☐ Irritability
☐ Anxiety or confusion

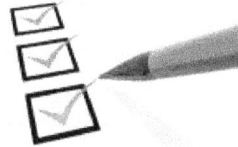

Sources: 131, 132, 133, 134, 135, 136,137,138,139

Look at the list above. Did you check everything that you recognize in your life? After you have done so, copy the symptoms to your "Your Action Plan Workbook" (chapter 12). Copy your symptoms and write down Vitamin B3 in the Nutrients column.

### 6.1.6    <u>Vitamin B6 – Phenomenal Pyridoxine</u>

Pyridoxine is of crucial importance in the production of hormones and neurotransmitters (especially serotonin and norepinephrine), therefore for the health of the entire nervous system.

Women benefit from supplementation with vitamin B6 because it improves premenstrual syndrome and helps prevent anemia. Funny enough, it is also used to treat ADHD, because it has the same relaxing effect that B3-Niacin does, but it brings even more to the table. It is recommended for people with high levels of lipids in the blood, like cholesterol and triglycerides, but also for those who suffer from muscle cramps and carpal tunnel syndrome.

If you are taking medications, you might need a higher amount of vitamin B6, in order to help the liver cope with all the extra work it is undertaking. Proper brain function is dependent on vitamin B levels; this is why it plays a key role in mental and emotional health[140,141]. Moreover, there is important evidence that shows the implication of B6-Pyridoxine in reducing the risk of developing heart disease[142,143].

Did you ever wonder what you can do to remember your dreams better? Well… most people don't expect this, but you could consider adding some Vitamin B6-Pyridoxine to your diet, because it has been proven to help in this rather strange matter.

### Deficiencies

Now that you know how important it is for your health, let's see some of the symptoms that derive from B6-Pyridoxine deficiency. Remember to mark them with a pencil.

Signs and symptoms of B6-Pyridoxine deficiency:

- ☐ Muscle weakness
- ☐ Chronic fatigue
- ☐ Attention deficit
- ☐ Eczema or dermatitis
- ☐ Muscle cramps
- ☐ Anemia
- ☐ Numbness in hands or feet
- ☐ Nausea
- ☐ Migraines and headaches
- ☐ Inability to remember recent events
- ☐ Increased irritability
- ☐ Depression

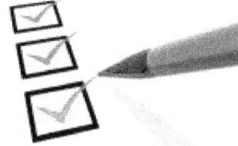

Look at the list above. Did you check everything that you recognize in your life? After you have done so, copy the symptoms to your "Your Action Plan Workbook" (chapter 12). Copy your symptoms and write down Vitamin B6 in the Nutrients column.

### 6.1.7    Vitamin B9 – Flabbergasting Folic acid

Folic acid is important for all mammals alike, especially humans. It is highly involved in the synthesis of the DNA, along with vitamin B12 and vitamin C.

Although it should be present originally in many locally grown dark leafy vegetables, currently the levels are dramatically reduced (see chapter: But where did our food go?)and cooking reduces it even more.

Vitamin B9 deficiency can cause anemia, colitis, memory loss, depression, pain and other conditions. Pregnant women have an increased requirement for folic acid, because it assists the normal development of the child's nervous system. A deficiency could result in either birth defects or miscarriages.

### *Deficiencies*

Look at the list below to see what symptoms you have experienced. Mark those symptoms with a pencil.

Signs and symptoms of B9-Folic acid deficiency:

- ☐ Insomnia
- ☐ Muscular fatigue or general weakness
- ☐ Poor appetite
- ☐ Delayed growth
- ☐ Digestive discomfort
- ☐ Mental fatigue
- ☐ Anemia
- ☐ Memory loss
- ☐ Depression
- ☐ Colitis
- ☐ Gingivitis
- ☐ Mouth or stomach ulcers
- ☐ Shortness of breath
- ☐ Premature grey hair

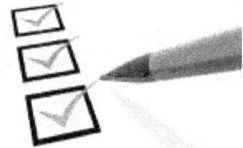

Check the list above. Did you mark everything that you recognize in your life? Copy those symptoms to your "Your Action Plan Workbook" (chapter 12) and write down Vitamin B9 in the Nutrients column.

### 6.1.8 Vitamin B12 – Confounding Cobalamin

This vitamin is not only important for the synthesis and repair of our DNA, but it is also a sensitive vitamin, and its absorption can be impaired by certain factors. Our stomach produces something called "intrinsic factor". This substance is used to facilitate B12 absorption. Without this, you would not be able to absorb it.

Sadly, as the years pass, our stomach loses the ability to produce enough intrinsic factor. This is why elderly people need more B12 (or better absorbing combinations), as higher amounts offer a greater opportunity for absorption.

A deficiency of B12-Cobalamin, can cause pale skin, fatigue, anemia, easy bruising and bleeding, an upset stomach and even diarrhea or constipation.

> **Lack of B12 leads to coronary artery diseases and strokes**

The worst part is that if you are not getting enough of this vitamin, your homocysteine levels will increase. This increases your risk of developing coronary artery disease or a stroke.

People who avoid eating animal products are especially prone to vitamin B12 deficiency, because these are the only items that contain it naturally. Also, people who suffer from eating disorders or other illnesses that impair absorption are at an increased risk of cobalamin deficiency.

Cobalamin is also important in improving mental acuity, especially in elderly people.

### Deficiencies

Now that you know how important it is for your health, let's see some of the symptoms that derive from B12- Cobalamin deficiency.

Signs and symptoms of vitamin B12- Cobalamin deficiency:

- ☐ Dandruff
- ☐ Pale skin
- ☐ Anemia
- ☐ Diarrhea or constipation
- ☐ Easy bruising or bleeding
- ☐ Sore red tongue or mouth
- ☐ Tingling sensation or numbness in toes and fingers
- ☐ Irritable
- ☐ Depression
- ☐ Diarrhea
- ☐ Fatigue[144]

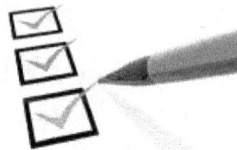

Mark the symptoms that you recognize in the list above and copy them to your "Your Action Plan Workbook" (chapter 12). Next to it, in the column Nutrients, write B12.

### 6.1.9    Vitamin C – Amazing Ascorbic Acid

The importance of vitamin C was, is and will be so debated that you might begin to consider it a myth. Even as children, we were told to eat foods rich in vitamin C and to take vitamin C supplements, in order to stay healthy and not catch colds. Surely, your grandmother must have filled you up with hot tea packed with lemon juice?

So, what do you think? Are you already aware of the importance of Vitamin C?

**Let's see the facts.**

Citrus fruit, and vegetables are full of vitamin C, but this vitamin is very volatile and it oxidizes quickly, rendering it useless. One study proved that if you heat lemon juice at a 30 degree Celsius temperature, in less than a minute, all the vitamin C will be useless due to oxidation. And it doesn't stop here. Even chopping food with an iron knife will make it useless. Apparently, your grandmother was wrong, but at least, all that tea wasn't harmful, and you stayed hydrated. Vitamin C plays a vital role in protecting cells and tissues from damaging oxidation[145].

Joking aside, let's try to understand why vitamin C is so good for us, and why we should have plenty every day.

We get vitamin C from foods we eat, but with all the preparation of foods and juices, the amount that enters our body, and the amount that is actuality absorbed is ridiculously small.

The need for vitamin C varies every day, from person to person, and it is influenced by many factors. One of the reasons most people have a vitamin C deficiency, is the fact that the body is unable to store it. If you take more than you need, it will simply be eliminated through urine, but at least you provide your bodies with everything it might need.

Your body needs vitamin C in order to repair damaged tissues and grow new ones, it is involved in the creation of collagen, and this is why many cosmetic products contain it. Collagen is not important only for your skin, it is also found inside joints, ligaments, and blood vessels. You will be surprised to find out that you actually need vitamin C to repair bones and teeth and to heal any wound.

> **Lack of Vitamin C leads to impaired brain development**

Vitamin C belongs to that class of vitamins we all know and love, antioxidants, and you already know how important they are in preventing disease and premature ageing.

We have discussed free radicals and antioxidants in another chapter. This is a very important issue that needs lots of attention. Re-read the chapter:

"Free-Radicals, Oxidative stress and antioxidants" if you need to.

For now let's see what else vitamin C does for us.

An extreme deficiency of vitamin C, will lead to Scurvy, a disease that is almost eradicated when there is sufficient ascorbic acid available. Smokers are more exposed to such deficiency because nicotine "eats" more vitamin C.

An insufficient amount of vitamin C in the blood can lead to a series of conditions like build-up of plaque on blood vessels, high blood pressure, some types of cancer, but in most cases the manifestation is not so brutal, and only a few symptoms develop, like: dry skin, splitting hair, gingivitis, bleeding gums, and the most common of them all - the inability to fight off infections.

Besides that, the American Journal of Clinical Nutrition reported in 2009 that a vitamin C deficiency could lead to impaired brain development[146].

Maybe the most interesting fact about this vitamin is that some scientists believe that it is so potent that it can actually cure cancer. Research is still underway, but many studies have proven that high doses of Vitamin C act on cancer cells, helping the body destroy mutating cells.

Most mammals have the ability to produce their own vitamin C and to regulate its amount, but humans lost this ability during evolution. It isn't lost forever, in a few thousand years we might gain it back, because we still have the gene to do it, but it's inactive.

Another experiment, published in the October 2006 issue of the Journal of Nutrition, demonstrated the importance of vitamin C even further. Scientists genetically manipulated mice. These manipulated mice were no longer able to create their own vitamin C. These mice were injected with influenza virus, along with other mice that were still able to make their own vitamin C. The results were astonishing. All mice that were vitamin C deficient, experienced massive lung tissue damage, and all the normal mice recovered from the flu[147].

Goats make their own vitamin C. An adult goat that weighs about 70kg will create more than 13,000 mg a day. This is when the goat is healthy. When the goat is faced with stress it produces manifold of that[148,149]. It is probably safe to say, that man needs more than what he can get from food.

If we were to talk about everything vitamin C does for you, we would have to write an Encyclopedia. It is important in every function of your body. It supports immunity, it is vital in wound healing. It also is a main ingredient in the formation of collagen, which is found in all tissues from bones and blood vessels to skin and ligaments.

Many people suffer from a vitamin C deficiency. The more exposed you are to free radicals, the more vitamin C is used to fight them, and the less of it is used for all its other purposes. Smokers and people who take medication on a daily basis, like contraceptive pills, need a higher amount of ascorbic acid.

### Deficiencies

Look at the following lists of symptoms. Which ones do you recognize? Mark those that you recognize with a pencil.

Signs and symptoms of vitamin C-Ascorbic acid deficiency:

☐ Frequent colds
☐ Inflammation or bleeding of the gums
☐ Slow healing of wounds
☐ Plaque buildup in blood vessels
☐ Weight gain
☐ Decreased immune response – frequent infections
☐ Delayed healing time for infections
☐ Nose bleeds
☐ High blood pressure
☐ Dry skin that keeps exfoliating
☐ Easy bruising
☐ Dry and splitting hair
☐ Adrenal fatigue

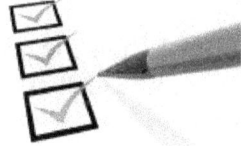

Look at the list above. Check all that apply then copy the symptoms to your "Your Action Plan Workbook" (chapter 12) and write down Vitamin C in the Nutrients column.

Surprise short quiz:

Do you know which the best source of vitamin C is?

☐ Oranges
☐ Lemons
☐ Pineapples
☐ Bell peppers
☐ None of the above

Did you guess?

It's none of the above. Actually, a particular type of cherry contains an incredible amount of vitamin C. It is called Acerola cherry, but we will discuss more about it later.

### 6.1.10   Vitamin D3 – Cool Cholecalciferol

Vitamin D3 is yet another vitamin which is still a mystery for most people. You probably know already something about the basics, but let's go one step further.

One of the basics that most people realize is that Vitamin D is very important for your health and that sunbathing helps to create vitamin D. That is true, but needs some vital clarification.

There are two different types of vitamin D, and they are totally different. D2 (Ergocalciferol) and D3 (Cholecalciferol). When you compare the difference there is only one conclusion to make:

**Use D3 , Avoid D2**

This is because on one hand D3 is 87% more potent in health effects. On the other, more serious side, D3 has shown to decrease mortality rate by 6% and D2 has shown to increase mortality rate by 2%. Although these numbers are low, it shows that D2 is something to avoid.

Vitamin D3 is one of those vitamins that isn't really a vitamin. Did you expect that? It is actually a hormone, and a very important one. It is known for its ability to strengthen your bones[150], but what it does stretches far beyond those limits.

The human body has the ability to create its own vitamin D3, when a big proportion of your skin is exposed to sunlight. The problem is that in order for the process to be efficient, you'd have to expose yourself to sunlight, almost naked, in the middle of the day, when the sun is highest in the sky, with no protection.

Even if you had the time and the means to do that on a daily basis, it could be dangerous. This type of extensive sunbathing will give you sunburn. Almost nobody does this and that is why nowadays about 90% of the population suffer from vitamin D3 deficiency.

You need to get your vitamin D3 in other ways to keep strong bones and immunity. Back in 2009, the International Osteoporosis Foundation warned that the vitamin D3 deficiency was on the rise causing serious bone-health problems[151].

Before talking about where to get an appropriate amount of vitamin D3, let's take a look at some facts, and understand why this hormone/vitamin is so important.

Take a look at this picture, describing how vitamin D3 influences many processes.

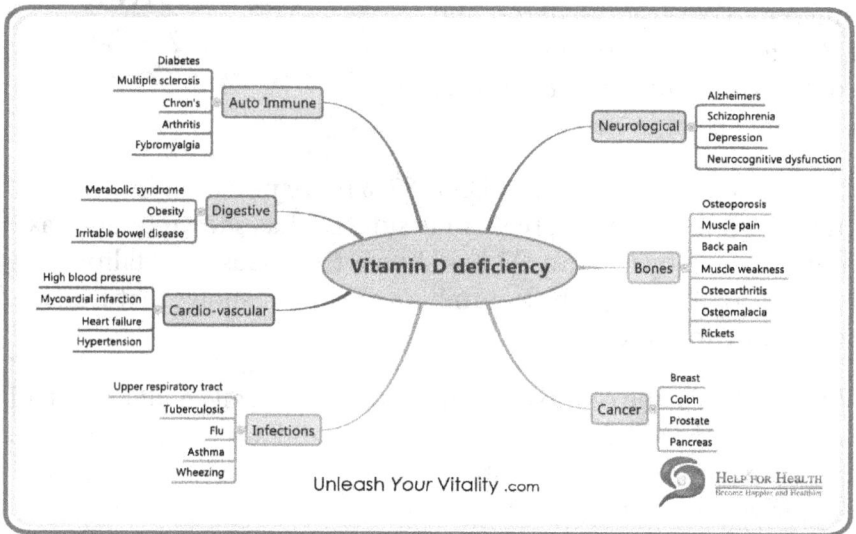

Diabetes
Multiple sclerosis
Chron's
Arthritis
Fybromyalgia
Auto Immune

Alzheimers
Schizophrenia
Depression
Neurocognitive dysfunction
Neurological

Metabolic syndrome
Obesity
Irritable bowel disease
Digestive

Osteoporosis
Muscle pain
Back pain
Muscle weakness
Osteoarthritis
Osteomalacia
Rickets
Bones

**Vitamin D deficiency**

High blood pressure
Mycoardial infarction
Heart failure
Hypertension
Cardio-vascular

Upper respiratory tract
Tuberculosis
Flu
Asthma
Wheezing
Infections

Breast
Colon
Prostate
Pancreas
Cancer

*Unleash Your Vitality* .com

HELP FOR HEALTH
*Become Happier and Healthier*

Can you see how important it is, and the extent that it influences symptoms? Think about the fact that every tissue in your body has receptors for it, even your brain.

Research has shown that people who suffer from heart disease and heart failure, almost always have insufficient levels of vitamin D3[152]. Also, having such a deficiency gives you a 80% higher chance of developing Diabetes[153]. A study was conducted in order to prove the importance of this vitamin, and for this they administered obese people with a high blood sugar level, a placebo or vitamin D3. The results were incredible. Those with vitamin D3 supplementation managed to lower their blood sugar, controlling the progression of the disease.

Another interesting study linked vitamin D3 deficiency to cancer[154,155]. People who live at high altitudes and are forced to stay in sunlight most of the day have a very small incidence of most cancers, with the exception of melanoma. People with the highest levels of vitamin D3 have decreased their risk of cancer by 80%.

Probably the most interesting relationship that this vitamin has with your body is the fact that it modulates the immune response.

In your blood, there is a special kind of white blood cells, called Natural Killer Cells. These are the cells that attack and destroy intruders and they prevent the formation of tumors. When they detect a threat, they activate the vitamin D3 receptors and with the appropriate amount of vitamin D, the cells start doing their job.

The problem occurs when the cells don't get the right amount of vitamin D3, and they just sit there, doing nothing. The effect is that you will catch every cold, flu, stomach bug or whatever you encounter. As with everything else, supplementing your vitamin D3 levels is an issue of being proactive rather than reactive.

**Lack of D3 leads to diabetes**

This is not the whole story with vitamin D3. It is common knowledge that it is important in the growth, development and health of bone tissue. This is why proper levels of vitamin D3 are of vital importance in preventing osteoporosis and bone damage.

Furthermore, vitamin D3 supports the cardiovascular system and muscle tissue. Research suggests that people with a higher concentration of vitamin D3 in their blood, have a 50% greater chance of surviving breast cancer, than those with low levels,[156,157,158]. High vitamin D3 levels reduces the risk of diabetes by 50% and even reduces the chance of ever developing cancer by 80%.

## *Deficiencies*

Knowing this, what do you think? Should you supplement your vitamin D3 intake, according to your needs, or should you wait and see what happens without it?

Let's see what the symptoms for vitamin D-Cholecalceferol deficiency are. Remember to mark them with a pencil.

Signs and symptoms of vitamin D-Cholecalceferol deficiency:

- ☐ Catching the flu or other viral infections
- ☐ Bone pain
- ☐ Fatigue
- ☐ Diabetes
- ☐ Osteoporosis
- ☐ Fragile nails
- ☐ Fatigue
- ☐ Heart disease
- ☐ Problems with blood sugar
- ☐ Mood swings
- ☐ Muscle weakness
- ☐ Joint pain

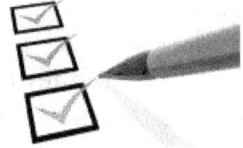

Sources: 159,160,161

Copy the marked symptoms above to your "Your Action Plan Workbook" (chapter 12) and write Vitamin D3 in the Nutrients column.

### 6.1.11 Excellent Vitamin E

This is another vitamin that seems to be all over the news nowadays, and you probably have heard about some of its properties. Are you curious to see what else it can do for you?

Vitamin E is a powerful antioxidant[162] to fight those free radicals. That is important for every cell in your body, more specifically for the cell's membrane. The part of your body that benefits the most from a vitamin E is your respiratory tract.

It can help in the prevention of heart and cardiovascular disease because it keeps LDL cholesterol from oxidizing. Keep in mind that cholesterol by itself is not bad for you, but when it oxidizes, it becomes toxic and builds up on the inside of the blood vessels, which can lead to heart failure.

Vitamin E is also a very efficient cancer fighter, due to the fact that it protects the DNA from suffering damage, which would lead to uncontrolled mutations, therefore cancer. It is even efficient in preventing melanoma if it's applied on the skin before being exposed to ultraviolet radiation. This is one of the main reasons why most sunscreens contain vitamin E.

Vitamin E also enhances the amount of insulin that the pancreas is able to produce, being very useful for those who suffer from diabetes.

Even athletes benefit from supplementation with vitamin E, because it helps the muscles fight against oxidation, and calms down the cramps.

### Deficiencies

Now that you know how important it is for your health, let's see some of the symptoms that derive from vitamin E deficiency. Mark the symptoms you recognize below with a pencil.

Signs and symptoms of vitamin E deficiency:

- ☐ Hair loss
- ☐ Nausea
- ☐ Angina (severe chest pains)
- ☐ Muscle cramps and weakness
- ☐ Muscle spasms
- ☐ High cholesterol
- ☐ DNA damage
- ☐ Numbness, tingling or burning sensations
- ☐ Clumsiness or instability
- ☐ Fertility problems
- ☐ Hormonal imbalance
- ☐ Dry skin

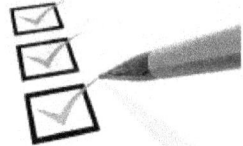

Sources: 163

Copy the marked symptoms and write Vitamin E in the Nutrient column of your "Your Action Plan Workbook" (chapter 12).

### 6.1.12   Kickass Vitamin K

Vitamin K is one of those vitamins everybody forgot about. Most people know that it is important in blood clotting, but that's about it. In fact, there is much more to this vitamin than meets the eye.

Vitamin K works alongside vitamin D3 to support healthy regeneration of bone tissue[164] and supports kidney and cardiovascular functioning. For this reason, deficiencies in vitamin K lead to osteoporosis and other bone loss diseases.

There are two important types of natural vitamin K: vitamin K1 and K2. They are both healthy. However vitamin K2[165] (MK-7) is better absorbed, and more efficient because it remains available in your intestines for a longer period of time. K2 is also much more expensive so that is why it is often not used in supplements.

Besides supporting your bones and teeth, Vitamin K is also shown to prevent a number of diseases, like inflammation of the prostate, and cardiovascular diseases.

If you are a woman, you probably would like to know the fact that a proper amount of vitamin K will help you diminish the menstrual flow. Isn't this something you wish you knew a long time ago?

### *Deficiencies*

Now that you know how important it is for your health, let's see some of the symptoms that derive from vitamin K deficiency. Mark the symptoms you recognize below with a pencil.

Signs and symptoms of vitamin K deficiency:

- ☐ Easy bruising
- ☐ Bleeding from the nose
- ☐ Blood in the urine or stool
- ☐ Heavy menstrual flow
- ☐ Easy broken bones
- ☐ Calcification of the arteries
- ☐ Osteopenia and osteoporosis
- ☐ Slow healing wounds

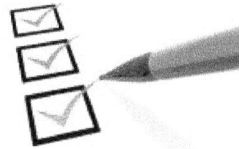

Copy the marked symptoms and write Vitamin K in the Nutrient column of your "Your Action Plan Workbook" in chapter 12.

### 6.1.13   Your Key Points to Remember

# Exercises

✓ *Did you mark all the symptoms that you recognized?*

✓ *Did you fill in those symptoms in your action plan including the vitamins associated to it?*

# Key points

✓ *The body cannot create vitamins, you need to eat them.*

✓ *Vitamins play a vital role in health and disease prevention*

✓ *Vitamin A is important in maintaining good eyesight, creating red blood cells and in the regeneration of tissues*

✓ *Vitamin B is a group of many different vitamins*

✓ *B Vitamins have a wide range of purposes, they are important in liver function, in the nervous system, in skin repair, preventing of inflammation, diabetes and cancer*

✓ *Vitamin B1- Thiamine creates energy from food*

✓ *20% of US citizens have a Vitamin B1deficiency*

✓ *Vitamin B2 – Riboflavin is a potent antioxidant, it is light sensitive: when in contact with light it loses its power.*

✓ *Vitamin B3 deficiency used to cause the serious disease pellagra*

✓ *Vitamin B3 helps in tissue regeneration, especially the pancreas*

✓ *Vitamin B3 improves mood and feelings of happiness*

✓ *Vitamin B6 is also essential for positive emotions like happiness, it has the same relaxing effect as B3 and reduces muscle cramps.*

✓ *Vitamin B9-Folic acid is reduced dramatically in your foods*

✓ *Vitamin B9 can cause depression, memory loss anemia and a range of digestive problems*

✓ *Vitamin B12 is important in repair of your DNA, it improves your mental acuity, especially when growing older*

✓ *Vitamin C helps in the creation of cells, fortifies the immune system and prevents cancer*

✓ *When you smoke or take medications you need additional vitamin C*

✓ *Vitamin C reduces the effects of the flu dramatically, when you have enough of this vitamin you recover much faster*

✓ *Vitamin D3 helps your bones stay strong, prevents infections, diabetes and cancer*

✓ *Vitamin D is created when you expose yourself to sunlight. Most of the population is seriously deprived of this important vitamin*

✓ *Only supplement with D3, Avoid D2 at all costs*

✓ *Vitamin E is an important antioxidant that also helps your tissues regenerate and your hair, nails and skin to stay strong and healthy, while lowering blood pressure and cholesterol*

✓ *Vitamin E increases insulin levels, which reduces diabetic symptoms*

✓ *Vitamin K regulates the way your blood coagulates, but it is also important in the proper absorption of calcium*

✓ *When supplementing go for K2, it is the better form*

## 6.2  Marvelous Minerals

We regard supplements only as vitamins, but there are so many other things needed in order to stay healthy. Another important part of a balanced nutrition is represented by minerals, which are the foundation that create our body. Our bones are made from a combination of minerals, and they have to stay strong to sustain all our body, all our movement and all our actions.

However, minerals aren't found only in our bones, they are an important part of the entire system, and they sustain our life, without us even noticing it.

So where can we find those important minerals? Minerals originate in the earth, and they take centuries to form. Since the soil is losing more and more minerals, we can no longer find them inside our food.

When was the last time you felt light-headed? Did you think it was just because you work too much, or because you are tired? Did you stop to consider the fact that you could have an iron deficiency?

Did you have muscle cramps that awakened you from your sleep? Did you think that it could be from an imbalance in the calcium-magnesium proportion in your body, and that you need to correct that imbalance?

Do you feel stressed, anxious and sometimes depressed? Yes, life can be difficult at times, but maybe you just need a few extra milligrams of magnesium, because it controls so many things, even your mood.

So, let's see what each mineral is important for, and what they can do.

### 6.2.1    Caring Calcium

People think of calcium as chalk, a white substance that is only useful for the bones in their bodies. The truth is that it is also very important in many other structures. It is used by the muscles to stop lactic acid build up. It is also used by your heart, brain, cardiovascular system, nervous system and even respiratory system.

Did you ever experience a severe drop in your calcium levels? It starts with dizziness, continues with tremor, and moves on to symptoms that mimic a heart attack. In fact, many people arrive at the emergency room, stating that they are having a heart attack, when what they actually need is extra calcium.

Calcium is important even for maintaining body weight. The British Journal of Nutrition conducted a study which showed that obese women who started taking a 1,200 milligram supplement every day and dieting at the same time, lost 13 pounds, while the ones who took the placebo, without any calcium, only lost 2 pounds[166].

Furthermore, there is more than one form of calcium out there and not all of them are easily absorbed by the body. If you want the best forms, and you most certainly do, you should look for supplements that contain calcium citrate or

> **Wrong Calcium Magnesium ratio could be fatal**

calcium maleate. Any other calcium form is just cheaper and more profitable for the manufacturer.

Another important aspect of calcium is that it prevents fluoride in water being absorbed in your bones, so a calcium supplement is a protective agent against fluoride poisoning (see chapter on Fluoride).

Finally, calcium does make your bones, teeth and nails strong, but you must always consider a supplement that is perfectly balanced, and also contains an appropriate quantity of vitamin D, magnesium and vitamin K2.

Recent research shows the fact that doctors who recommended calcium supplementation alone did more harm than good[167]. Calcium alone can actually be dangerous because it imbalances the electrolytes in your blood, which can cause heart problems, and it can also be deposited on your blood vessels instead of your bones. The same study showed the supplementing calcium alone doubled the number of heart attacks.

This is why it is of utmost importance to have a 1:1 calcium-magnesium ratio. Considering the fact that 80% of adults and 40% of children are calcium deficient, it is no surprise that the market offers a wide variety of calcium supplements, but only a few of them are made with the client's health in mind. So, always try to find the special few.

### Deficiencies

Knowing this, what do you think? Should you supplement your calcium levels? Let's take a look at what the symptoms related to calcium deficiencies are. Mark the symptoms below with a pencil when you recognize them.

Signs and symptoms of calcium deficiency:

☐ Dizziness
☐ Weight loss or weight gain
☐ Muscle pain and cramping
☐ Frail bones
☐ Tooth decay and cavities
☐ Brittle or misshaped nails
☐ Thyroid problems
☐ Joint swelling and pain
☐ High blood pressure
☐ High cholesterol
☐ Chronic fatigue
☐ Insomnia
☐ Spastic contractions of muscles
☐ Menstrual pain
☐ Bone pain
☐ Tingling fingers, toes or lips

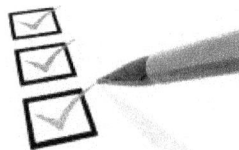

Now look at the list above, did you check everything that you recognize in your life? Copy the symptoms to your "Your Action Plan Workbook" (chapter 12) and write down Calcium in the Nutrients column.

### 6.2.2    Magnificent Magnesium

Everyone talks about how important it is to get enough calcium, but why is there so little public information on magnesium? Is it less important for the human body? Definitely not!

So, what does magnesium do in our body? It is a major ingredient in the production of the cell's membrane, in the production of energy and in muscle activity. It even offers protection against free radicals while allowing your heart to pump blood in the most efficient way, preventing arrhythmia.

A magnesium deficiency can cause certain problems, which in time, become hard to ignore. It can lead to blood clots that increase the risk of stroke and heart attack, it raises the secretion of adrenaline, which puts the whole body under stress, and it can even increase the level of cholesterol in your blood, leading to plaque on your arteries.

Magnesium is best known for its stress-relief proprieties, and this function shouldn't be taken lightly, because a stressed organism is an organism unable to fight diseases, and it is exposed to premature ageing.

Its properties extend further than that, inside the body it is the
active ingredient that "tells"
calcium where to go.
Without its help, calcium
would be deposited in a
variety of places, like on
blood vessels, and it

> **80% of people are lacking
> magnesium. This leads to
> heart attacks.**

wouldn't be able to go where it's really needed – inside the bones.
This is why it is very important to have good calcium-magnesium
balance. Which is the right proportion? Studies show that the best
way to achieve balance is by having a 1:1 calcium-magnesium ratio.

According to the U.S. Department of Agriculture and the Institute
of Medicine, most people are deficient in essential minerals.
Actually, 80% of people of all ages have a magnesium deficiency,
which raises the risk of bone fractures, osteoporosis, depression
and even heart attacks.

Besides this, magnesium prevents the absorption of fluoride in
your body and protects you against poisoning (more on this in the
chapter on Fluoride).

There are many forms of magnesium, but the ones which are
best absorbed and tolerated by the human body are Magnesium
amino acid chelate, magnesium taurinate, magnesium citrate and
magnesium glycinate.

One of the worst forms to use is magnesium oxide (oxide =
rusting), which has the lowest absorption rate, at only 4%.

### Deficiencies

Look at the following lists of symptoms. Which ones do you
recognize? Mark those that you recognize with a pencil.

Signs and symptoms of magnesium deficiency:

☐ Dizziness
☐ Mood swings
☐ Bad absorption of calcium
☐ High stress levels

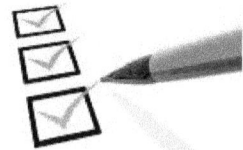

☐ Kidney stones
☐ Depression
☐ Insomnia
☐ Anxiety
☐ Muscle cramps
☐ Apathy
☐ Fatigue
☐ High blood pressure
☐ Headaches or migraines
☐ Nausea or vomiting
☐ Poor memory
☐ Muscle weakness or cramps
☐ Muscle spasms or twitching
☐ Arrhythmia
☐ Rapid heart beat
Sources: 168,169,170,171,172,173,174,175

Mark the symptoms that you recognize in the list above and copy them to your "Your Action Plan Workbook" (chapter 12). Next to it, in the column Nutrients, write Magnesium.

### 6.2.3    Idyllic Iron

Iron is one of the most important minerals that runs through your blood and without it, you wouldn't be able to stand and breathe. Why? Iron is used in the production of red blood cells. It is a major part of hemoglobin: the particular part of a red blood cell that carries oxygen.

So, when your iron levels drop, you became anemic, which is not the prettiest of conditions, because it gives you dizziness, blurry vision, lack of energy and a sense of confusion.

Iron is also used by the body to convert glucose into energy; meaning that in order to "burn" what you eat, you need iron. Besides that, it is used in the production of certain enzymes, which help in the creation of new cells. This is an important process, especially if you are recovering from a disease.

Women need more iron than man, because during menstruation, when they lose blood, along with this blood, important iron is lost, this is also why they are more prone to anemia.

### Deficiencies

Knowing this, how do you rate on your iron levels? Should you supplement it? Look at the deficiency below and mark those that you recognize with a pencil.

Signs and symptoms of iron deficiency:

- ☐ Anemia
- ☐ Tiredness
- ☐ Lack of focus
- ☐ Pale skin
- ☐ Muscle pain
- ☐ Headaches
- ☐ Dizziness
- ☐ Irritability
- ☐ Cold hands and feet
- ☐ Lack of energy
- ☐ Low immune functioning (example frequent colds)
- ☐ Shortness of breath
- ☐ Blood in stool
- ☐ Food cravings for inedible items (ice, plants, clay, dirt)
- ☐ Insomnia or disturbed sleep
- ☐ Lack of concentration
- ☐ Confusion
- ☐ Poor memory
- ☐ Short attention span

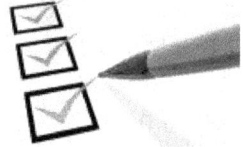

Look at the list above, and check all that apply then copy the symptoms to your "Your Action Plan Workbook" (chapter 12) and write down Iron in the Nutrients column.

### 6.2.4    Sensational Selenium

Selenium is an essential trace mineral, and it is indispensable for health, but in the not-so-distant past, it was considered toxic. This is why the public is not well informed on the benefits of having enough selenium in the diet.

Like other antioxidants, selenium prevents cell damage, but it also has the unique ability of improving thyroid function. This allows the level of thyroid hormones in our blood to stay balanced.

It is also important in the development and growth of bone tissue, meaning that it protects against fractures and osteoporosis, both of which are common in postmenopausal women.

Selenium works alone, or along with vitamin E, to shield you from disorders like cataracts, heart disease and cancer. Research shows that it's extremely useful for women with fertility problems, and it also prevents miscarriage[176].

> *we can no longer extract selenium from our food*

The effect on the immune system has also been studied, and it was found that selenium works by strengthening phagocytes (a special "division" of white blood cells), and this was proven to be very important for those suffering from AIDS[177].

Nevertheless, used inappropriately it can become toxic, this is why when choosing a supplement, you must be sure that it has the right concentration of this mineral, and that it comes from natural sources. Sadly, we can no longer extract selenium from our food, since the soil has been depleted, this important mineral can no longer be consumed the "traditional" way.

### Deficiencies

How are your selenium levels? Should you supplement? Look at the deficiency below and mark those that you recognize with a pencil.

Signs and symptoms of selenium deficiency:

☐ Hypothyroidism
☐ Mood swings
☐ Frail nails
☐ Hair loss
☐ Greater susceptibility to stress
☐ Arthritis
☐ High blood pressure
☐ Lethargy/ fatigue
☐ Depression
☐ Weight gain
☐ Heavy menstruation
☐ Dry skin
☐ Whitened fingernail beds

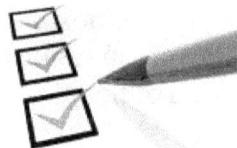

Sources: 178,179

Look at the list above. Did you check everything that you recognize in your life? After you have done so, copy the symptoms to your "Your Action Plan Workbook" (chapter 12). Copy your symptoms and write down Vitamin B1 in the Nutrients column.

### 6.2.5 Zany Zinc

Zinc is a mineral that is important for all life alike, it is found in humans as well as other animals and most plants. This is due to the fact that it is used in many functions. Inside the human body, it is found (or should be found) almost everywhere, inside bones, muscles, organs, and cells.

It is needed for cell division, which is the way cells multiply, this is why pregnant women need it the most, to aid the baby in developing properly and at the normal, healthy pace.

Zinc is also important for men, because it protects the prostate from inflammation and other typical illnesses, like infections spreading from the urinary tract to the prostate.

You probably know that this mineral is important in the immune function. Do you want to know why it is so valuable? Zinc acts directly on the T-cells (these are white blood cells specialized to fight certain viruses and bacteria). If the zinc level is low, they will be unable to recognize the "villain" and you can get the same symptoms over and over again.

Another interesting fact that you might like to know is that zinc is related to how you perceive smells and tastes. An improper level of zinc can make you perceive taste and smells differently. This doesn't seem like a big deal, but if you are a chef, or you should smell a gas leak, zinc suddenly becomes the most important mineral in your system.

### *Deficiencies*

Look at the following lists of symptoms. Which ones do you recognize? Mark those that you recognize with a pencil.

Signs and symptoms of zinc deficiency:

☐ Loss of appetite
☐ Frequent infections
☐ Skin lesions
☐ Hair loss
☐ Lack of smell or taste
☐ Frequent flu and other infections
☐ Skin ulcers
☐ Slow wound healing
☐ Low levels of testosterone
☐ Impotence
☐ Mental lethargy
☐ Depression
☐ Unexplained weight-loss
☐ Diarrhea
☐ Night blindness

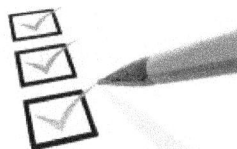

Sources: 180

Copy the marked symptoms and write Zinc in the Nutrient column of your "Your Action Plan Workbook" (chapter 12).

6.2.6  Your Key Points to Remember

# Exercises

✓ *Did you mark all the symptoms that you recognized?*

✓ *Did you fill in those symptoms in your action plan including the minerals associated with it?*

# Key points to remember

✓ *Minerals not only make our bones strong, they govern many different biochemical processes to maintain your health*

✓ *Minerals originate from soil*

✓ *Lack of minerals in the soil creates lack of minerals in you, which leads to symptoms*

✓ *Minerals are an essential ingredient of life itself*

✓ *Every mineral is important, and lack of any element can cause great damage*

✓ *Minerals don't just influence bone health, they affect hormones, and organs as well*

# Calcium

✓ *Calcium makes your bones strong and reduces muscle soreness*

✓ *Calcium is important to aid weight-loss and protects against fluoride poisoning*

✓ *Use only calcium citrate or calcium maleate, other forms are just fillers*

✓ *Calcium and magnesium need to have a 1:1 proportion to be protective of your health*

✓ *Supplementing calcium alone increases risk of heart attack*

✓ *80% of adults have calcium deficiencies*

# Magnesium

✓ *Magnesium is important for muscle activity, including your heart muscle*

✓ *Magnesium reduces general stress levels*

✓ *Magnesium and calcium form a symbiotic relationship. Magnesium tells the calcium to go to the right places*

✓ *Magnesium deficiencies lead to similar problems as calcium deficiencies*

✓ *Select Magnesium-amino-acid-chelate, magnesium-taurinate or magnesium-glycinate but not magnesium-oxide*

# Iron

✓ *Iron is important when you are recovering from any disease*

✓ *Selenium supports the thyroid function*

✓ *Selenium combined with vitamin E is shown to have effects on eye diseases, heart diseases and cancers*

# Zinc

✓ *Zinc helps you taste and smell more effectively*

✓ *Zinc is important in cell-division, especially during pregnancy*

✓ *Zinc helps in remembering past bacterial infections to protect the body in the future.*

## 6.3 Other Important Elements

### 6.3.1 Oh My! Omega-3

You have certainly heard about this one. It is everywhere in the media and many doctors say that foods containing it are among the healthiest foods in the world.

So, nothing new here, but do you know what it really is?

Besides Omega-3 there is also Omega-6. We are not going into depth with Omega-6, and this is why. Omega-3 and Omega-6 should be balanced in your system. However the current diet in most countries has a high surplus of Omega-6. For every gram of Omega-3 in your regular diet you can find 20 (!) grams of Omega-6. In order to balance this out again, you need to supplement Omega-3. Forget about other Omega numbers.

**Only supplement: Omega-3 EPA/DHA**

Omega-3 is a special kind of fat. It's called a polyunsaturated fat. Why is this different fat healthy?

Well, there are a series of reasons, but the most important one is the fact that they interact with your body as fatty acids.

Your body isn't able to make fatty acids, but it depends on them.

There are 3 main types of Omega-3 and you need to know them to make the proper choices in your selection later on. They are:

✓ *ALA (alpha-linolenic acid, found in plant oils)*

✓ *EPA (eicosapentaenoic acid, found in fish)*

✓ *DHA (docosahexaenoic acid, also found in fish).*

The primary sources of EPA and DHA are cold water fatty fish, whereas the primary source of ALA is plant based, like flaxseed, chia, hemp, walnuts, etc.

ALA is converted inside your body to EPA and DHA, which then can be used for many different functions. Only a very limited amount of the ALA is actually converted into the usable element EPA and DHA. In healthy young people- where the conversion is optimal, only 8% of ALA is converted to EPA and 0-4% is converted to DHA. This makes ALA a very ineffective source of getting essential Omega-3 fatty acids.

When you want to achieve the same health benefits from using plant based ALA as you could get from marine based EPA/DHA, then you would need to eat 12.5 times the amount of ALA to get the same amount of EPA, and even 500 times the amounts of ALA to get the same amounts of DHA.

Taking 1gram of either marine (EPA/DHA) based omega-3 compared to 1 grams of plant (ALA) based Omega-3, this is the amount your body can use: From the marine based, the body uses 1 gram, from the plant based, the body only uses 0.02-0,08 grams. So better spend your money wisely on the most effective forms.

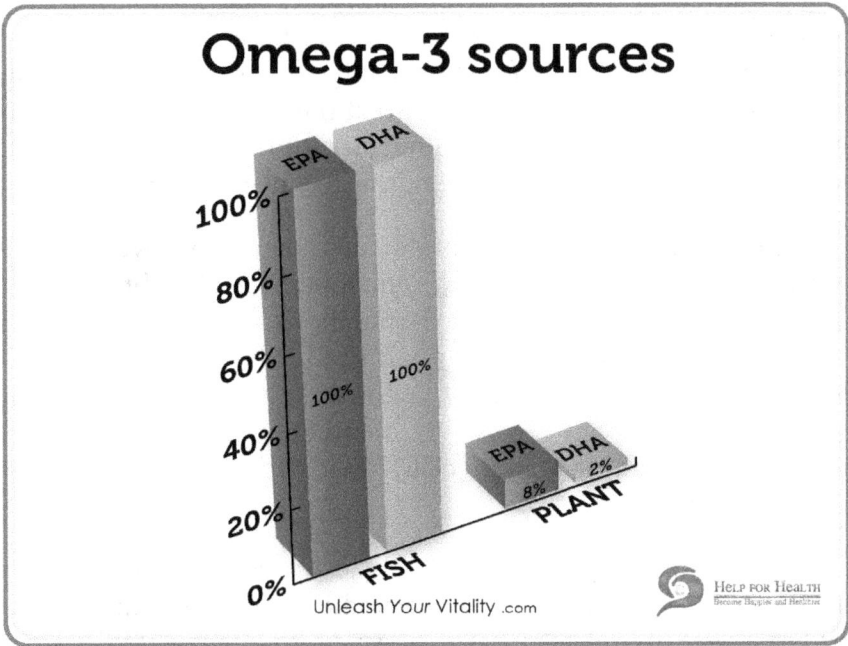

Omega-3 sources

EPA  DHA

100%

80%

60%   100%   100%

40%                          EPA  DHA  2%

20%                               8%   PLANT

0%   FISH

Unleash Your Vitality .com

HELP FOR HEALTH
Become Happier and Healthier

When looking at the research you will notice that most healthy benefits of Omega-3 are attributed to the EPA/DHA sources of omega-3. Cardiologists recognize the benefit of EPA/DHA supplements whereas for ALA supplements there is no supporting evidence.

EPA/DHA is also referred to as marine based Omega-3, or Omega-3 fish oil to differentiate from the other less effective plant based sources.

From this moment on when I discuss Omega-3, I am talking about EPA/DHA or marine based fish oils.

EPA/DHA help in regulating cholesterol levels. A clinical study published in the Archives of Internal Medicine focused on comparing two groups of people. The first group took statin drugs to control high cholesterol levels, and the other group only took fish oil capsules. The purpose of the entire study was to measure the effects on mortality . The results were amazing. The group taking statin drugs had a decreased mortality rate of 10%, and the group taking only fish oil decreased the mortality rate by 23%, when compared with the placebo. That is an extremely good result, especially taking into consideration that there were no side-effects whatsoever for the fish oil. Actually, fish oil alone has twice the benefits of statin drugs and none of the disadvantages.[181]

EPA and DHA, which feed the brain and thereby improve and maintain a healthy brain function. Moreover Dr. A.J. Richardson, from Oxford University, showed that marine based Omega-3 doesn't just help in the nourishing of brain cells, but it also improves blood flow to this sensitive area.

**EPA/DHA feeds the brain**

This same nutrient that feeds the brain also lowers blood pressure and helps build new cells inside the cardiovascular system, helping the heart, and the entire circulatory system to stay healthy.

The American Heart Association suggests using marine based Omega-3 to prevent heart disease and for other cardiovascular benefits.

Most people suffer from inflammation, even if they are unaware of it. It's the price we have to pay for our modern life. Stress creates inflammation, drugs create inflammation, too much food, too much alcohol, too little rest and we all know that inflammation leads to diseases such as heart disease, cancer[182], diabetes, arthritis and a host of other medical problems.

Omega-3 fish oil prevents inflammation from happening at its core. It feeds and supports cells, and even protects the DNA, which needs fatty acids to slow down the telomere shortening rate.

One of the causes of damaged DNA is the shortening of the so-called telomeres. Telomeres are the caps at the end of DNA strands, the shorter they are the more you have aged. The longer they are they more youthful you are. People with the highest levels of Omega-3 fish oil have the longest telomeres. Omega-3 protects these telomeres and thus supports healthy ageing[183]

A study monitored 3,000 people for as much as 16 years, and it showed that those consuming high levels of Omega-3 fish oil had decreased the risk of premature ageing by 27%[184].

Even the effect on diabetes is very interesting to notice. Over the course of 20 years they followed 2,000 men. Those men with the highest Omega-3 levels had their risk of developing diabetes decreased by over 30%.[185]

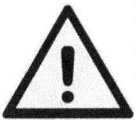

IMPORTANT NOTE: When selecting a brand for your Omega-3 fish oil supplements, quality and cleanliness becomes very important. Many fish oil supplements were contaminated in the past with high levels of toxins. You must be sure that the supplements you are taking are clean and safe. More on this in the chapter "Warning 7 – Missing 100% natural and toxin free indications?"

### Deficiencies

Knowing this, how about taking some extra Omega-3 fish oil, do you think you would benefit from that? Let's take a look at what the symptoms of Omega-3 deficiency are. Remember to mark them with a pencil.

Signs and symptoms of Omega-3 EPA/DHA deficiency:

☐ Fatigue
☐ Poor memory
☐ Dry skin
☐ Mood swings
☐ Depression
☐ Inflammation
☐ Chronic pain
☐ Cold hand or feet
☐ Soft or brittle nails
☐ Dandruff
☐ High cholesterol
☐ Attention deficit or hyperactivity
☐ Inability to concentrate
☐ Irritability
☐ Joint pain
☐ Anxiety
☐ "Short fuse" – fast and highly emotional outbursts
☐ Poor sleep
Sources: 186,187,188,189

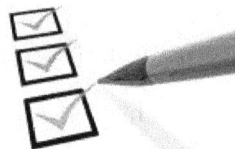

Look at the list above, and check all that apply then copy the symptoms to your "Your Action Plan Workbook" (chapter 12) and write down Omega 3 in the Nutrients column.

### 6.3.2    Commendable Coenzyme Q-10

Coenzyme Q-10 is another actively discussed nutrient. Most people consider it to be just another supplement, when in fact it is the spark of life without which the body would be unable to generate energy. It is fundamental, but often neglected.

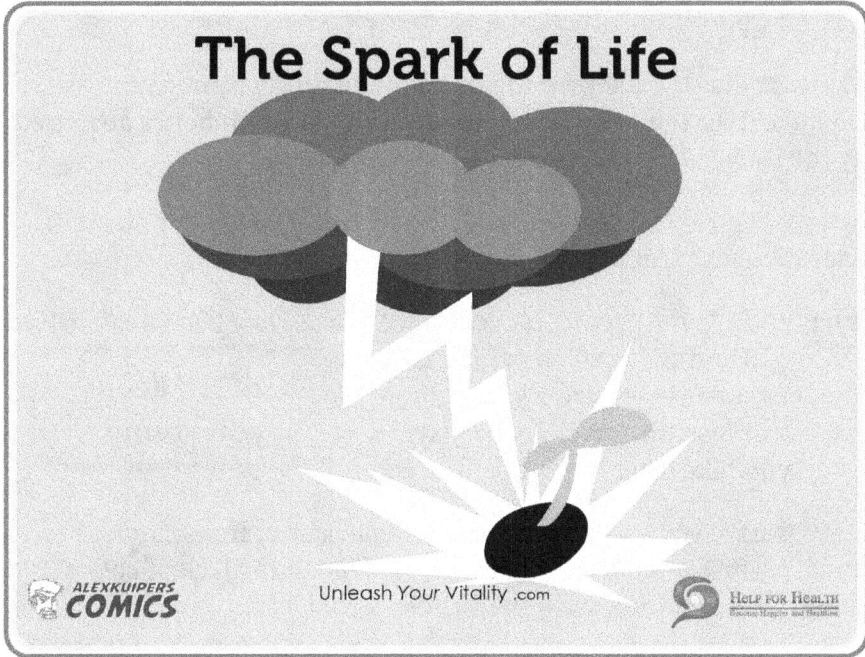

It is like the spark plug in your car that ignites the gas. Without this spark the car will not run.

Coenzyme Q-10 is an oil-soluble vitamin-like substance, found in all cells of the body.

Do you know what is needed to generate 95% of your energy? You've guessed it, it's coenzyme Q-10.

Do you know which part of your body uses more of the energy produced by it? The bigger the organ, the more energy it uses. So, your brain, heart and liver benefit most from coenzyme Q-10.

There are two forms of Coenzyme Q-10, Ubiquinone and Ubiquinol. Inside your body the Ubiquinone is converted to the Ubiquinol form.

Most supplements contain Ubiquinone. What is the difference between these two? Ubiquinone is the oxidized form of CoQ10 and it is very poorly absorbed by your body[190].

Many studies have shown that taking Ubiquinol is much more effective than the other version: because it is much better absorbed by the body[191].

Now, let's go ahead and see why it is so important to supplement your diet with CoQ10.

It has anti-ageing properties. When cells age, they become deprived of CoQ10 and they can't produce as much energy as they are supposed to. Also, cells lose this precious coenzyme, when you take drugs to treat a disease.

> **CoQ10 keeps you young**

Studies have shown that people who take statin drugs can lose as much as 40% of their original CoQ10. Due to the lack of coQ10 there will be an increase in bad cholesterol levels.

All muscles use CoQ10 to create energy, and this includes your heart and lungs. When your CoQ10 reserves become low, you will lose muscle strength, so if you are experiencing muscle weakness, you probably need to supplement. Interestingly this is a known side effect of statins, which can be reduced by increasing CoQ10 intake.

CoQ10 lowers blood pressure by relaxing blood vessels. If you are taking blood pressure lowering drugs and using a high quality CoQ10 supplement, you might want to talk to your doctor about lowering the dosage of your medication.

Other benefits of Ubiquinol include:

- ✓ *It is necessary for energy production, cellular energy that is, and that is the base of life*

- ✓ *Your brain, heart and other important organs will have more energy, therefore they will function better, making you feel more energetic*

- ✓ *Coenzyme Q10 also acts as an antioxidant, protecting you from free radical damage*

- ✓ *Prolongs the life of patients suffering from terminal cancer*[192]

Sources: 193,194,195,196,197,198,199,200,201,202,203,204,205,206,207

We are all exposed to the wear and tear of daily life and energy levels seem to reduce over time. CoQ10 helps the entire body by acting inside the cell, and helping it generate more energy. The body's ability to produce CoQ10 declines with age. Other nutritional deficiencies and even medication also lower the levels of CoQ10, therefore making it necessary to supplement for optimal energy production[208]. If you want to take your vitality to the next level combine your CoQ10 supplement with Bioperine, because studies showed that it increases the coenzyme's absorption by 30%[209].

Studies even have shown that consuming additional Ubiquinol increases the functioning of the heart[210] and brain. It makes you smarter[211]!

*Ubiquinol makes you smarter*

### Deficiencies

What about CoQ10- Ubiquinol, how can you benefit from taking more? Let's take a look at what the deficiencies are. Remember to mark them with a pencil.

Signs and symptoms of Ubiquinol deficiency:

☐ Mental fatigue
☐ Difficulty concentrating
☐ Mood swings
☐ Decreased ability to handle stress
☐ Fibromyalgia
☐ Extreme fatigue
  (waking up tired, feeling exhausted after walking for a few minutes)
☐ Gum disease
☐ Periodontal disease
☐ Headaches , migraines and nausea [212,213]
☐ Frequent cold or flu
☐ Arteriosclerosis
☐ Heart problems (angina, arrhythmia, heart failure)
☐ High blood pressure
☐ High cholesterol
☐ Obesity, inability to lose weight
☐ Stomach or duodenal ulcers
☐ High levels of blood sugar
☐ Kidney failure
☐ Frequent colds

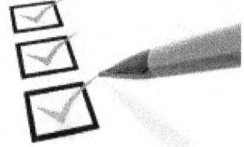

Look at the list above. Did you check everything that you recognize in your life? After you have done so, copy the symptoms to your "Your Action Plan Workbook" (chapter 12). Copy your symptoms and write down CoQ10 in the Nutrients column.

### 6.3.3    Your  Key points to remember

# Exercises

✓ *Did you mark all the symptoms that you recognized?*

✓ *Did you fill in those symptoms in your action plan including the vitamins or minerals associated with it?*

# Key points

✓ *Marine based Omega- 3 (EPA/DHA) is far more beneficial for your health than plant based (ALA) Omega 3*

✓ *Your body needs to convert plant based ALA to the usable EPA/DHA from*

✓ *EPA/DHA helps reduce the effects of ageing and reduces cholesterol levels*

✓ *EPA/DHA is suggested by the American Heart Association to prevent heart diseases and cardiovascular diseases.*

✓ *You have about 20 times the amount of Omega-6 compared to Omega-3 in your diet, that is why you only need to supplement Omega-3*

# CoQ10

✓ *CoQ10 is the sparkplug of life*

✓ *CoQ10 produces 95% of your energy*

✓ *Always select the Ubiquinol (with the L) form, avoid the Ubiquinone (NONE) form or non-specified forms*

✓ *The body needs to convert the Ubiquinone form to the Ubiquinol form to be used by the body*

✓ *CoQ10 lowers blood pressure and cholesterol*

✓ *Combine Ubiquinol with Bioperine to supercharge the effects*

## 6.4   Summary

We've covered the basics of vitamins and minerals, and we've shown you a few of the important nutrients that your body needs to stay healthy and fit. Now we will continue to present ways to improve your life, because just knowing what you need is not enough. You must learn how to balance those nutrients, where to get them from, what to look out for and which are the best sources.

Before you start reading the next chapter, take a few moments to reflect on what you've learned so far and you are starting to comprehend the extent of the situation.

✓  *What is your opinion on this new information?*

✓  *What is your opinion on all those vitamins and minerals?*

✓  *Do you think that you've been misled so far, and that you could have been healthier if you knew what you know now?*

✓  *What do you think about the fact that nobody teaches you these things?*

✓  *Do you feel like you should have learned it in school, in order to be able to maintain your health?*

✓  *Do you think that you are getting enough vitamins from your food?*

✓  *Are you already feeling the effects of deprivation of these important nutrients?*

If you have not yet done the exercises in this chapter and filled in your symptoms and nutrients, than please do so now. This will form the basis of your Personal Nutritional Plan that we are building. It will also give you a clearer picture of your current situation and your current needs.

Does your family know that they need more vitamins in order to grow and live the way they want to? Do your friends know? Do you still have questions about this subject? If you need to know more, if you want to learn more, and most importantly, if you want to take control over the way your body functions, please go online and discover all the scientific breakthroughs.

Share what you have learned, and let other people know that is important to stay healthy.

Our society is so focused on nutrition, and what to eat in order to lose weight, to look prettier, to have a "commercial" image, that many people have developed an obsession over it. It isn't wrong to eat the right things, to stay away from the wrong fats and from the chemicals that infiltrated our food, but it is extremely important to get enough nutrients, because they are the building blocks of our body.

**Food cannot provide enough nutrition, you need to supplement**

Food alone can no longer provide for us, the way it used to. This is the price we had to pay for our rapid development. This doesn't mean that there is nothing left to do. Scientists have struggled to find ways of nourishing the body, and they did, they discovered how to combine nutrients in the most dynamic of ways, and now you can benefit from that knowledge, and improve your life considerably.

# *Your Amazing Insights and Actions*

Date: __ / __ / _____

## What are your insights and learnings from this section?

Now we have come to the conclusion of this chapter. Write down your main insights about what you learned and about yourself.

## What are you going to do differently starting today?

Insights alone will not unleash your vitality. You need to take actions. What are the actions you are going to do in order to implement these insights in your life?

# Getting these nutrients
## How can You get these vital nutrients?

We have established that food no longer contains the necessary nutrients and without these nutrients you will develop serious symptoms. However, something can be done to change that for you. When you take your life and health seriously there are ways to prevent these symptoms, but you need to take action and change your habits.

---

*"Your body is a temple, but only if you treat it as one."*
*~ Astrid Alauda*

---

However, before we can delve into creating an action plan together, we are going to discuss some nutrient-rich foods that might save your life.

## 7.1   Superfoods For a Super Sensational You

Personally, I always regarded this as a nice interesting quote
and I kind of believed that it was true. However now that I have
done some serious research into the effects of certain foods and
nutrients, this is no longer a belief… this is truth. Universal truth.

> *"Let food be thy medicine and medicine be thy food"* ~
> *Hippocrates*

Even if food itself fails to provide enough nutrients, this doesn't
mean that we can't extract nutrients from it. There is a special class
of foods that are called "superfoods". This name is controversial,
but there is a point to it. Certain fruits and vegetables contain more
vitamins and minerals than others. When you take a deeper look at
some of the foods that I have selected, you will start noticing that
they have amazing properties.

So, what superfoods are there, and what do they do?

Let's dive in and see what you can do to change your health and
step into the world of people with vibrant vitality.

## 7.2 Acai Berry

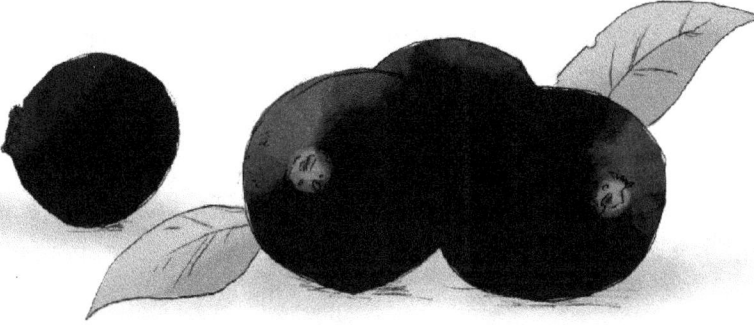

Acai Berry

ALEXKUIPERS COMICS — Unleash Your Vitality .com — Help for Health

This is a berry, and we all know that berries are healthy, but this one is really special. The acai berry grows in the Amazon forest, and there it extracts minerals from a soil that isn't yet demineralized. It is rich in antioxidants and has been used for hundreds of years by the indigenous people because of its immune-stimulating and energy enhancing proprieties.

It contains the same antioxidant found in red wine, anthocyanin, which is well-known for its heart-protecting qualities. The fact that the acai berry doesn't contain alcohol makes it perfect for those suffering from high blood pressure.

The acai berry reduces oxidative stress better than most fruits due to its high Oxygen Radical Absorbency Capacity. It also provides rich amounts of vitamins B and some important minerals, which are critical in preventing and reducing inflammation, but also in raising energy levels.

This berry also contains a specific type of carbohydrate, called polysaccharide, which has been found to stimulate the T cells, meaning that it can help you rebuild your immunity.

Probably the most known fact about the acai berry is that it helps in weight-loss. This is true, due to its effect over fat and on the metabolism, but the effect it has on the cardiovascular system is much more important than the effect on weight.

### Benefits

Take a look at the following benefits for the acai berry. Mark those benefits that are important to you with a pencil:

- [ ] Increases energy
- [ ] Assists in weight-loss
- [ ] Improves immune system
- [ ] Accelerates fat metabolism
- [ ] Strong antioxidant
- [ ] Protects the heart
- [ ] Anti-inflammatory
- [ ] Anti-ageing
- [ ] Boost sex drive
- [ ] Lowers cholesterol
- [ ] Lowers blood pressure
- [ ] Detoxification digestive system
- [ ] Prevents mental imbalance in menopausal women

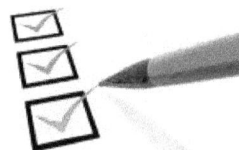

Did you check the benefits that are most important to you? Copy those benefits to your "Your Action Plan Workbook" (chapter 12). Then decide how important this benefit is to you (0= not important, 10 = vital importance). Fill in this number in the column Need. Then in the last column fill in the fruit, acai berry in this case.

## Copy your benefits to the action plan !

## 7.3    Acerola Cherry

# Acerola Cherry

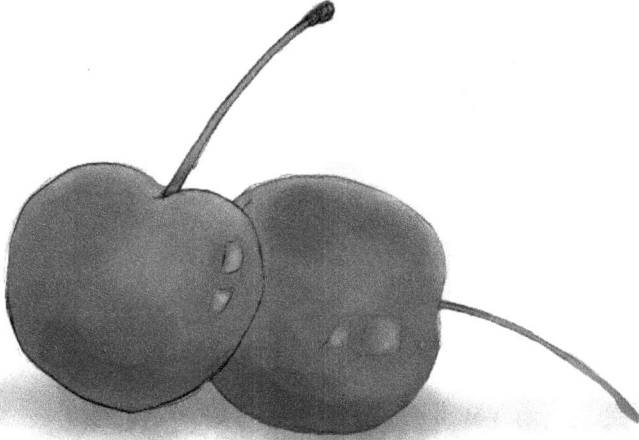

ALEXKUIPERS
COMICS

Unleash Your Vitality .com

HELP FOR HEALTH

Acerola cherry is a fruit that is found all over Central and South America. It is not commonly consumed, but that doesn't mean that it isn't full of flavor. It has already been used for hundreds of years in the Amazon and Latin America for health promotion and medicinal uses. Recently, it became more popular for Westerners due to its remarkable health effects.

What makes this cherry so special that it is found in the superfoods list? It is one of the richest fruits in vitamin C. One single cup of fruit contains as much as 1,644 milligrams of vitamin C, while a cup of oranges contains no more than 95 milligrams. So it is up to you, take 1 cup of these potent berries, or 17 oranges. It is a very strong antioxidant[214].

Do you remember how important vitamin C is for your health? It boosts your immune system, provides extraordinary defense against free radicals, protects your heart and keeps your bones and teeth strong.

So, next time that you are thinking about vitamin C, forget lemons and oranges, and remember the acerola cherry.

### *Benefits*

Take a look at the following benefits for the acerola cherry. Mark those benefits that are important to you in the list below with a pencil:

☐ Regulates blood sugar
☐ Reduces effects of obesity
☐ Prevents cold and flu
☐ High source of vitamin C
☐ Increases muscle strength
☐ Heals wounds faster
☐ Strong antioxidant
☐ Lowers risk of heart disease
☐ Enhances memory function
☐ Anti-inflammatory
☐ Anti-fungal
☐ Prevents diarrhea
☐ Reduces fever
☐ Creates strong elastic skin

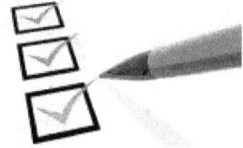

Did you check the benefits that are most important to you? Copy those benefits to your "Your Action Plan Workbook" (chapter 12). Then decide how important this benefit is to you (0= not important, 10 = vital importance). Fill in this number in the column Need. Then in the last column fill in the fruit, acerola cherry in this case.

## Copy your benefits to the action plan !

## 7.4 Bergamot

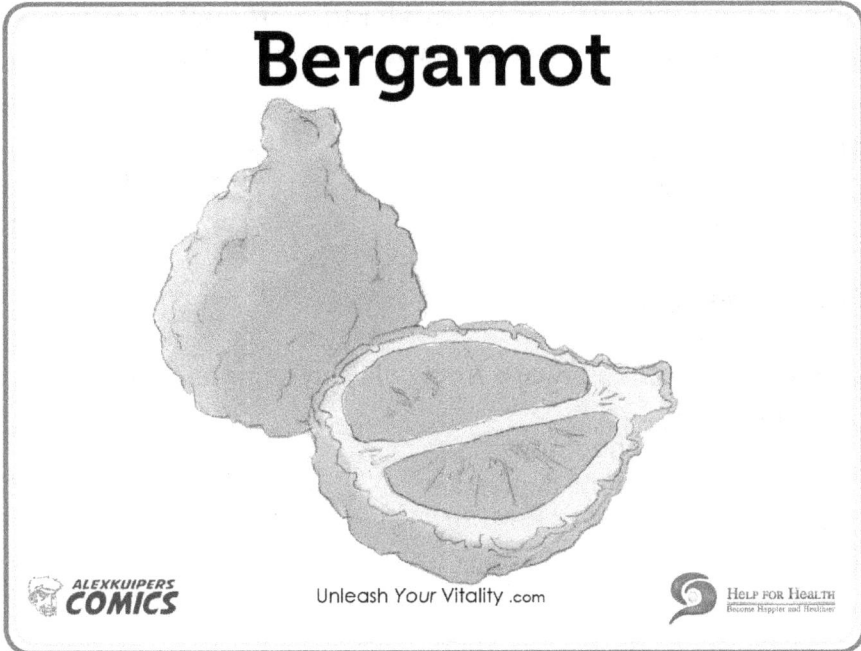

Bergamot is a fruit that looks like a lime. It comes from Calabria, a region in Italy and has been used for its properties for more than 200 years. But it brings more to the table than its sibling. It is mostly known for the oil that is extracted from it, but there is more to it than meets the eye.

It was shown that it is able to lower LDL cholesterol (the bad kind), while raising the HDL (good cholesterol). This fact is extremely useful for those suffering from cardiovascular disease, but also for those looking to prevent blood lipids from increasing.

### *Benefits*

Take a look at the following benefits for the Bergamot. Are there any benefits that are important to you? Mark them with a pencil:

- ☐ Lowers cholesterol
- ☐ Acts as a substitute for statins[215]
- ☐ Protects against heart disease
- ☐ Alleviates bacterial infections
- ☐ Strong antioxidant
- ☐ Improves digestion
- ☐ Reduces nausea
- ☐ Speeds up healing process from cold sores, mouth ulcers and herpes
- ☐ Improves skin conditions
- ☐ Elevates mood/ anti-depressant
- ☐ Relieves pain
- ☐ Increases energy

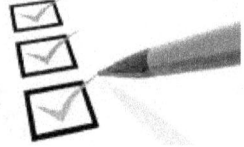

Look at the benefits that you marked. Copy them to your "Your Action Plan Workbook" (chapter 12), and fill in the columns with how much you need this benefit and the fruit (Bergamot).

## Copy your benefits to the action plan !

## 7.5 Black Pepper

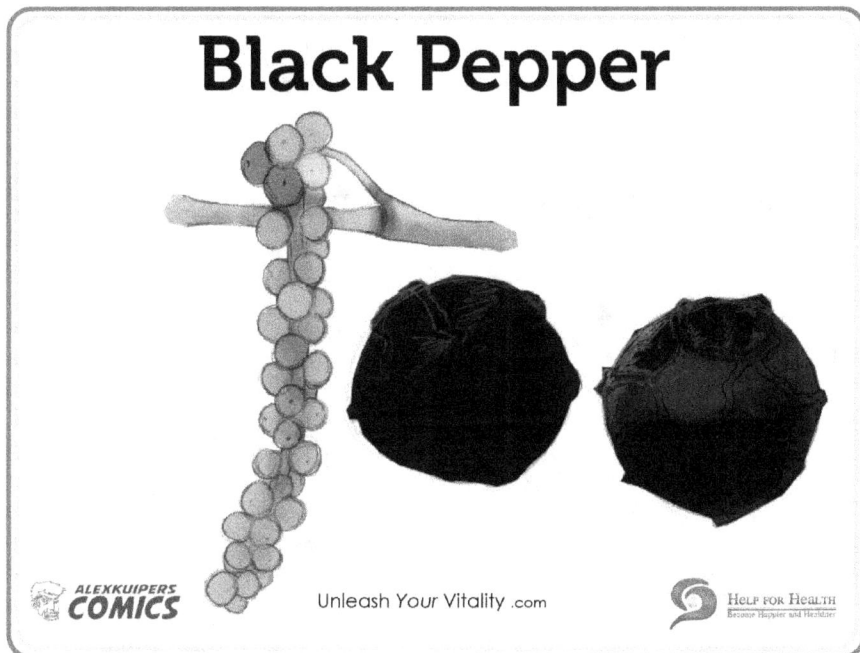

**Black Pepper**

ALEKKUIPERS COMICS

*Unleash Your Vitality* .com

HELP FOR HEALTH

Bioperine® is an exceptional pure natural extract derived from black pepper (piper nigrum). The active ingredient is piperine. Although both black pepper and Bioperine® contain piperine, there is a huge difference between these two. Regular plain black pepper contains only 3-9% of the valuable piperine, whereas Bioperine® contains 95-99% pure piperine. This is why the special Bioperine® is much more potent than plain black pepper.

Piperine helps greatly enhances the absorption of nutrients in the body such as co-enzyme Q10, selenium, curcumin, vitamin B6 and Vitamin C.

It acts like a turbo booster for these nutrients. Piperine increases the uptake of every nutrient dramatically[216,217,218,219] meaning you benefit more from the same quantity.

For example: When you take 180 mg of vitamin X without Bioperine® your body absorbs 100mg and excretes 80mg. Now when you add Bioperine® to the same product your body absorbs 160mg (and only excretes 20mg). So you get a greater effect from the same supplement.

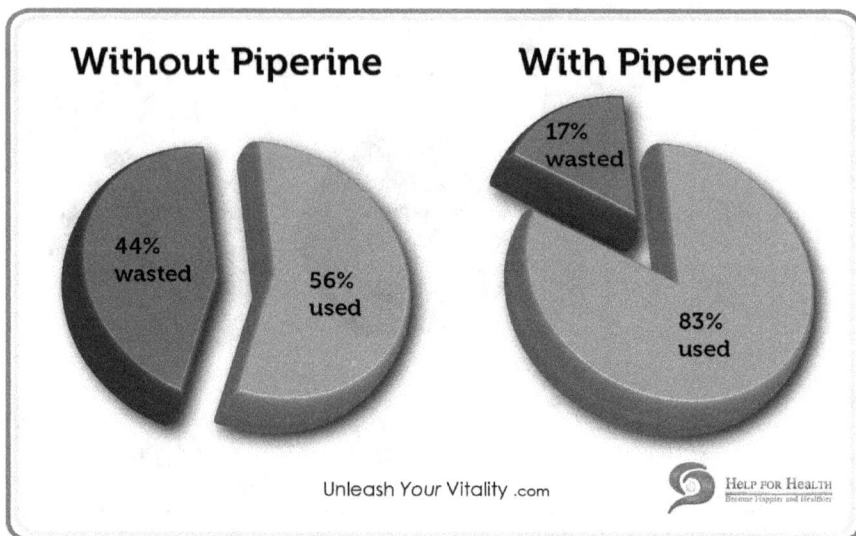

**Without Piperine**

44% wasted

56% used

**With Piperine**

17% wasted

83% used

Unleash Your Vitality .com

HELP FOR HEALTH

These increases in absorption happen with most nutrients, however there are nutrients whereby the effect is much higher. Take Curcumin for example, when piperine is added to that the absorption skyrockets by 2000% !! [220]

Due to this supercharger effect you should always consider supplementing your diet with additional piperine. It will greatly enhance the nutrient absorption of whatever you eat.

In and of itself it also has an anti-depressant effect and enhances the cognitive functions of the brain. Besides that, it also helps to fight colon cancer. Piperine has the ability to increase the blood supply to the gastrointestinal tract, and has been shown to help accelerate metabolism. Moreover, it provides an anti-inflammatory and anti-arthritic effect.

*Benefits*

Although piperine does not have many benefits of its own, it is a supercharger for all nutrients that you take. Just take a look at the following benefits, and mark the ones that are most important to you:

☐ Supercharges uptake of all nutrients
☐ Improves immune system
☐ Increases metabolism
☐ Reduces arthritis
☐ Especially supercharges Co-enzyme Q10, selenium, curcumin, vitamin B6 and Vitamin C (look at their individual benefits)
☐ Anti-cancer
☐ Anti-inflammatory
☐ Anti-depressant
☐ Enhances cognitive functioning

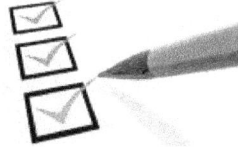

Look at the benefits that you marked. Copy them to your "Your Action Plan Workbook" (chapter 12), and fill in the columns with how important this benefit is to you and note the element; Bioperine®.

# Copy your benefits to the action plan !

## 7.6  Black Seed

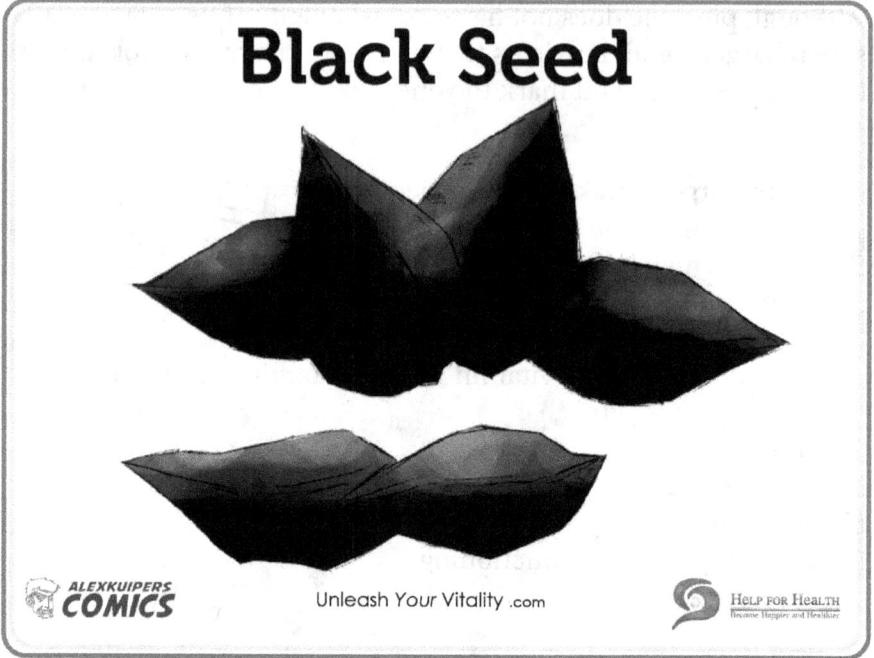

# Black Seed

ALEXKUIPERS
COMICS

Unleash *Your* Vitality .com

HELP FOR HEALTH
Become Happier and Healthier

Black seed (also known as Nigella Sativa) originates from western Asia and is the seed of a plant that grows to 20-30 cm tall. From this plant, the small sharp shaped and deep black seeds are used.

These seeds are commonly referred to in Arabic as "blessed seeds" and according to ancient Arabic scriptures will heal everything except death. Even in the days of ancient Egypt, the power of the black seed was known. The Egyptian pharaohs where entombed with a carefully selected set of black seeds to assist them in the afterlife.

The taste is quite strong, sharp and bitter; you can compare it a bit to a black peppery taste. Because of this feature you can easily determine when it is used in a product. It gives any product a very distinctive taste.

Traditional medicine typically uses it for respiratory illnesses, stomach and intestinal problems, circulatory, liver and kidney diseases.

Over 600 studies have been published showing the remarkable results of this black seed. These include usages as cancer therapy, antibiotics, anti-inflammatory and general immune boosting properties. The list of situations for which it might be beneficial is so long that there are only a few issues that it cannot help with.

> *"Use the black seed, which is a healing for all diseases except death"*
> *~ Arabic scriptures*

### Cancer

Black seed possesses a strong anti-cancer property. Scientists were able to reduce the tumor cells by 52%, which makes it a very potent anti-cancer agent[221]. In another study they showed that black seed reduced malignant and benign tumors, and reduced metastasis in various organs[222], including lung, prostate, pancreas, colon[223]. This, all without side effects. The scientists even called this chemo-preventative therapy.

> *"These findings demonstrate... inhibit colon carcinogenesis ... with no evident adverse side effects"*[224]

### Liver

If you are struggling with poor liver functioning, due to medication or alcohol consumption, or if you want to speed up detoxifying your body, then the black seeds have many benefits to clean the liver and to help liver function[225,226.]

### Diabetes

Black seed has been used successfully to heal treat diabetes. Only 2 grams a day resulted in a stable decrease in glucose levels[227] and an increase in pancreas functioning. Black seeds promote glucose metabolism and thus promote the functioning of pancreatic cells to prevent diabetes[228]. At the same time, it decreased weight gain triggers and reduced overall weight, which resulted in reduction of diabetes[229] and obesity[230]. Black seed is one of the very few substances being researched to prevent and revert both type 1 and type 2 diabetes and it has none of the traditional diabetes medication side effects like nausea, vomiting, diarrhea, weakness and stomach upsets.

### High Blood pressure

You can reduce your blood pressure by using a few grams of black seed for as little as two months[231,232]

### Superbugs

With the global use of antibiotics, a new brand of bacteria is developing, the superbug. These superbugs are resistant to most, if not all known antibiotics. This is a huge health problem in the world and superbugs are rapidly becoming a global health risk[233]. Some of these resistant superbugs are impossible to treat and include strains of HIV, malaria, gonorrhea, tuberculosis, staphylococcus and even the common influenza.

### Black seed can help slow down or stop MRSA[237]

In a Harvard study they calculated that MRSA alone caused about 20,000 deaths[234] in the USA in 2005. That is more than HIV and tuberculosis combined! Yet many people are still not fully aware of the dangers of the deadly MRSA.

People who are infected with one of the many strains of superbugs have much longer hospital stays and require a more complicated treatment. Many times there is not even a treatment available and people don't recover at all. Some reports even mention that about 50% of the people who are infected with a resistant microbe will die from it.

**Hospitals host dangerous superbugs**

One of the most researched properties of the black seed is its anti-bacterial function. In a study[235] the researchers compared 147 strains of superbugs that were resistant to existing antibiotics. Even though they were resistant to other antibiotics, 97 of them could be treated with black seed.

The most important superbug that is threatening our health is the MRSA (Methicillin Resistant Staphylococcus Aureus). MRSA terrifies hospitals and nursing homes. People in hospitals or elderly people are not only more exposed to the MRSA but they are also more susceptible to it because of generally weakened immune systems and invasive procedures like surgery and intravenous tubing.

According to the CDC people are at risk who:

✓ *Have a health condition*

✓ *Have been in a hospital or nursing home*

✓ *Have been treated with antibiotics*

✓ *People who have NOT been to a hospital or nursing home (?)*

This makes almost everybody susceptible to the antibiotic-resistant MRSA infection.

Specifically studies showed that black seed has a potent anti-bacterial effect on all tested strains of MSRA[236], where modern medicine has no effect, black seed shows reduction of the MSRA activity.

Other studies show similar effect on resistant staphylococcus[238], resistant Helicobacter Pylori[239] and other multi-drug resistant microbes [240]. At the same time, it is a potent anti-fungal. None of the tested fungus and molds could exist in the presence of these nutrients[241].

*"[black seed] confirmed to suppress harmful intestinal bacteria in animals and humans"* [242]

## *Benefits*

Black seed has tremendous benefits, take a look at the following and mark those benefits that are important to you:

☐ Reduces Diarrhea[243]
☐ Relieves asthma[244,245]
☐ Relieves bronchial problems
☐ Reduces influenza & nasal congestion
☐ Reduces hair greying/ hair loss
☐ Kills MRSA (and other superbugs)
☐ Increases energy to reduce apathy and fatigue
☐ Prevents autism
☐ Reduces diabetes
☐ Reduces liver problems
☐ Assists detox programs
☐ Anti-inflammatory[246,247,248,249]
☐ Reduces effects of Helicobacter Pylori Infection
☐ Reduces fungal infections
☐ Reduces Impotence and Increases fertility[250]
☐ Works against stomach ulcers[251,252,253]
☐ Lowers blood pressure
☐ Prevents post-surgical adhesions
☐ Suppresses breast and liver cancer growth

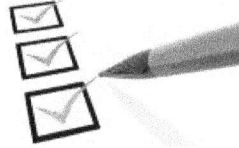

Look at the benefits that you marked. Copy them to your "Your Action Plan Workbook" (chapter 12), and fill in the columns with how important this benefit is to you and note superfood; black seed.

# Copy your benefits to the action plan !

## 7.7 Chaga

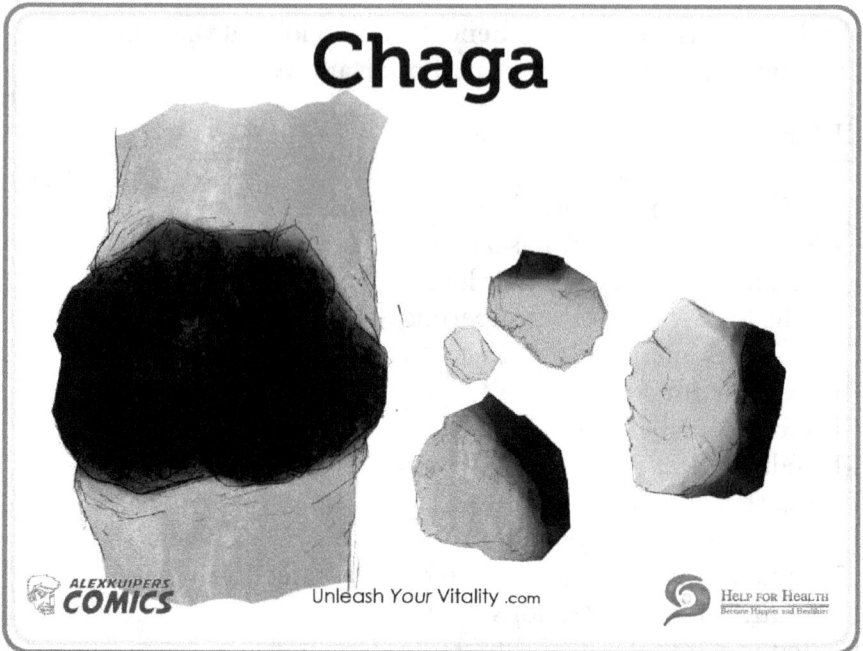

The chaga mushroom, also known as Inonotus obliquus, grows on birch trees. It looks like burned cracked charcoal on the tree. It is deep black on the outside and light brown on the inside. On average they grow to be a 20-30 cm in diameter and can reach a weight of 15 kilograms. They have a rough bark-like surface with a unique shape.

The chaga grows mostly in the very cold birch forests of Russia, Canada, Eastern and northern Europe and the northern parts of the United States. Although the properties of the different areas where it grows are similar, the potency greatly differs from location to location.

It has a very interesting symbiotic relationship with the tree it grows on. If the birch tree bark gets damaged, the chaga repairs the damaged bark. Even more amazing is that sick trees will heal when chaga is inserted manually.

The Siberian people have used chaga since the 16th century to prevent the onset of degenerative diseases, increase physical stamina and improve longevity. Because of its powers, chaga is considered to be a medicinal mushroom by many people. It is also referred to as the "Gift from God", "Mushroom of Immortality" and "King of Herbs".

Although many popular writings discuss chaga's very high levels of antioxidants, it is not always the case. The valuable properties really depend on where it grew and how the final product was created. High quality chaga has over 30 times higher levels of antioxidants levels than other forms. Like with many herbs, it depends on many different factors, only one of them being the location. Unfortunately due to the popularity of chaga, many unfavorable low-quality products are currently available on the market.

As far back as 1950, Russia started researched and experimented with chaga. Their results were used for competing athletes and astronauts to enhance their physical and mental capacity.

The most common usages however, include chronic fatigue syndrome, flu and stomach problems. But even cancer and HIV[254,255] are mentioned as possibly responding well to treatment with chaga. Due to its eminent powers, research is focusing on its possible usages for many other different types of ailment.

### *Cancer*

Different researchers showed the value of chaga in the case of cancers[256]. The use of this medicinal mushroom not only inhibited tumors from growing[257,258,259] but also assisted in cancer reduction[260,261,262,263,264].

It has been suggested that chaga has a significant anti-tumor effect[265, 266], which could make it a candidate for a new anti-cancer agent (for increasing cell-death) without affecting healthy cells[267].

The possible anti-cancer properties are nicely demonstrated
by a study that showed in 67% of mice with cancer, the disease
disappeared after being fed with chaga[268], all signs of cancer were
gone.

> **"Extracts have a strong anti-cancer effect and may be useful as
> an ingredient in functional anti-cancer food"** [269]

Some Finnish and Japanese studies confirmed the effectiveness of
chaga in tumor treatment[270,271, 272]

### DNA Protection
The strong antioxidant[273,274] workings of the chaga also function as
a protective agent against DNA damage. When testing for DNA
protection properties, they noticed that the chaga group had 40%
less DNA damage than the control group[275]. The chaga prevents
against different types of DNA damage as well[276,277].

### Diabetes
In the diabetes research, scientists observed a strong hypoglycemic
effect. Chaga showed a significant decrease in blood glucose levels
(31% reduction)[278, 279,280.] This is very promising news for people with
diabetes or fluctuating blood glucose levels.

### IBD- Inflammatory Bowel Diseases
Inflammatory bowel diseases, such as Crohn's disease and ulcerative
colitis were reduced by counteracting oxidative stress[281] with chaga.
This suggests that chaga can be used in any case where oxidative[282]
stress (too many free radicals) is playing a part.

### *Benefits*

Take a look at the following benefits for the chaga. Mark those benefits that are most important to you with a pencil:

- ☐ Reduces chronic fatigue
- ☐ Relieves stomach problems
- ☐ Increases athletic performance
- ☐ Kills viruses[283]
- ☐ Reduces inflammations[284]
- ☐ Increases immune system[285,286]
- ☐ Reduces Inflammatory bowel diseases
- ☐ Anti-cancer
- ☐ Normalized blood glucose levels / diabetes
- ☐ Lowers cholesterol levels[287]
- ☐ Reduces stomach ulcer[288]
- ☐ Works against pneumonia and lung disorders

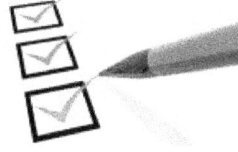

Did you check the benefits that are most important to you? Copy those benefits to your "Your Action Plan Workbook" (chapter 12). Then decide how important this benefit is to you (0= not important, 10 = vital importance). Fill in this number in the column Need. Then in the last column fill in Chaga.

## Copy your benefits to the action plan !

## 7.8 Chamomile

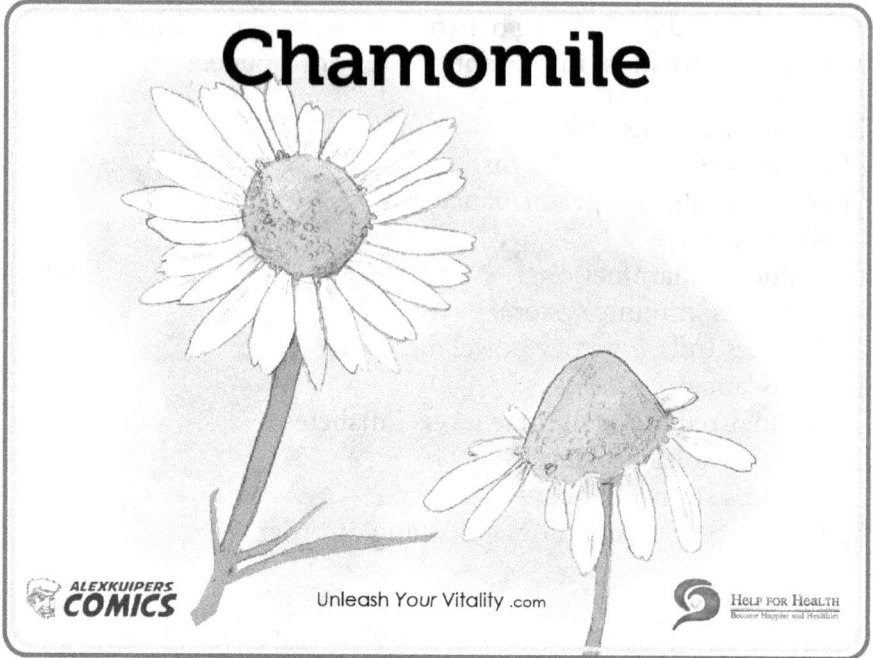

Chamomile is considered a medicinal plant actually, and even if it is not a superfood, it definitely is a super plant. It has been used throughout history to prevent anxiety[289,290], stomach cramps and other digestive problems[291]. Only in the last decade, scientists started to take it seriously.

In one study the strong antibacterial effect of Chamomile was noticeable in the urinary tract[292].

The department of Hospital Pharmacy, from the University of Toyama[293], in Japan led a study that clearly showed drinking chamomile tea after every meal helps those who suffer from diabetes to maintain blood sugar within acceptable levels.

Furthermore, as with most superfoods, Chamomile is packed with antioxidants, and you already know that these are very important for your health.

*Benefits*

Take a look at the following benefits of chamomile. Mark the benefits that are most important to you:

☐ Improves relaxation
☐ Relaxes cramped muscles
☐ Detoxification of the intestine
☐ Speeds up wound healing
☐ Aids in healing from psoriasis and eczema
☐ Reduces allergic symptoms
☐ Stabilizes blood sugar
☐ Antibacterial on the urinary tract
☐ Reduces stomach cramps / soothes upset stomach
☐ Reduces digestive problems
☐ Strong anti-inflammatory
☐ Improves sleep
☐ Reduces menstrual cramps
☐ Reduce anxiety, stress or depression
☐ Reduces headaches

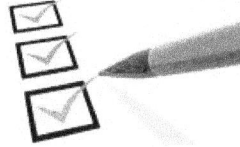

Sources: 294,295,296

Look at the benefits that you marked. Copy them to your "Your Action Plan Workbook" (chapter 12), and fill in the columns with how important this benefit is to you and the Chamomile as superfood.

## Copy your benefits to the action plan !

## 7.9 Cordyceps Mushroom

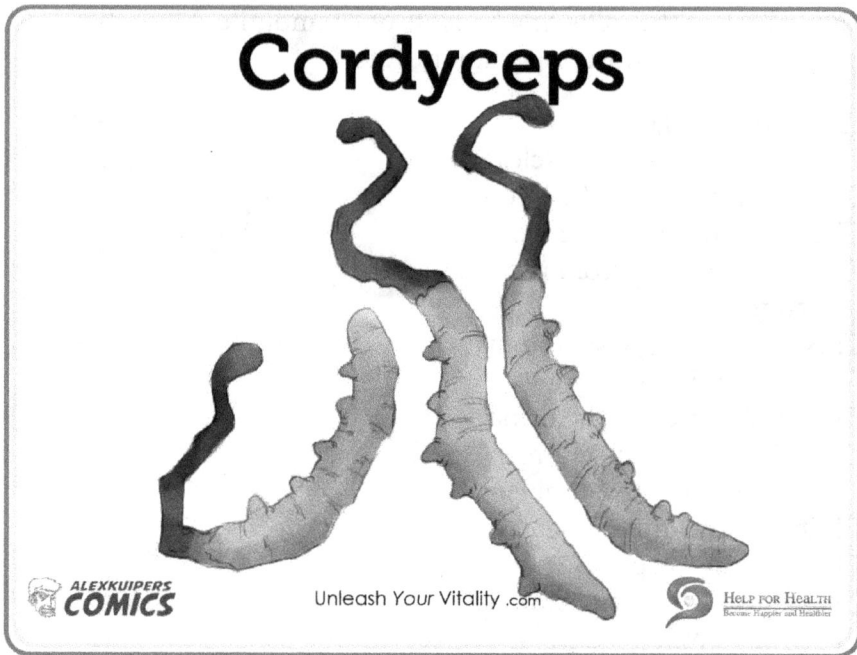

The Cordyceps sinensis mushroom is a powerful traditional medicine that first appeared in Tibetan medical texts in the 15th century. It is one of the exotic Chinese medicinal herbs that has been used for fatigue, kidney and respiratory diseases. Because of its scarcity and huge demand, the price was very high (worth more than silver). Only the super-rich could afford it.

Traditional Chinese medicine uses the Cordyceps to strengthen the kidney and lung meridians. Healers still use this mushroom for many ailments including bronchitis, diabetes, cough, erectile dysfunction, longevity and cancer[297]. Current research verifies the traditional usages. According to Dr. Cornelia de Moor, Lecturer in RNA Biology, Cordyceps reduces the inflammation in airways during an asthma attack.

It also enhances cellular energy promotion. During a 3 week double-blind, placebo controlled trial, Chinese researchers were investigating the effect on endurance, resistance and fatigue. The results were stunning. After only 3 weeks, there was a 73% increase in endurance measured[298,299]. Besides the increase in endurance, other research confirmed that lactate clearance was greatly improved, resulting in less muscle aches and faster recovery[300]. This is why people who use it on a regular basis tend to feel more concentrated and physically fit.

A Japanese study showed the relaxation of the major artery (aorta) after administering Cordyceps. The diameter increased 40%. This is of great value to people with heart conditions or stressed arteries.

Cordyceps also has beneficial effects on the release of adrenal hormones, which also increases fitness and energy, and symptoms of adrenal fatigue.

Japan and China are studying Cordyceps for its effect on sexual dysfunction and sexual performance in men and woman. In ancient medicine, it was already used as a stimulant for the sex hormones. Recently studies showed the effect in treating impotence and other sexual dysfunction in men and women.

*Overall, scientific evidence of the Cordyceps mushroom looks very promising and provides great benefits.*

### Benefits

Take a look at the following benefits for the Cordyceps mushroom. Mark those benefits that are most important to you with a pencil:

☐ Increases energy production
☐ Increases respiratory functioning
☐ Increases concentration
☐ Relieves bronchitis
☐ Reduces coughing
☐ Increases longevity
☐ Relief from asthma
☐ Supports cardiovascular health
☐ Improves sexual functioning/ reduces sexual disorders
☐ Reduces kidney disorders
☐ Prevents nighttime urination
☐ Lowers cholesterol
☐ Improves breathing
☐ Increased fitness
☐ Increases endurance
☐ Faster muscle recovery
☐ Reduces muscle aches

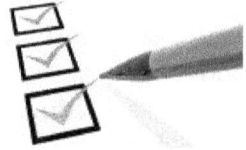

Look at the benefits that you marked. Copy them to your "Your Action Plan Workbook" (chapter 12). Then complete the column with how important this benefit is to you and the Cordyceps as superfood.

## Copy your benefits to the action plan !

## 7.10 Curcumin

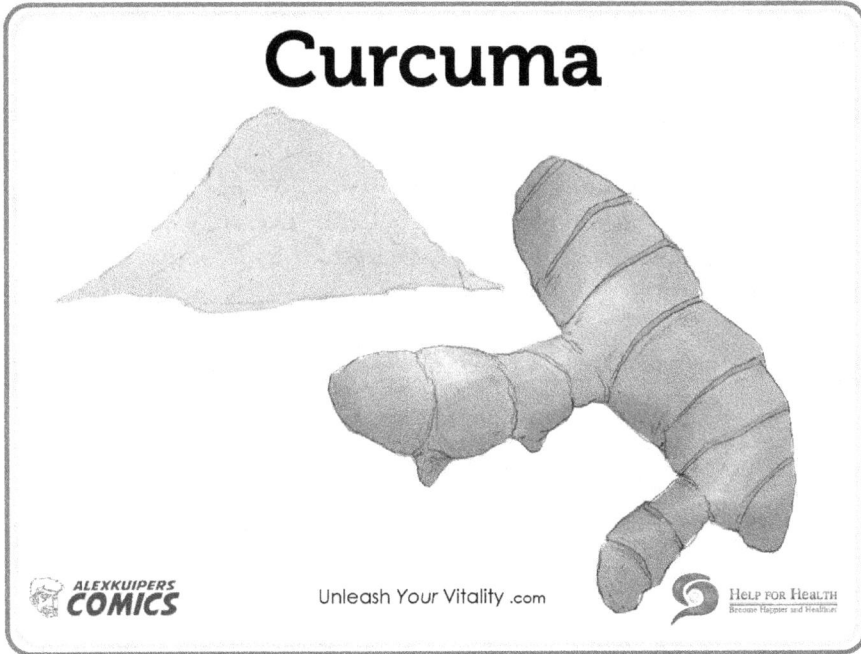

Curcumin (also known as Turmeric) has been used for more than 4,000 years, not only in traditional Indian and Chinese medicine, but also as a spice for its flavoring properties. Only during the last few years, after intensive studies, the true power of Curcumin was recognized.

This spice is rich in fiber and antioxidants, which will help you keep your digestion under control. It has a variety of essential vitamins, such choline, niacin, riboflavin pyridoxine. The root also contains approx. 22.9 mg of vitamin C, a very powerful antioxidant that will help your body's immunity.

It protects and cleans the liver and prostate of toxins, prevents prostate cancer, skin cancer, and esophageal cancer. It is also able to improve Irritable bowel syndrome symptomology.

In India, where people consume masses of Curcumin, there is a much lower rate of prostate cancer (5 out of 100,000) than in other countries (9,116 out of 100,000). This finding is confirmed by several research papers that discovered that Curcumin could stop prostate cancer from developing[301,302]

One of its effects is that it plays a role in apoptosis (normal cell death) in which it could slow down or even reverse tumor growth. For this role, the spice is being researched for its effective use in cancer treatment[303,304].

> *"It has been known for long that Curcumin*
> *has a strong anti-cancer effect"*
> *~ Dr Heger*

Unfortunately, the absorption levels of Curcumin in the body is extremely low. It was only recently discovered that when Bioperine is added, the absorption levels skyrocket. It is estimated that when Bioperine is added to the Curcumin, the health effect is increased by 2,000 times. In that case 1mg of Curcumin combined with Bioperine can be compared to 2000mg of regular Curcumin.

### *Benefits*

Take a look at the following benefits of Curcumin. Mark those benefits that are important to you with a pencil:

☐ Improves digestion
☐ Reduces arthritis pain
☐ Reduces indigestion, bloating, gas
☐ Reduces Inflammatory bowel diseases
  (Crohn's and ulcerative colitis)
☐ Anti-cancer
☐ Strong antioxidant
☐ Detoxifies the body
☐ Reduces inflammation
☐ Reduces stomach ulcers
☐ Prevents diabetes
☐ Reduces bacterial and viral infection
☐ Lowers cholesterol
☐ Improve liver function
Sources: 305,306,307

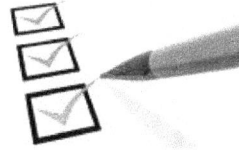

Look at the benefits that you marked. Copy them to your action plan your "Your Action Plan Workbook" (chapter 12). Then complete the column with how important this benefit is to you and the Curcumin as superfood.

## Copy your benefits to the action plan !

## 7.11   Elderberry

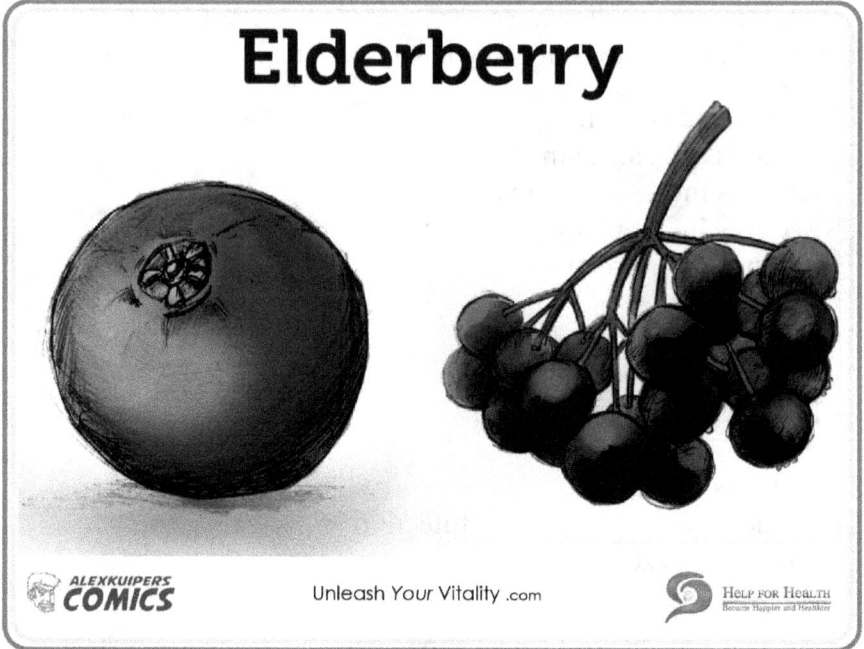

Elderberry is a common plant worldwide. In some parts of the world, its flowers are used to make a beverage called "Shokata" and in others to make marshmallows.

Nevertheless, the power that the fruit contains has been vastly overlooked. The berries have an impressive antioxidant potency and they also offer protection against viruses and bacteria. That is why many people eat them to fight a cold or the flu[308,309]. Like most berries they pack impressive amounts of vitamins A, C and B.

Elderberry has been shown to enhance the immune function, but also regulate it. This is due to special compounds called Cytokines, which are proteins that interact directly with the immune system.

One of the other amazing features is that Elderberry regulates blood pressure and increases physical and emotional wellbeing. It makes you more emotionally stable and happy.

### *Benefits*

Take a look at the following benefits for the Elderberry. Are there any benefits that are important to you? Mark them with a pencil:

☐ Lowers cholesterol
☐ Assists weight-loss[310]
☐ Reduces swelling
☐ Increase physical and emotional wellbeing
☐ Reduces nasal and chest congestions
☐ Reduces asthma and hay fever symptoms
☐ Support healthy blood glucose levels / diabetes
☐ Anti-viral functions
☐ Reduces sinus infections
☐ Reduces bronchitis
☐ Increase urine flow
☐ Improved blood circulation
☐ Improves the immune response
☐ Reduces flu and cold symptoms like: fever, headaches, sore throat, fatigue, cough
☐ Relieves constipation

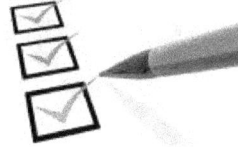

Look at the benefits that you marked. Copy them to your "Your Action Plan Workbook" (chapter 12). Then complete the column with how important this benefit is to you and the Elderberry as superfood.

## Copy your benefits to the action plan !

## 7.12 Goji Berry

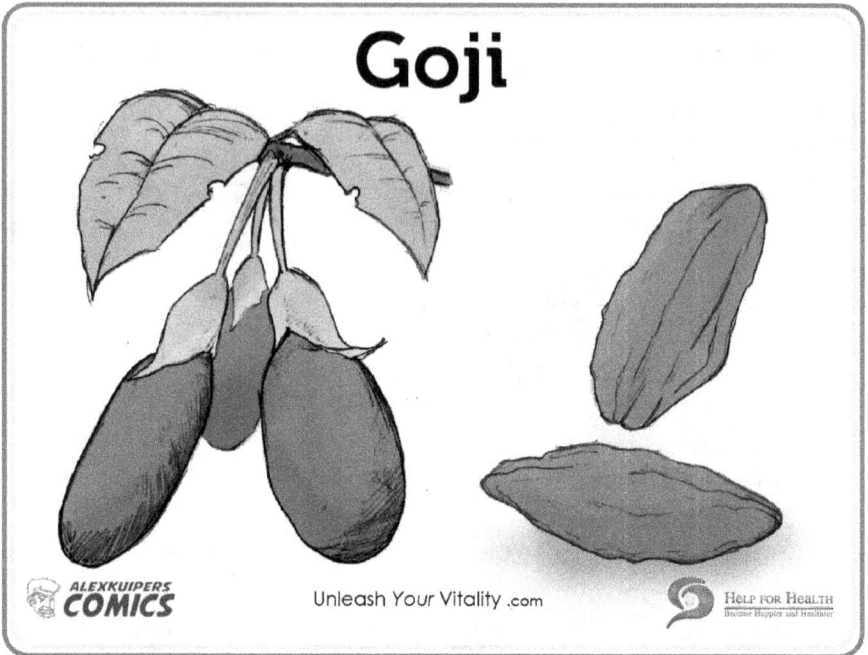

Goji Berry (the fruit of Lycium barbarum) is another member of the berry family, which is found in the subtropical regions of Asia and in the Himalayas. They are famous for their richness of nutrients and health benefits.

In Tibet and China they are used as a traditional medicine, and Tibetans consider it a national treasure, referring to it as: "the key to eternal youth" due to its massive amount of antioxidants. They have been regarded as sexual enhances, a real aphrodisiac.

The levels of vitamin C are very high in Goji berries; containing 500 times the amount found in an orange. They also provides many amino acids, of which 8 are essential amino acids, meaning that your body will absorb them properly, and put them to good use.

The other great and important factor it brings to your system is the amount of trace elements and minerals, which are truly impressive. It contains generous amounts of calcium, copper, iron and selenium.

A research study published in the Chinese Journal of Oncology[311] showed that people who suffered from cancer and were given a Goji berry supplement, responded to treatment better.

### *Benefits*

The Goji berry has some very interesting benefits. Take a look at the following list and mark the most important ones:

☐ Prevents prostate cancer
☐ Improves eyesight[312]
☐ Increases mental wellbeing
☐ Antioxidant
☐ Aphrodisiac
☐ Enhances calmness
☐ Increases athletic performance
☐ Improves sleep

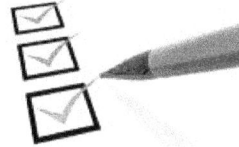

Look at the benefits that you marked. Copy them to your "Your Action Plan Workbook" (chapter 12). Then complete the column with how important this benefit is to you and the Goji Berry as superfood.

## Copy your benefits to the action plan !

## 7.13 Grape Seed Extract

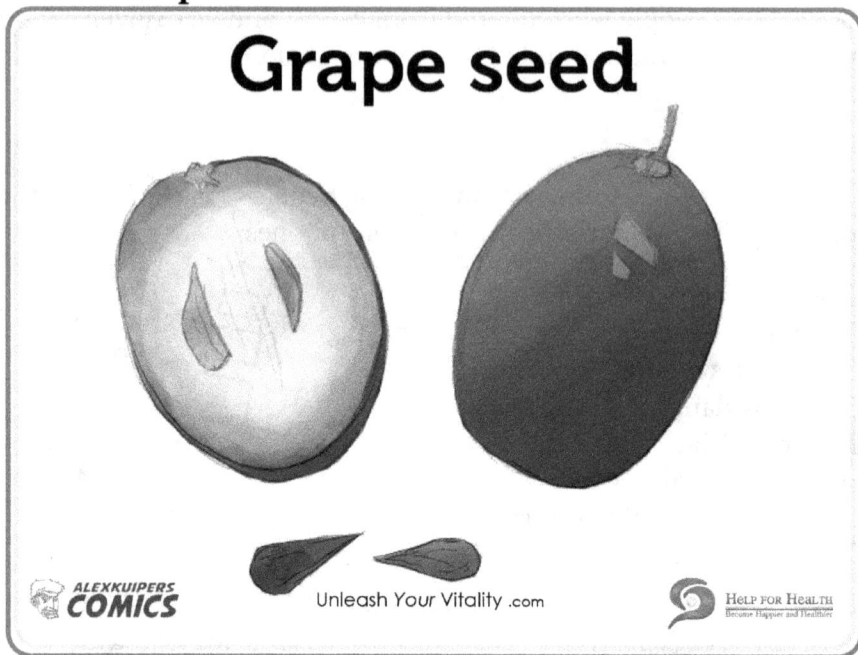

Grape seed

ALEXKUIPERS COMICS

Unleash Your Vitality .com

HELP FOR HEALTH
Become Happier and Healthier

Grapes are valued all over the world for their richness in antioxidants. Ancient Egyptians already consumed grapes more than 6,000 years ago. Grape seeds concentrate all the nutrients in grapes inside their tiny capsules.

Many researchers focused on the medicinal benefits of grape seed extract. One of these studies analyzed the blood of healthy patients before and after taking grape seed extract, and found that it largely increased the amount of antioxidants[313].

As you know people who smoke need additional antioxidants. Besides the antioxidants there are tremendous benefits for cholesterol levels for smokers. A study[314] looked into the effects of grape seed in healthy smokers over the age of 50, and it concluded that after 4 weeks of supplementation, the cholesterol levels lowered. Therefore, it is safe to assume that grape seed extract has a protective effect for the heart and blood vessels.

Swelling and pains of many types can be treated with the anti-inflammatory effects of the Grape seed extract.

Grape seed extract is one of the strongest antioxidants available today, and if it is combined with vitamin C, it becomes even more effective. It is one of the few antioxidants that are able to penetrate the BBB (Brain-Blood-Barrier), so it can provide the brain with a local antioxidant effect.

Today extracts of the grape seed are being used for treatment a range of health conditions related to free radical damage, including cancer, diabetes and heart disease. Combining grape seed extract with calcium increases bone density and prevents fractures[315].

### _Benefits_

Take a look at the following benefits for grape seed extract. Mark the benefits that are most important to you with a pencil:

☐ Very potent antioxidant
☐ Stimulates immunity
☐ Lowers cholesterol levels
☐ Prevents Alzheimer's[316]
☐ Reduces diabetes
☐ Reduces hemorrhoids
☐ Supports the healing of small aches and pains, swelling, cuts and burns
☐ Antioxidant for the brain
☐ Increases circulation (reduces cold hands and feet)
☐ Reduces swelling by injury
☐ Speeds up wound healing
☐ Improve bone strength
☐ Prevents cognitive decline
☐ Increases energy/ reduces fatigue
Sources: 317,318

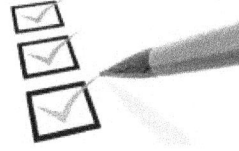

Look at the benefits that you marked. Copy them to your "Your Action Plan Workbook" (chapter 12). Then write in the column how important this benefit is to you finalize the columns with Grape seed extract as superfood.

## Copy your benefits to the action plan !

## 7.14   Green Coffee Bean

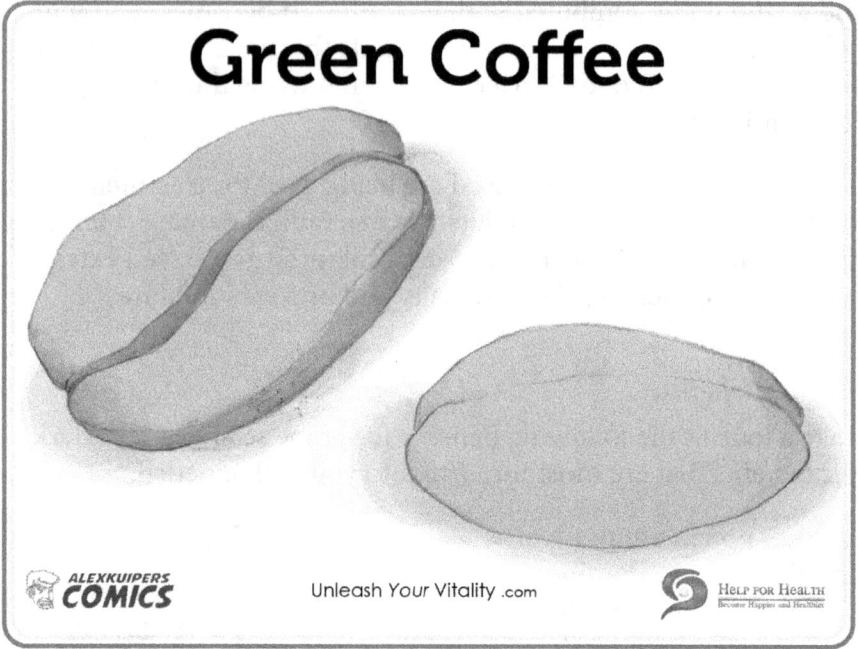

The Green Coffee Bean is one of those things everybody heard of, but not so many people understand the mechanism behind it. A lot of people love coffee, and appreciate the fact that it keeps them awake all day, and sometimes all night. It is even considered the number 1 drug in the world, but green coffee has some other benefits that might be beneficial to you.

Green coffee is the bean before roasting for use of coffee. The green bean has not been exposed to any thermic process. Therefore all its nutrients are kept intact.

One particular nutrient that remains unharmed is chlorogenic acid, which has been studied by scientists. It was reported that it has laxative effects that helps in weight-loss, while also delivering health benefits for those suffering from heart disease and diabetes. An interesting fact about this compound is that it has antihypertensive effects, which is rather odd, considering the fact that drinking coffee usually has the opposite effect.

Green coffee it is often used for weight-loss because it directly influences the way the body metabolizes glucose. It decreases the absorption rate of sugar, therefore releasing it into your blood at a slower rate.

Green coffee also contains many antioxidants, which, as we have already seen, protects you from free radical damage, helping your cells to live a longer life.

### *Benefits*

Take a look at the following benefits of the green coffee bean. Anything you like? Mark those benefits that are most important to you:

- ☐ Assists weight-loss
- ☐ Balances blood sugars/ diabetes
- ☐ Reduce sugar cravings
- ☐ Reduces constipation
- ☐ Anti-inflammatory
- ☐ Reduces stress
- ☐ Heart disease prevention
- ☐ Purifies and detoxifies your body
- ☐ Improves liver function, especially its property of processing fat[319]
- ☐ Reduces blood pressure[320]
- ☐ Increases metabolism

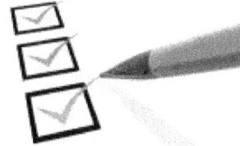

Look at the benefits that you marked. Copy them to your "Your Action Plan Workbook" (chapter 12). Then complete the column with how important this benefit is to you and the Green Coffee Bean as superfood.

## Copy your benefits to the action plan !

## 7.15   Green Tea

# Green Tea

ALEXKUIPERS
COMICS

Unleash Your Vitality .com

HELP FOR HEALTH
Become Happier and Healthier

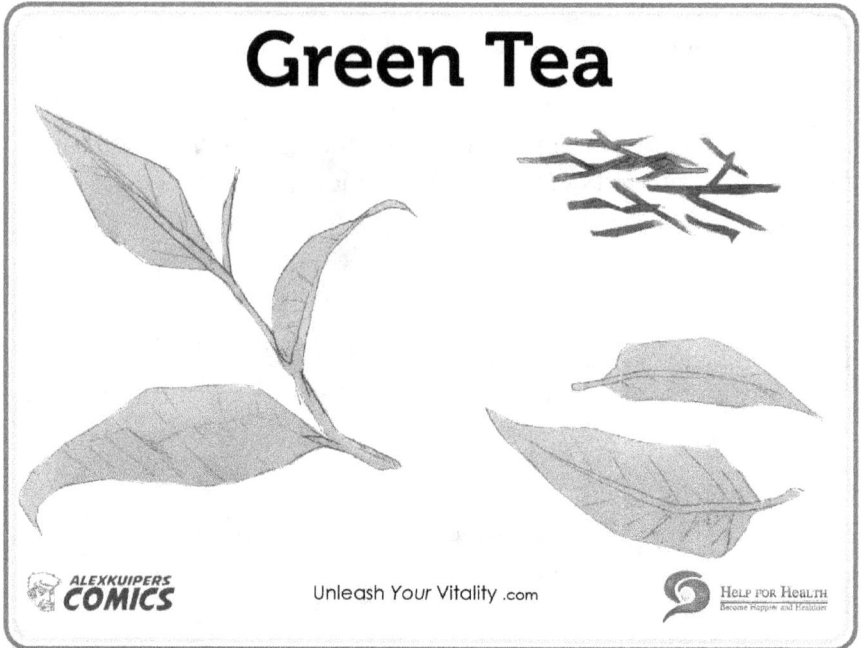

Green tea is another old-fashion herbal remedy, and it has been consumed for thousands of years in China and India for its medicinal benefits. Green tea is made from non-fermented tea leaves and has the highest concentration of antioxidants of all teas.

What is it about it that makes it so important for our health and the second most consumed beverage in the world after water?

It contains an incredible level of antioxidants, but besides this fact, it contains one special ingredient called L-Theanine, an amino acid that derives from Glutamic Acid – a neurotransmitter found in our brains. This L-Theanine helps you relax by reducing general stress levels and plays a preventive role in cancer.

An experiment was led by the Laboratory of Nutrition Biochemistry, in Japan, and it showed how this amino acid works. After taking L-Theanine, dopamine levels in the brain increased. Dopamine is a neurotransmitter that affects human emotions, so it created a well-being sensation.

Some laboratory studies showed great effect with green tea and stomach cancer. The polyphenols in the tea tended to prevent the stomach cancer from growing further[321]. Also in pancreatic[322] and esophageal cancer,[323] green tea has proven to have positive effects. A Japanese study researched women in various stages of breast cancer. Those who drank the most green tea had the least amount of cancer metastases[324].

Moreover, recent studies suggest that green tea helps increase the metabolic rate, and therefore it is of great help in weight-loss[325,326,327], but also in the prevention of atherosclerosis, due to its quality of preventing LDL cholesterol from oxidizing.

If you relax for 35 minutes after drinking a cup of green tea, the production of alpha brain waves is stimulated. The alpha waves are those you experience right before you fall asleep. It is during this period that you are most relaxed. In fact, combining relaxation and green tea together, you will obtain a mental state similar to meditation, but you will still be awake and active.

### Benefits

Take a look at the following benefits of green tea. Mark the benefits that are most important to you:

☐ Lowers cholesterol levels
☐ Protection against heart disease
☐ Anti-bacterial
☐ Fights free radicals
☐ Increases dopamine
☐ Increases wellbeing feeling
☐ Reduces stress
☐ Anti-cancer
☐ Assists weight-loss
☐ Boosts immunity levels
☐ Regulates fat metabolism
☐ Inhibits the development of cell cancer, especially colon, rectal, urinary, bladder, esophageal and stomach cancer
☐ Speeds up weight-loss
☐ Alzheimer's prevention – protect your brain in old age
☐ Improves brain function, it makes you smarter
☐ Increases focus
☐ Stabilizes blood sugar
☐ Lowers blood pressure
☐ Physical performance improvement

Sources: 328,329,330,331,332,333

Look at the benefits that you marked. Copy them to your "Your Action Plan Workbook" (chapter 12). Then complete the column with how important this benefit is to you and the Green Tea as superfood.

## Copy your benefits to the action plan !

## 7.16 Hawthorn

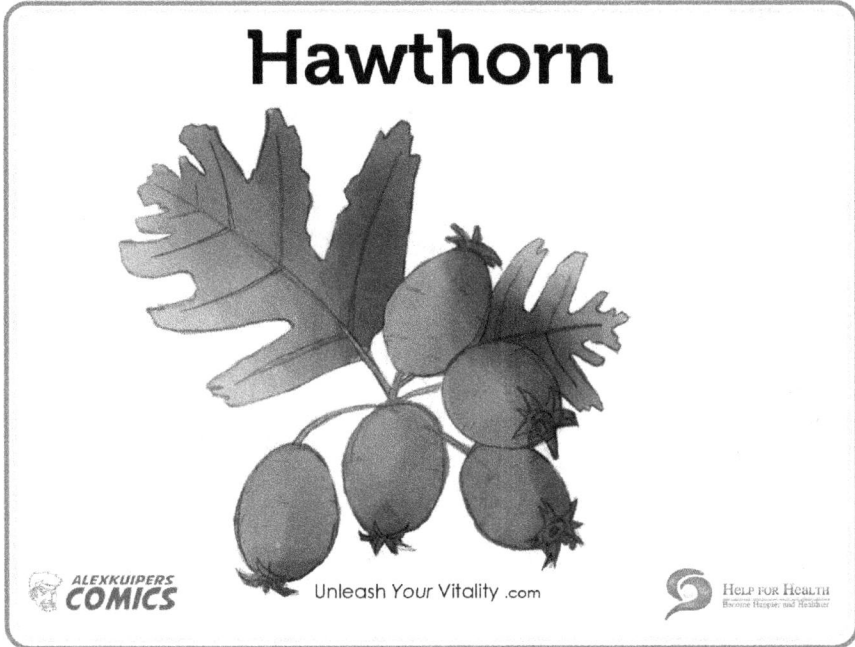

Hawthorn is a plant which has already provided us with health benefits for centuries. In the early 1800s, doctors used it to treat circulatory problems like heart rhythm and blood pressure, and this is what encouraged modern scientists to research its properties.

Hawthorn is mostly valued for its ability to restore the tone of the heart, and for this reason it is administered to patients who suffer from heart failure. It acts by relaxing the blood vessels around the heart, allowing it to pump blood the proper way, thus minimizing stress on organs that otherwise wouldn't get the right amount of oxygen and nutrients.

A large study unveiled the fact that hawthorn supplement helped 952 patients suffering from heart failure. According to the results of the study, after 2 years of daily administration, clinical symptoms decreased and those who also took prescription medication were able to decrease the dose of those prescription medicines[334,335,336] .

According to the Maryland Medical Center, Hawthorn also helps those suffering from angina and high blood pressure.

Moreover, the plant is rich in antioxidants and vitamins capable of fighting free radicals and lowering cholesterol levels.

### Benefits

Take a look at the following benefits for hawthorn. Mark those benefits that are most important to you:

- ☐ Lowers blood pressure
- ☐ Increases energy
- ☐ Stimulates the immune system
- ☐ Improves circulation
- ☐ Reduces chest pains
- ☐ Strong antioxidant
- ☐ Lowers cholesterol
- ☐ Improves digestion
- ☐ Reduces stomach pain
- ☐ Relaxes the arteries of the heart and provides more blood to the heart
- ☐ Increases urine output
- ☐ Reduces diarrhea
- ☐ Reduces anxiety
- ☐ Stabilizes high and low blood pressure

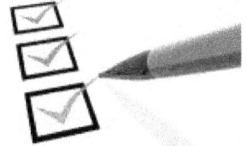

Sources: 337,338,339

Look at the benefits that you marked. Copy them to your "Your Action Plan Workbook" (chapter 12). Then complete the column with how important this benefit is to you and the Hawthorn as superfood.

## Copy your benefits to the action plan !

## 7.17   Maitake Mushroom

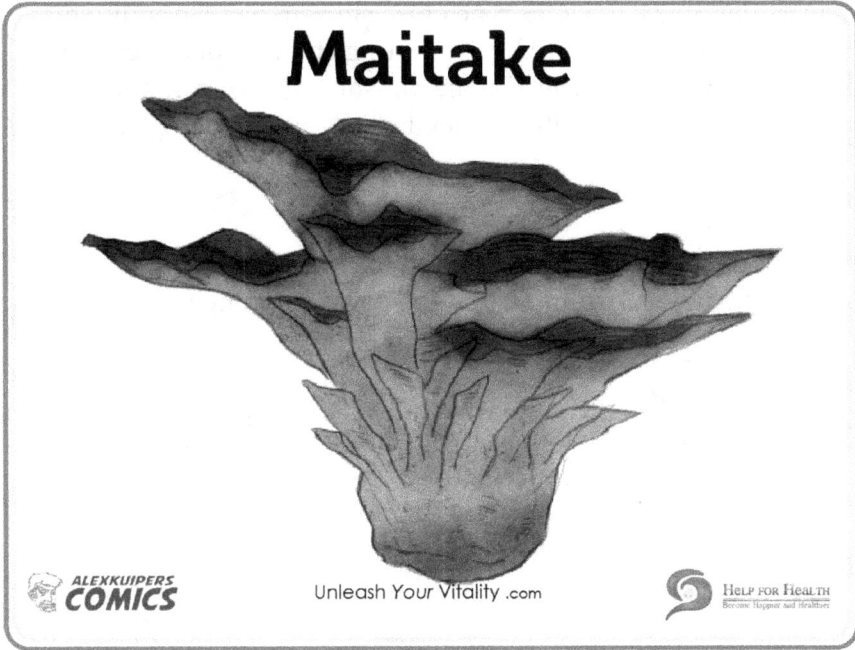

Maitake (also known as Grifola frondosa) is a mushroom native to Japan. In Asian countries it is commonly consumed as food, but it is also appreciated for its positive effects on health.

Studies showed that it has the capacity to activate specific cells in our immune system: cells that fight cancer cells and slow the progression of cancer cells. The ability to increase the immune function with Maitake seemed to prevent the spreading of cancer[340,341]. Maitake is now being investigated for its anti-cancer properties[342]. It tends to reduce the side effects of chemotherapy, like hair loss, pain and nausea. It also relieves the pain of terminal cancer.

Studies[343] led at the Kobe Pharmaceutical University, in Japan, suggest that this particular type of mushroom has the ability to improve lipid metabolism by preventing cholesterol increase in both blood and liver. The Maitake mushroom also contains an alpha glucosidase inhibitor, which helps lower blood sugar.

### Benefits

Take a look at the following benefits for the Maitake. Mark those benefits that are most important to you with a pencil:

- ☐ Lowers cholesterol
- ☐ Lowers blood sugar/ diabetes
- ☐ Offers active protection against cancer[344]
- ☐ Immune system enhancer
- ☐ Reduces side effects of chemotherapy
- ☐ Reduces chronic fatigue
- ☐ Reduces hepatitis
- ☐ Relieves hay fever
- ☐ Lowers high blood pressure
- ☐ Assists weight-loss

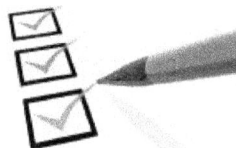

Look at the benefits that you marked. Copy them to your "Your Action Plan Workbook" (chapter 12). Then complete the column with how important this benefit is to you and the Maitake as superfood.

## Copy your benefits to the action plan !

## 7.18  Mangosteen

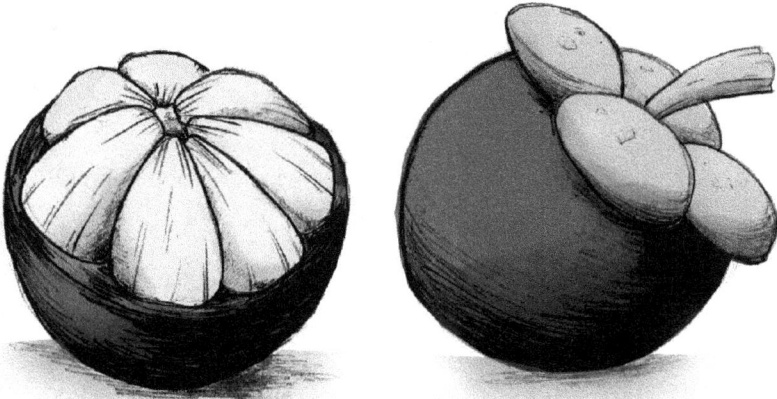

Mangosteen is a fruit that has been an important part of traditional Asian medicine for centuries. It is filled with essential nutrients necessary for the growth and development of cells and tissues. Despite the name, Mangosteen is not related to the mango fruit.

Mangosteen has a polyphenol compound called Xanthone. This particular ingredient makes it a strong anti-inflammatory, anti-allergic and gives a big breath of fresh air to those suffering from cardiovascular disease. Xanthones are similar to bioflavonoids but are much rarer in nature.

Mangosteen is also filled with antioxidants[345,] preventing free radical damage and premature ageing. Not only is it rich in antioxidants, but also in vitamin C, copper and magnesium providing a boost to the immune system, while protecting arteries.

*"Mangosteen is by far the most powerful anti-inflammatory I have ever seen in 30 years of practice. Research has proven this to be true, along with folk medicine history."*
~ *Dr. Kenneth J. Finsand*

## Benefits

Take a look at the following benefits for Mangosteen. Mark those benefits that are important to you:

☐ Reduces bladder infections
☐ Reduces eczema and acne
☐ Reduces inflammation
☐ Prevents premature ageing
☐ Stabilizes blood pressure
☐ Reduces cardiovascular symptoms
☐ Improves blood flow
☐ Reduces cholesterol
☐ Reduces urinary tract infections
☐ Reduces menstrual disorders
☐ Improves mental health
☐ Protects against viral and fungal infections
☐ Prevents weight gain
☐ Prevents and reduces diarrhea

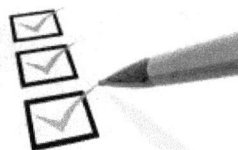

Look at the benefits that you marked. Copy them to your "Your Action Plan Workbook" (chapter 12). Then complete the column with how important this benefit is to you and the Mangosteen as superfood.

## Copy your benefits to the action plan !

## 7.19  Maqui Berry

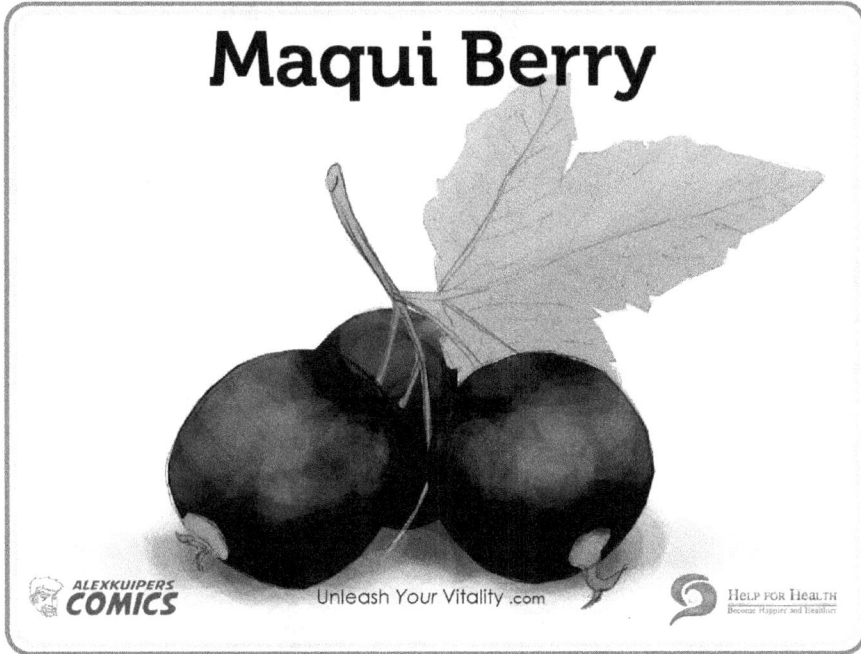

Maqui Berry is another berry that grows in South America. It was used for a very long time as a simple fruit, and for its juice, until it was found to have special qualities.

Studies found that this particular type of berry contains a special class of antioxidants called anthocyanins. This is a very potent antioxidant in fighting high blood pressure and obesity[346, 347].

In 2002, a study published in the Journal of Agricultural and Food Chemistry[348], revealed that Maqui berry extract helps in lowering the cholesterol levels and fights oxidative stress, while also aiding in the prevention of atherosclerosis.

Another study published in the Journal of Pharmacy and Pharmacology, showed the fact that the Maqui berry contains chemicals that help ease pain and reduce inflammation[349].

*Benefits*

Take a look at the following benefits for the Maqui berry. Mark those benefits that are most important to you:

- ☐ Increases energy/ reduces Fatigue
- ☐ Detoxifies the body
- ☐ Assists in weight-loss
- ☐ Reduces inflammation
- ☐ Lowers cholesterol
- ☐ Potent Antioxidant
- ☐ Prevents heart disease
- ☐ Anti-viral properties
- ☐ Cancer fighting antioxidants
- ☐ Improves insulin production
- ☐ Reduces pain
- ☐ Reduces blood pressure

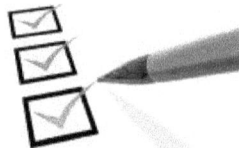

Look at the benefits that you marked. Copy them to your "Your Action Plan Workbook" (chapter 12). Then complete the column with how important this benefit is to you and the Maqui berry as superfood.

**Copy your benefits to the action plan !**

## 7.20 Noni

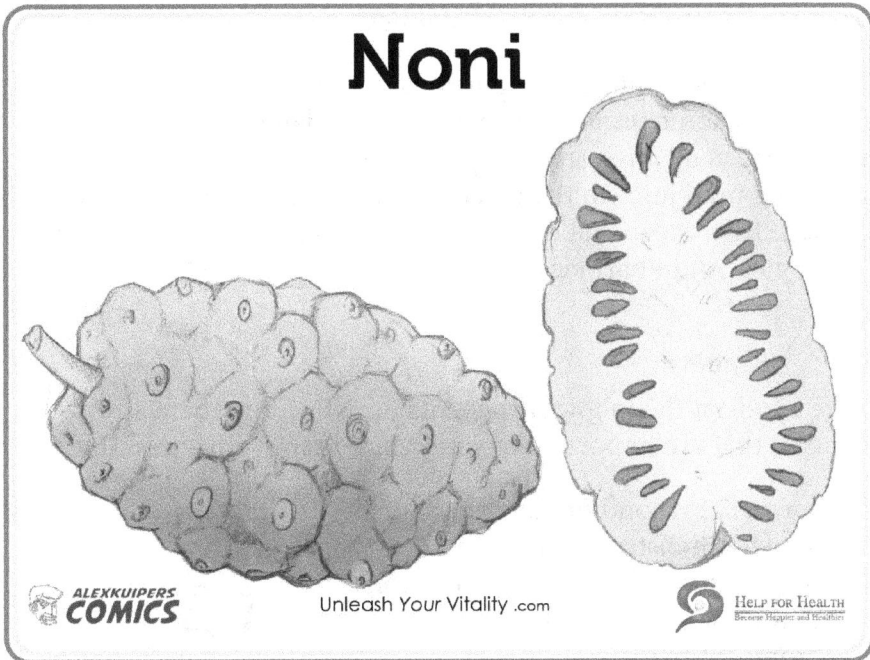

# Noni

ALEXKUIPERS COMICS    Unleash Your Vitality .com    HELP FOR HEALTH

Noni (also known as Morinda citrifolia) is a fruit found in tropical regions and has been used for a long time for its medical benefits. This is why researchers focused on testing its effects, in order to be able to provide people with a healthy and natural supplement, based on it.

Scientists are getting increasingly interested in the effects of this fruit. However, the actual active ingredient stayed a mystery for a long time. Ralph Heinicke found the active ingredient in 1985 and he extracted the active ingredient Xeroine[350, 351].

The Noni fruit has an impressive amount of antioxidants[352] and a balanced amount of minerals and vitamins, but this is not its most impressive feature.

It was proven to have antibacterial proprieties. An in-vitro study tested this idea, which found that noni juice is able to fight bacteria like E. coli[353] and Staphylococcus Aureus, which we all know, are found everywhere.

Another study demonstrated that noni juice can decrease pain[354] in a way similar to prescription analgesics.

Maybe the most interesting information about it is the fact that it can offer some protection against stroke damage. Research that took place at a University in Japan illustrated evidence that rats receiving noni juice in their water experienced less neurological damage than those that didn't. These findings, can be found in the "Biological and Pharmaceutical Bulletin" of 2009.

### Benefits

Take a look at the following benefits for Noni. Are there any benefits that are important to you? Mark them with a pencil:

- ☐ Normalizes blood pressure
- ☐ Reduces menstrual cramps
- ☐ Helps fight against urinary infections, relieves painful urination
- ☐ Strong antioxidant
- ☐ Anti-inflammatory
- ☐ Protects against stroke damage
- ☐ Anti-anemic
- ☐ Reduces coughs
- ☐ Stabilizes blood glucose levels / diabetes
- ☐ Reduces fever
- ☐ Reduces nausea and constipation
- ☐ Assists brain tissue regeneration
- ☐ Reduces bone or joint problems
- ☐ Reduces colds
- ☐ Increases mood and reduces depression
- ☐ Relieves digestive problems
- ☐ Relieves migraines and headaches

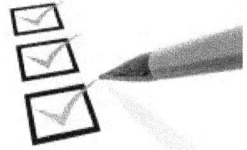

Sources: 355,356,357,358,359

Look at the benefits that you marked. Copy them to your "Your Action Plan Workbook" (chapter 12). Then complete the column with how important this benefit is to you and the Noni as superfood.

## Copy your benefits to the action plan !

## 7.21 Pomegranate

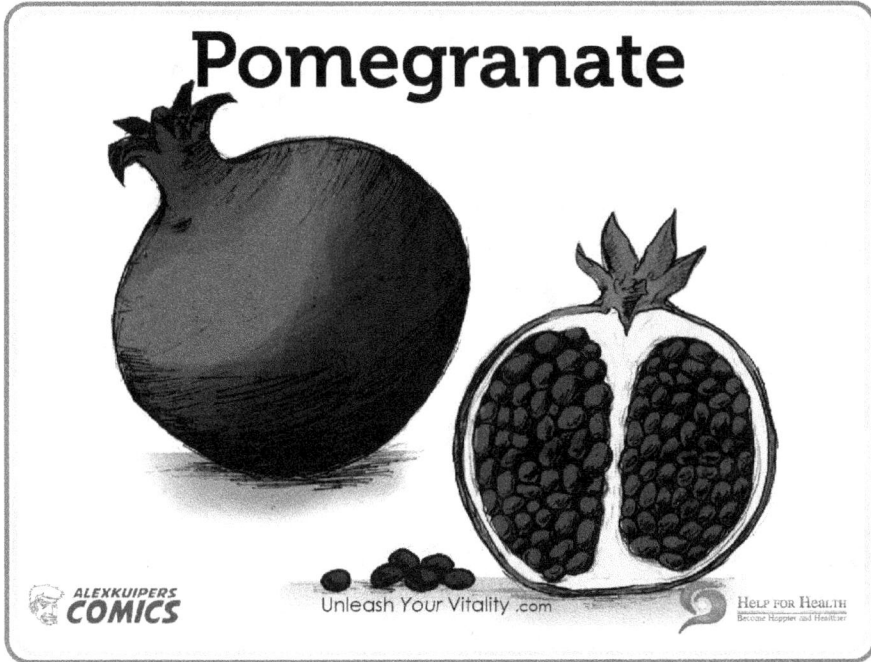

Pomegranate is said to originate from the Garden of Eden. That is probably not true… at least it wasn't mentioned in the Bible. Nevertheless, it has been used for its proprieties for thousands of years.

The fruit is rich in antioxidants[360], vitamin B5 and vitamin C. It offers cholesterol-lowering properties and reduces inflammation[361]. This anti-inflammatory effect prevents cholesterol from oxidization and adhering to the blood vessel walls, therefore protects against hardening of the arteries and reduces blood pressure.

In several studies it was noticed that drinking pomegranate juice reduced the PSA (Prostate-specific antigen) doubling times. Indicating it could be used in the case of slowing down prostate cancer[362,363] and even reverse it[364].

A more recent study has shown a particularly interesting feature of this fruit. The research was led in Edinburg and it showed that people who drank Pomegranate juice, had a marked increase in testosterone levels. In women this means that it helps in strengthening muscle and bones therefore, indirectly preventing osteoporosis.

What's the twist? Increased levels of testosterone also increase sex drive, making it basically a very healthy aphrodisiac. Some call it natural Viagra for both men and women.

### Benefits

Pomegranate has some great benefits. Take a look them. Mark the most important ones to you with a pencil:

- ☐ Increases memory
- ☐ Elevates mood and reduces depression
- ☐ Reduces menopausal symptoms
- ☐ Slows down and reverts prostate cancer
- ☐ Promotes cell death in cancer cells
- ☐ Reduces inflammation
- ☐ Bone strengthening/ reduces osteoporosis
- ☐ Reduces joint pain
- ☐ Lowers blood pressure
- ☐ Lowers cholesterol
- ☐ Reduces erectile dysfunction
- ☐ Prevents cholesterol damage
- ☐ Protects the arteries and the heart
- ☐ Increases sex drive

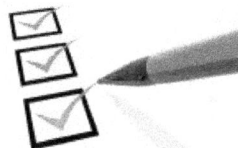

Look at the benefits that you marked. Copy them to your "Your Action Plan Workbook" (chapter 12). Then complete the column with how important this benefit is to you and the Pomegranate as superfood.

## Copy your benefits to the action plan !

## 7.22 Reishi Mushroom

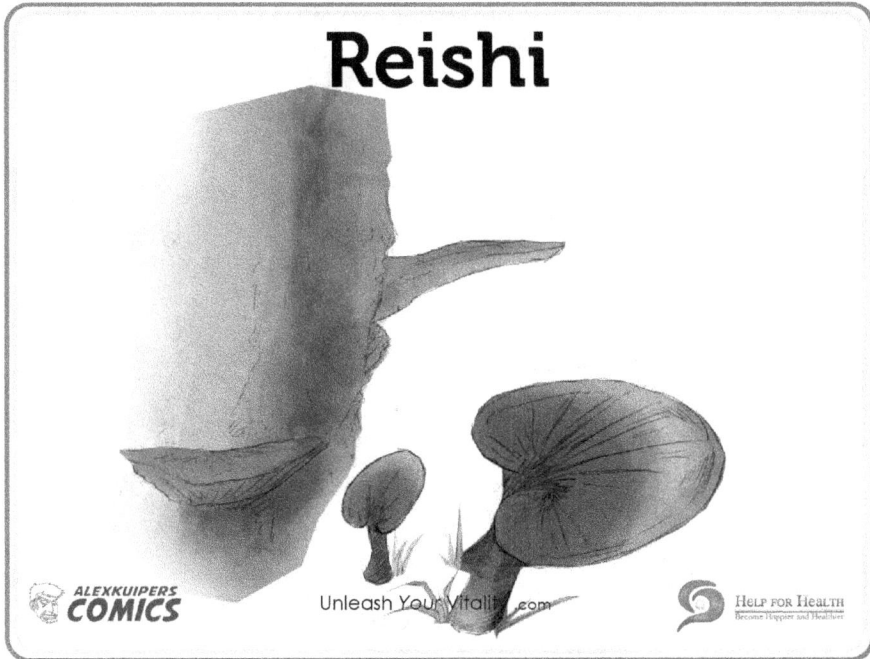

The Reishi mushroom, which is commonly known as Ganoderma lucidum, originates in Japan where it's been valued for a very long time due to its immune stimulating proprieties, but also for its effects on blood cholesterol and blood sugar levels.

It is rich in water-soluble polysaccharides, which interact with the immune system, telling it to be on alert. This is why people consuming this mushroom tend to be healthier than most other people[365].

The same active ingredient that boosts immunity helps lower cholesterol levels, but it has another secret ingredient, called Triterpenes that helps in lowering blood pressure.

Last, but not least, it contains an active ingredient that is able to ease allergic reactions. This happens because it inhibits histamine release.

### Benefits

Take a look at the following benefits for the Reishi. Are there any benefits that are important to you? Mark them with a pencil:

- ☐ Lowers stress levels
- ☐ Boosts immune system
- ☐ Lowers blood pressure
- ☐ Lowers cholesterol
- ☐ Reduces allergic reactions symptoms / histamine inhibitor
- ☐ Reduces inflammation
- ☐ Prevents cancer
- ☐ Prevents viral infections like the flu
- ☐ Reduces symptoms of asthma and bronchitis
- ☐ Improves kidney functioning
- ☐ Increases energy/ reduces fatigue
- ☐ Reduces stomach ulcers
- ☐ Improves sleep

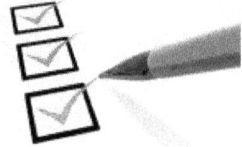

Look at the benefits that you marked. Copy them to your "Your Action Plan Workbook" (chapter 12). Then complete the column with how important this benefit is to you and the Reishi as superfood.

## Copy your benefits to the action plan !

## 7.23 Sea-Buckthorn

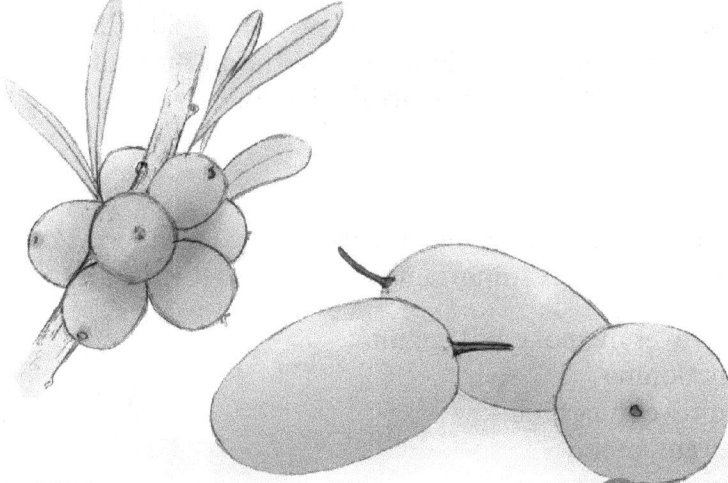

Sea-Buckthorn is probably one of the oldest and most impressive fruits used to improve health. It is found all over Europe and Asia and this might be one of the reasons for which there are well over 200 scientific studies that attest its benefits. Many people, including myself, never heard of it before.

For a small fruit, it has incredible amounts of vitamin C. 100 grams can provide up to 1600 mg of vitamin C, while the same amount of lemon juice will provide a modest 53mg. Impressive, Right?

There is even more to this fruit, it has lots of good fatty acids that protect your heart and cardiovascular system, and more than 60 different types of antioxidants.

Sea-Buckthorn also contains vitamins B, E and Beta-carotene and, a very interesting twist, it contains 5-HT, which is a form of serotonin, the neurotransmitter that has the ability to enhance mood.

One particular study[366] that researched the benefits of this fruit, involved supplementing the diet of 30 patients suffering from peptic ulcer with Sea-Buckthorn. After a month, the results were impressive 96.7% of the subjects had a 76.6 cure rate. This is a huge number for using just one supplement with no side effects and no additional drugs. The results are due to the anti-inflammatory and restorative effects it has on mucosal tissues.

*Benefits*

Take a look at the following benefits for Sea-Buckthorn. Are there any benefits that are important to you? Mark them with a pencil:

- Improves memory and cognitive functioning
- Improves digestion
- Elevates mood
- Prevents the common cold
- Loosens phlegm
- Antioxidant
- Heals mucosal tissue
- Relieves asthma
- Reduces angina
- Boosts immunity
- Lowers cholesterol
- Detoxifies the body
- Reduces acid reflux (GERD)
- Prevents and cures intestinal ulcers

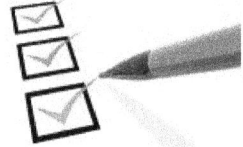

Sources: 367

Look at the benefits that you marked. Copy them to your "Your Action Plan Workbook" (chapter 12). Then complete the column with how important this benefit is to you and the Sea-Buckthorn as superfood.

## Copy your benefits to the action plan !

## 7.24  Shiitake Mushroom

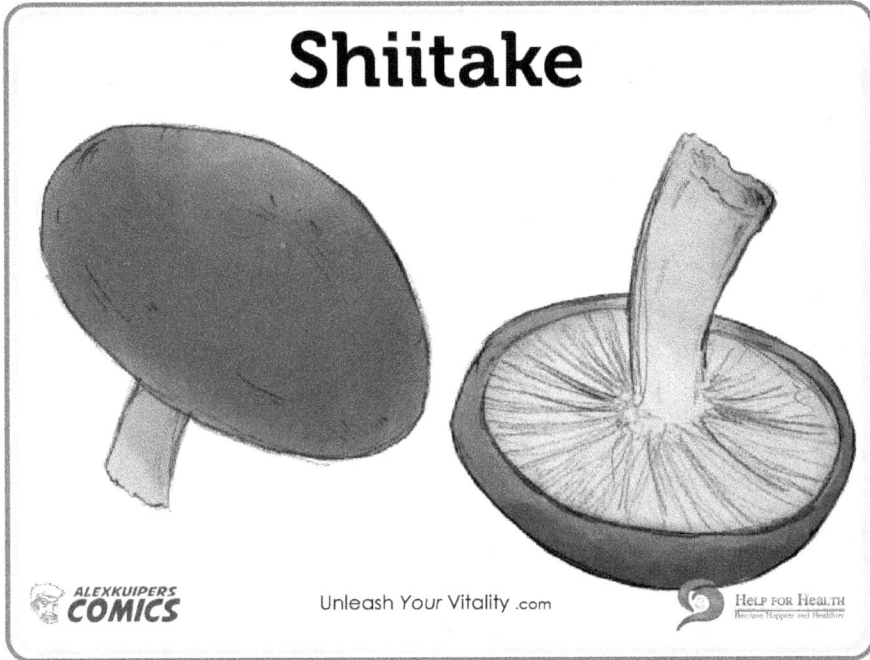

Traditional Asian herbalists have used the shiitake mushroom for thousands of years due to its extraordinary immune boosting proprieties[368]. Sometimes it is referred to as "King of mushrooms" and the "Elixir of life".

Laughed at for centuries, nowadays, modern science has proven that they were right all along. Studies suggest that it's not just rich in copper and zinc, but it also brings another very important benefit.

It was found to help fight cancer. It stimulates the immune system to produce more T-cells that automatically fight any cancer cells, and it also slows down the development of tumors.

During a study in mice Prof. Ikekawa noted that sarcomas disappeared in all 180 mice after administering this mushroom. The Shiitake mushroom contains substances that are now being used as treatment for stomach, intestine, liver, lung and ovarian cancers[369,370,371].

The fact that it boosts immunity is beneficial for those suffering from AIDS, but also for those who experience recurrent infections. Also, it helps stabilize cholesterol levels by acting directly on the liver.

In animal studies, shiitake was showed to decrease tumors and disable virus activity[372,373].

### *Benefits*

Take a look at the following benefits for the Shiitake. Are there any benefits that are important to you? Mark them with a pencil:

☐ Stimulates the immune function
☐ Prevents cancer
☐ Lowers cholesterol
☐ Reduces ageing
☐ Slows down tumor growth
☐ Protects against cardiovascular diseases
☐ Prevents and protects against viruses

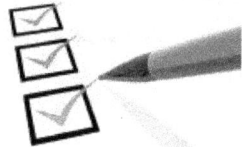

Look at the benefits that you marked. Copy them to your "Your Action Plan Workbook" (chapter 12). Then complete the column with how important this benefit is to you and the Shiitake as superfood.

## Copy your benefits to the action plan !

## 7.25 Zeolite

# Zeolite

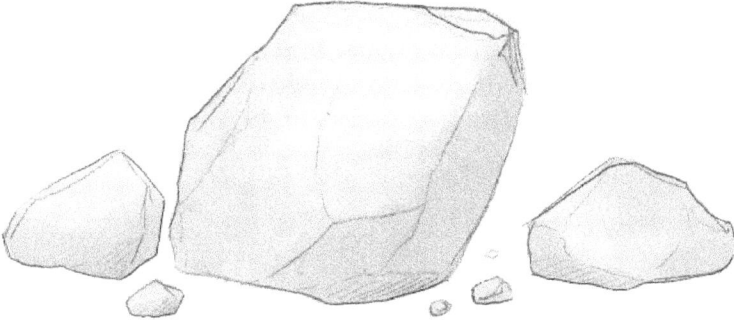

Zeolite is not as much a super-food, as it is a super-rock. Nature gave us everything we need in order to survive, and sometimes, the most useful of ingredients, are found in the most peculiar of places.

Zeolite is formed when water meats volcanic ash. It brings those minerals from deep down in the earth towards the surface. It contains a whole array of valuable minerals. Even if these minerals don't sound attractive, they are capable of doing something truly unique.

It is capable of absorbing toxins and trapping free radicals at the same time. The specific structure of Zeolite structure acts as a sponge to catch those toxins and eliminate them.

It doesn't do this only with poisons and free radicals; it is also able to extract heavy metals from the body. As you know we are exposed to many different chemicals, poisons and heavy metals. Zeolite is one of the best substances to help you detoxify and restore your entire system.

It is for these qualities that it is also of great benefit in water purification systems. So, if you are looking for a great water purification method, make sure that it has Zeolite as an active ingredient.

There is even a more potent version of Zeolite on the market today. By increasing the surface of the zeolite ,it performs better at trapping toxins. This process is called micronization. Look for that form of Zeolite when you want to detoxify your body or you need a water purification system.

### Benefits

Zeolite has some interesting benefits. Take a look at them, mark the most important ones with a pencil:

☐ Detoxifies the body
☐ Reduces alcohol hangovers
☐ Removes micro toxins
☐ Traps and removes virus components
☐ Balances body PH levels
☐ Purifies water
☐ Balances the immune system
☐ Removes fungal infections
☐ Removes heavy metals
☐ Removes free radicals
☐ Improves kidney function

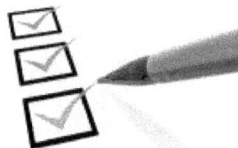

Look at the benefits that you marked. Copy them to your "Your Action Plan Workbook" (chapter 12). Then complete the column with how important this benefit is to you Zeolite.

## Copy your benefits to the action plan !

# 7.26 Summary

*"True healthcare reform starts with you, not others"*

Did you finish the exercise? It is really important that you have marked the benefits of the different foods in your action plan. We will work with this action plan to find the best solution for you.

After writing this chapter I was truly amazed about the value of these superfoods and the research to back this up. Sure, I was already a bit familiar with the health benefits of food, but I never realized the full extent of it.

Whenever I give a presentation about the scientific research behind these superfoods, people are amazed. They come to me with the most interesting stories about their personal experience and with questions about what superfoods are best for them. We will discuss that in next chapter. But if you need the quick answer, read the section called: What do I need for symptom X.

The foods we presented and the health promoting benefits are just a small subsection of what is available and they all have almost miraculous abilities to support your health. Some of them you might know, others might be new. They have all been shown to have amazing health promoting effects.

Even though these effects are sometimes debated, it is very important to remember that there are no side effects. That is the great thing about them, you can benefit from their "powers", without having to cope with negative side effects. So instead of using chemical medication, you might want to consider finding alternatives.

# WARNING NOTE:

These foods are becoming more known to the public and more products containing these foods are entering the market. This is not always a good thing. When you go to the store to obtain these foods you will be faced with multiple brands. Because of the commercialization of these products, there will be bad quality products on the market. You need to be aware of this.

Even though these are superfoods, many available from the stores are still chemically sprayed or grown on soil-depleted grounds. Finding the proper, clean and healthy variant of the specific type can sometimes be hard.

A research organization bought all products available that contained a certain superfood to determine their quality. Their results were shocking. They analyzed the levels of chemicals that were in the product, even though the label mentioned "organic". The researchers found that all except one had used chemicals whereby they were not allowed to call their product organic anymore (but it was still marked as organic). Many of the products contained chemicals above safety levels for human consumption. One product even exceeded the safety levels for human consumption by 700%.

*Remember, these were sold as health promoting supplements.*
*These products were actually dangerous for human health.*

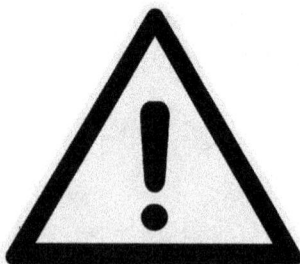

## 7.27 Your Key Points to Remember

Looking for the right supplements that are healthy can be a daunting task. The more commercialization, the harder it becomes. In the next chapter we are going to look further into how to choose the right supplements. You need to learn how to select those that are healthy and efficient, and how you can select the cleanest quality that will actually improve your health.

✓ *Superfoods are nature's safety plan*

✓ *Superfoods are super rich in nutrients (hence super foods)*

✓ *Superfoods are packed with antioxidants*

✓ *Superfoods help in building strong immunity*

✓ *Superfoods are efficient in treating disease and have no side effects*

✓ *The potency of superfoods depends on the type of fruit, where it is harvested and how it has been grown*

✓ *Superfoods can be hard to get and very expensive*

✓ *Commercialization of superfoods makes it harder to find pure healthy foods*

✓ *Superfoods can be dangerous if you do not have toxin free versions*

# *Your Amazing Insights and Actions*

Date: __ / __ / _____

## What are your insights and learnings from this section?

Now we have come to the conclusion of this chapter. Write down your main insights about what you learned and about yourself.

## What are you going to do differently starting today?

Insights alone will not unleash your vitality. You need to take actions. What are the actions you are going to do in order to implement these insights in your life?

# Call to action :
## Are you really ready?

Some people might tend to skip this chapter. Yes, they do want to learn a bit, but when it comes time to taking action they move on to the next book. A book is just some paper; you will only reach vibrant vitality when you implement it in your life.

## 8.1 Are you asking yourself, "Why bother?"

Before I continue, read the following reactions of people who changed their health by taking action. The have been anonymized to protect the privacy of those individuals.

And remember:

### Most diseases can be 100% prevented... if you take action now !

✓ *My son had to use hormone treatment for his eczema, for the last 10 years. Now it is gone. JvV.*

✓ *My child suffered from severe ADHD, now he can concentrate much better on school, without medication. J.*

✓ *For the last 25 years I suffered from eczema. I tried all kinds of pills and salves. Nothing worked sufficiently. After 4 days the itch disappeared forever. E.*

✓ *Over the last year I had many bouts of stomach ache and stomach complaints. Now my stomach is at rest. What a relief! G.*

✓ *Since I was 16 years old I suffered from chronic fatigue and could only work for 3 days a week. Currently I feel energetic and fit. After 24 years (I am 40 now) I finally have my life back. YeeHaa!! I.*

✓ *My dad was close to a burnout but did not want to admit that. Now he feels fit and energetic and even his eyes look more sparkly than ever. C.*

✓ *I no longer have headaches or migraines. A.*

✓ *My friend lost 21 kilos within a year, it never came back C.*

✓ *Currently I am 77 years or age with some small health issues. I can remember more and my muscles are more flexible. T.*

✓ *For the last couple of years I have pains in my joints of my hands. Now I have hardly any pains left. I am very happy with this result W.W.*

✓ *My father in law used to have an elevated blood pressure and diabetes 2 (including medication). Now his blood pressure is normal and his glucose levels are stable. W.W.*

✓ *...etc...etc...etc.*

We have many more such amazing testimonials.

But the main question is...what are you going to do? Are you going to take action and join these people?

We would love to hear from you. Either feedback directly to our email (see contact information at the back of the book), but even better, share your results on Facebook and on our site: http://www.UnleashYourVitality.com/results

Then you can inspire more people to do the same and change their health forever.

## 8.2 Taking a proactive approach to health

There is a very important difference between being proactive and being reactive. Being reactive basically translates into sitting and waiting until the worst has happened, and only then doing something about it. It is like firefighters, they only turn up when your house is almost burned to the ground. The work of doctors is also reactive. You visit them when you are already in trouble somehow.

When you are proactive, you are thinking of things in advance, you are preventing. Like installing a fire alarm, or thinking about and acting on what you can do to increase your general health and wellbeing (like reading and implementing the steps in this book).

Reactivity is the reason for which people are getting sick. Modern medicine provides a way of coping with disease by offering painkillers and expensive treatments. This is why most people don't focus on prevention, but a proactive person

**Are you proactive or reactive ?**

would never accept this compromise, and would always think ahead; preventing rather than treating.

There is a huge difference in proactive and reactive people and their history of illnesses. In my book "Healing Psyche", I explain how emotions and beliefs influence the cancer process. It also presents the evidence that proactive people are much healthier than reactive people.

In regard to your health, you must always be proactive. It's your wellbeing we are talking about, not something that can easily be replaced. Even if treating and curing a disease might seem easy. You must keep in mind that illness might scar you; it affects your mind, your body and your social environment. Preventing a disease is just like preventing a fire that could burn down your house.

You can compare the damage created by the fire with the effects of the disease, and that created by the water used to put it out, with the side effects of drugs. Compare all that damage caused by the fire and water to having prevented the fire. The choice is yours.

When you think about matters that are as important as your health, you must use all possible resources.

In a study[374] scientists researched the effect of nutritional support for long-term chronic patients. All clients were already involved for a long time in traditional symptomatic treatment of their ailments, without any relief whatsoever.

The patients were administered vitamin supplementation and that resulted in either full elimination of their long-term symptoms or remarkable relief from them. Vitamin treatment is safe and without any side effects. Remember these patients had severe symptoms for many years. Within 6-12 weeks, more than three quarters (85%) improved dramatically, just by vitamin supplementation alone.

> **Most diseases are 100% preventable, if YOU take action**

*It is up to you to take charge of your health.*

## 8.3 Nothing to lose - Are you ready?

There is lots of useful information in this book, and most of it will motivate you to start taking care of yourself, but will you keep it up? Will you be able to motivate yourself?

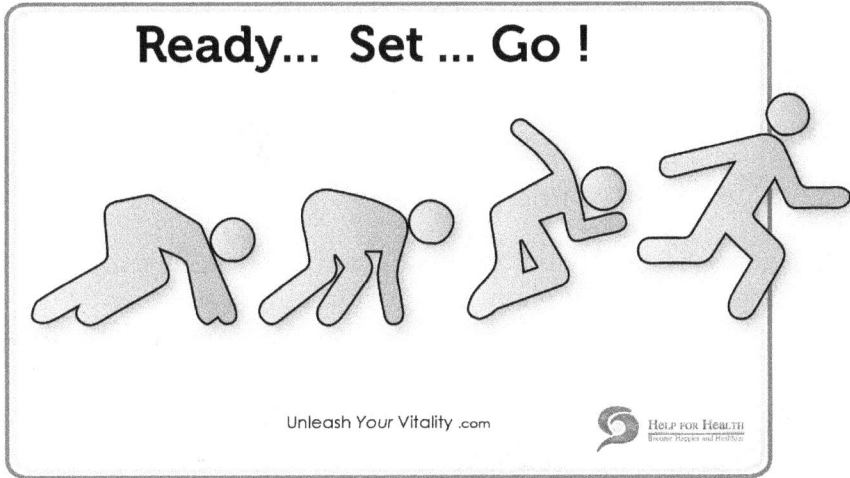

Ready... Set ... Go !

Unleash Your Vitality .com

HELP FOR HEALTH

Many people encounter ideas that have the potential to change their lives for the better, and most of them are enthusiastic at first, but they become less motivated with every day that passes. This is not such a bad behavior when it comes to business ideas or traveling, but when it comes to health issues, you must find ways to stay motivated because you will want to stay balanced, not to get sick.

One of the main troubles in supplementing your food with the proper nutrients is that it takes tremendous time and energy on your part to get, combine and prepare all those different types of food. When you have bought them they have a very short shelf life. The fruits itself are never certified, so you are still uncertain of the quality, type and if it contains toxins.

The easiest solution is to find a brand of highly certified supplements that provide all the nutrients you need. Having these supplements will make it much easier for you to change your health. But still you need to take action.

Almost every single person in the world wants to change something about his or her life. Most of these people make a commitment that they will start doing something about it. This commitment usually begins with the phrase "Starting Monday I will …." Or "Next year I will do …, until I obtain the results I want". Does that sound familiar?

The fact that you want to start improving your life is the first step, but you need to keep taking all the other steps too. When you start changing your life, and then stop for a variety of reasons, you will be forced to start again from the bottom.

Sadly, there isn't a pause button for life, so when you commit to something, you have to follow it through until you see the results you want. This requires will power and a focus on your health goals

---

*"Great ideas need landing gear as well as wings."*
*~ C.D. Jackson*

---

### Get in line – stay in line

Imagine it like this. You have set a clear goal and that is to get your life and health back in control, like a booth at the carnival where you can collect your prize.

Now you get in line to collect your prize. You need to wait a little until it is your turn. Every person no matter what their status is and how long they worked to reach their ultimate rewards started at the end of the line.

Even people who made remarkable changes in their life and health, lost tremendous weight or recovered from serious illnesses had to start at the end of the line. Remember that.

Finally, at the booth they can collect their rewards. All those remarkable recoveries started at the same place as you did, the end of the line. They stayed in the line until they reached the point to collect their rewards and their vibrant vitality.

Let's take a look at how many people (even people reading this book) work the queue. Take for example a new year's resolution, a goal to lose weight, stop smoking or eat enough nutrients. Many people get in line. It is quite a long lone.

The first week people manage to pick the right foods at the supermarket and eat the right supplements. The second week it also goes very well, so they are on track and closing in on the booth to collect their rewards.

The third week there is a party, or they go on a holiday or something else happens and they drop out of line. Just for a short moment.

No worries, you can always get back in line right?

Yes, but where do you need to go in the line... at the end... You cannot jump the queue; you need to start all over again.

In order to actually collect your rewards and reach your vitality goal you need to do only 2 things:

1. *Get in line*

2. *Stay in line*

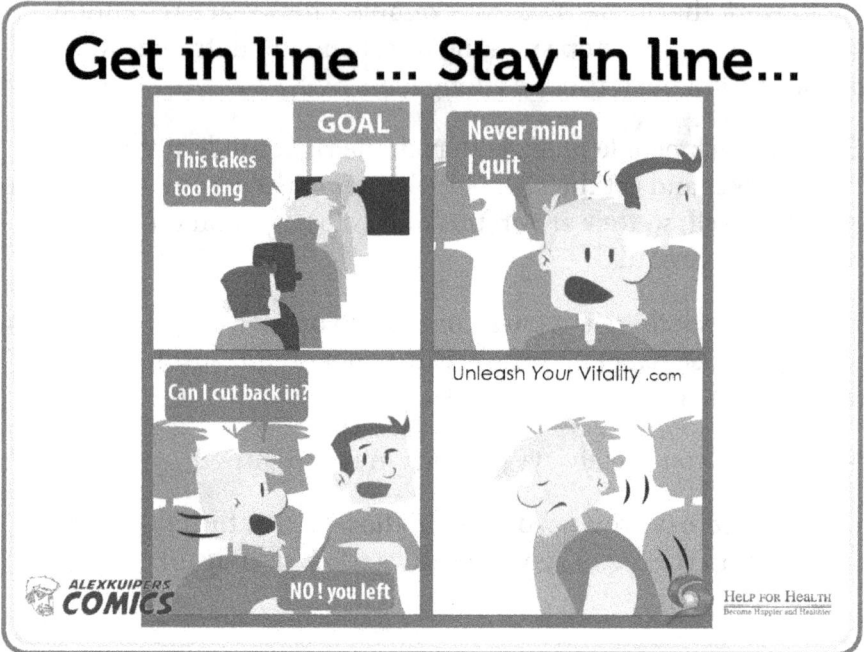

If you recognize this pattern, draw a big exclamation mark next to the image to remind yourself. Copy the image and place it somewhere where you can see it daily.

You can also download it and print it out. Just go to:
http://www.UnleashYourVitality.com/resource/

# Get only the BEST
## Because You're Worth It - How to select the best of the best

When it comes down to supplementing your health and finding the best quality supplements that you can trust, you face a forest of confusion. You need to pay attention to every detail.

The supplements market is very unregulated, and for this reason some manufacturers are allowed to deceive the customer. Well, it isn't lying when you are just hiding bits of information. Or is it?

---

*"Quality is more important than quantity.*
*One home run is much better than two doubles."*
*~ Steve Jobs*

---

This is a huge problem for the average health conscious consumer like yourself. If you pick the wrong calcium for example you increase the risk of a heart attack. If you pick a regular fish oil that is not cleaned well you increase your exposure to toxins and poison yourself.

So, when you decide to buy a supplement online or in a drug store, pay attention to some extremely important details. You don't want to realize that you've been taking a supplement that is made out of chemical ingredients and might harm your health.

One on the ways you can do that is by checking the label. It might be time consuming, but we are talking about your health. Most supplements aren't made according to the Good Manufacturing Practice (GMP). This translates into not telling you everything, so they can write anything down on the label to try to sell it to you. You will learn more about GMP in subsequent sections.

This chapter will teach you how to select the best and cleanest quality products; products that you can rely upon and use safely to supplement your health.

## 9.1    The dark side of supplements

But if it is on the label it is ok, right?

I can look at the list of ingredients, so I know
I am safe?

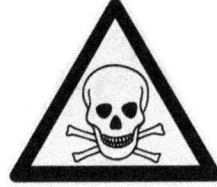

Let's take a look at some research to see
where the dangers are and what to look out
for.

Researchers from the University of Guelph in Ontario[375] reverse
engineered several herbal supplements. They researched the
products to see what ingredients were inside and then compared
that to the label. The results are shocking:

- ✓ *59% of the products contained plant species that were not listed on the label*

- ✓ *33% contained contaminants and fillers that were not listed on the label and could be dangerous*

- ✓ *32% of the samples contained absolutely none of the herbs listed on the label, but instead contained some other plant species*

- ✓ *9% of the samples were complete junk—they contained only rice or wheat*

Imagine going to the store and there are 10 different brands, they
all have nice packaging, and promise to increase your health. The
above statistics show that at least 2 or 3 contain illegal steroids.
About 6 will have unlisted ingredients, and 3 will have none of the
listed ingredients in the product. Of course these numbers do not
add up, because a product might be contaminated and also not
have the listed ingredient.

The result: You think you're buying something that increases your health, but there is a high chance that you are poisoning your body.

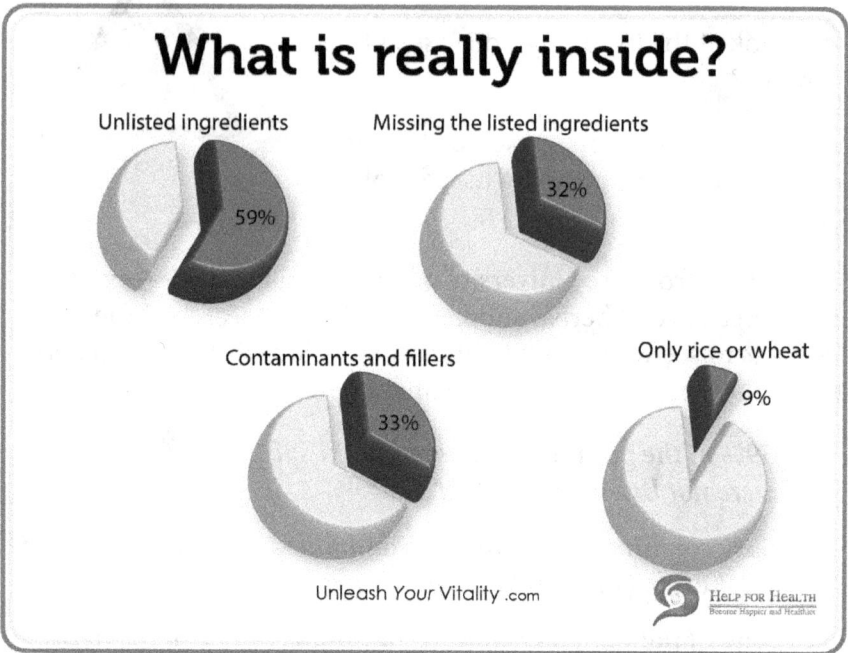

# What is really inside?

**Unlisted ingredients** — 59%

**Missing the listed ingredients** — 32%

**Contaminants and fillers** — 33%

**Only rice or wheat** — 9%

Unleash *Your* Vitality .com

Help for Health
*Become Happier and Healthier*

---

*It is not what is on the label what you should be worried about.*
*You should be worried about what is NOT on the label*

---

In another study, it was noted that about 15% of the researched supplements to support energy, weight control and joint support were contaminated with illegal steroids that were not on the label[376,377]. For products bought in the UK, it was even close to 20% contamination (1 out of every 5 products contained harmful substances). Other studies confirm these findings whereby they reviewed regular multivitamin supplements and found steroids, illegal stimulants, prescription drugs, heavy metals and bacteria[378,379,380,381,382,383].

Do you think those companies learned from their fraudulent behavior? Think again!

Even though many companies have been warned in the past, in February 2015 another scandal became apparent. The Center for Biodiversity Genomics conducted further study to see what the actual ingredients in some supplemental products were..

**Many products have false or incomplete labels**

Nothing had improved! Some companies are still not labeling their products correctly.

Contamination, substitution and and, more importantly, present consider: the products purchased revealed the foll

Gingko Biloba: Negative. No gingko b "oryza"(x4)(commonly known as rice), whatsoever.

St. John's Wort: Negative. No St. John identified any DNA, and it included all n

Ginseng: Negative. No ginseng DNA v pinus strobus, wheat/grass, and citrus sp

Garlic: Positive. All 20 tests yielded DN

Echinacea: Negative. Five tests identifi Fourteen tests detected no plant DNA of

Saw Palmetto: Qualified negative. Onl positive results were principally from on sample demonstrated no plant DNA, and was positive for DNA from the primrose

## Official Report:

Ginko Biloba: NEGATIVE

St. John's Wort: NEGATIVE

Ginseng: NEGATIVE

Garlic: POSITIVE

Echinacea: NEGATIVE

Saw Palmetto: NEGATIVE

".. *NOT* providing the public with authentic products...

Studies conducted by the Centre previously alerted the dietary supplement industry to the fact that it is not providing the public with authentic products without substitution, contamination or fillers. It is disappointing that over a year later the General's researcher reached similar conclusions, demonstrating that the industry has failed to clean practices.

HELP FOR HEALTH
Become Happier and Healthier

Unleash Your Vitality .com

This resulted in an official indictment for those several main retailers, the names you would recognize and might be the ones where you shop weekly. I surely hope you did not buy their supplements hoping that they will help you. The stores were accused of selling fraudulent and potentially dangerous herbal supplements.

In this case 80% of the products did not contain any of the herb listed on the labels. They only contained than cheap fillers like rice, asparagus and houseplants. In some cases they even contained substances that are dangerous to people with allergies. Some contained wheat despite the claim being wheat-and gluten-free.

*"It is an unbelievably devastating indictment of the industry!"*
*~ Dr. Pieter Cohen, assistant professor at Harvard Medical School and an expert on supplement safety.*

The current verification of safely and accurate labeling is just an honor code. There is no regulation whatsoever by the FDA or any other organization. Supplements are, by law, considered safe until the authorities prove otherwise.

This research only starts after many claims of serious injuries, sometimes even death. Only then the products are pulled off the shelves.

One of the many examples is an outbreak of hepatitis due to tainted supplements. Hereby, 72 people in 16 different states were infected, three people required a liver transplant and one person even died.

And you were thinking of buying their supplements to become healthier.

You are FAR better off NOT taking any supplements than taking low quality or contaminated supplements. However, if you want to increase your health and wellbeing, high quality supplements can no longer be ignored, but at least know you will know what to look for.

This is exactly why vitamins and minerals sometimes get bad publicity. So you really need to be on the lookout for high quality supplements.

## 9.2 Clarity on Quality Labels

There are some voluntary quality labels that a manufacturer can apply for. Only when the supplement manufacturer reaches the required levels of excellence will they be awarded with that quality label.

The following quality labels are really important to recognize. They will ensure safety, cleanliness, quality and effectiveness of the supplements:

✓ *OTC*

✓ *USP*

✓ *NSF*

✓ *GMP*

✓ *FDA*

### 9.2.1   OTC

This is the certificate you must look for, when you want to choose a supplement. OTC stands for Over the Counter drug, and it is important to know that the company that produces nutritional supplements has this certificate.

It means that the entire facility has been verified and audited extensively. The manufacturer has the equipment and knowledge to create products that meet very high quality standards, the products are not just safe, but also they do exactly what they are meant to do.

Many companies have struggled to obtain this certificate, and didn't manage to do so, but you must look only for those few special ones who succeeded, because they can actually provide you with what you really need… The Very Best Quality Available.

### 9.2.2   USP

USP stands for United States Pharmacopoeial Convention and it gives certificates that attest the fact that certain products are free of toxic residue and are actually absorbable by the body.

### Cleanliness

This is very relevant as the FDA estimates approximately 50,000 adverse reactions occur due to contaminated or wrong dietary supplements. Almost daily, the FDA takes products off the market because they were found to be dangerous for your health. Often the FDA is too late because people have already suffered from poisoning, even cases of death have been reported[384,385]

Recently scientists researched all brands of quinoa (also considered a superfood) sold in stores. What they found shocked even me. They found chemicals over 700% the maximum allowed for food safety. So 10ug was the maximum allowed levels of chemicals for the product to be SAFELY consumed by humans. Anything above this level is considered dangerous. They actually found levels of 70ug !

> **Only buy the cleanest products without contaminants**

The product was immediately pulled off the market. However, it had already been sold in stores for months, and people bought it because they thought it was healthy. Only by accident they found these dangerous products. That is why you need to be so aware of the quality.

If this product had been USP certified, it would have never reached any consumer.

For example in 2008 researchers inspected a certain type of Indonesian herbal tea (Jamu Traditional Super Mandau) after a woman experienced severe abdominal pain, nausea and diarrhea. After careful lab inspection, they found western prescription medication inside the tea. Therefore, it is highly important that you only get those items that are very well checked.

There are several cases known where herbal supplements were spiked with illegal medication or chemicals without labeling; this could pose a serious threat to your health[386,387,388,389,390]. Reports have shown that this could lead to hospitalization or even worse.

For example, when you are shopping for Omega-3 fish oil supplements, you need to realize that they are from fish. Fish can be polluted with mercury and even though fish oil is healthy, mercury is highly toxic. When you have a USP certificate on a supplement, you know that it's clean and free of toxic waste.

In fact, this is one of the most important certificates you should look for in a product. It wasn't long ago that many important supplement brands were sued because their products contained toxic waste. Laboratory studies confirmed the fact that widely consumed products containing Omega-3 fish oil, contained up to 10 times the maximum amount of PCB (Polychlorinated biphenyl), and this increases the risk of cancer by the same number of times. Ten products were tested in this lawsuit and all the results were alarming.

So, be aware and always be on the lookout for products that might contain dangerous contaminants.

### Absorption

Besides the cleanliness of the product, the USP also tests the absorption rate.

This American certification is used worldwide to establish how well the supplement is dissolved in your digestive tract. If the quality of the dissolution is poor, the nutrients will never reach your blood stream. In that case, you will be basically throwing money in the toilet.

The supplements that enter your body need to be decompressed inside the digestive tract. If this dissolution is not optimal, they will do nothing for you, and you'll just be investing in

**USP guarantees that the nutrients are absorbed**

expensive urine. Supplements need to be able to go from your mouth, to your blood and cells.

During a study by Prof Shangraw, it was noticed that most of the supplements on the market were not dissolving at all, meaning they were unable to deliver their nutritional value to the body. According to Prof Shangraw "There is no great public harm being done in terms of safety. It`s a question of people getting what they pay for". However, if people were aware and selected USP certified supplements, they would actually protect their health.

The USP certificate also brings a guarantee that the supplement, be it tablet or be it capsule, has a high dissolution quality. There are many companies that fail to receive this certificate, or never apply for it because of this particular reason.

No matter what a supplement, or tablet of any kind contains, it must be able to be absorbed by your body, and for this reason it needs to dissolve properly. This is what the USP certificate brings to the table, the guarantee that the nutrients you are buying will actually reach your cells and are safe to use.

### *Unfortunately less than 1% of the available supplements on the market bear this label and are safe to use.*

### 9.2.3    NSF

The NSF used to be known as the National Sanitation Foundation, and it is an organization that focuses on providing services concerning the public health and safety.

It gives certification regarding the equipment used, and in order for a facility to receive its certification, there are a few steps that it needs to take.

The equipment used must undergo a physical evaluation to make sure that it is in conformity with food safety standards. All products certified by the NSF have to be tested end evaluated and also, the entire facility must be audited annually, to ensure that they keep the equipment at a high standard.

If the supplements you intend to use are NSF certified, you can be sure that the equipment used to make them was strictly evaluated, and they are safe from that point of view.

Also, the NSF is used as a third party laboratory, the best in the world, that is. Meaning that, after a company has tested products, these are sent to NSF for another round of tests, just to make sure that they are in perfect shape.

The final products are tested by this third party, which verifies the cleanliness and claims of the final product.

### 9.2.4    GMP

GMP stands for Good Manufacturing Practice, and it is a certificate given to companies that respect a very strict set of standards. It refers to every aspect involved in the production starting with the material and the equipment and ending with the personnel.

This certificate ensures that the final product is safe for human consumption, and for that the entire facility is verified. In order to gain this certificate, a company must have:

1. *Perfect hygiene*

2. *A controlled environment that prevents cross contamination*

3. *Processes that are clearly defined and controlled*

4. *Written procedures and instructions*

5. *Trained personnel,*

6. *Records of the entire process of manufacture and distribution*

7. *The ability to recall any product when it is desired*

There are two kinds of GMP, therefore confusion is created and some companies take advantage of this fact.

There is:

✓ *Food grade GMP (relatively useless)*

✓ *Pharmaceutical grade GMP (valuable)*

### Food grade GMP

The food grade GMP that we talked about certifies supplement manufacturers and food. The good manufacturing practice that refers to foods only attests the fact that the product meets food safety and quality legal requirements.

However, and this might come to you as a shock, to be certified for the food grade GMP, the label does not have to match the product inside. It is acceptable when the label just mentions the main ingredients. This means that only about 30% of the label needs to match the actual product. So, what is on the label is only what they want to sell to you, the rest could be right about anything, ranging from fillers, to toxins or illegal substances.

**Most ingredient labels lie to the consumer**

This leads to great misunderstanding and problems. In the case of Omega-3, many manufacturers left some oil chemicals like PCB and other contaminants inside their product because it was very expensive to remove. However, they did not mention it on the label.

### Pharmaceutical grade GMP

The supplements that you want and need are those which respect the pharmaceutical grade GMP, because this means that they list on the label every single item used to create the pill or capsule.

For your safety and wellbeing, always make sure that you choose a supplement that is produced by a company that treats its products as pharmaceutical grade products. This will assure you that the label corresponds 100% with the ingredients inside. So, if there are contaminants inside, they MUST be listed. This will ensure that you can select the cleanest product available.

You want to buy your products from a company that treats its products with the same care and safety as if they were drugs, not food. This way you will know that the supplements are coming from a safe and controlled environment. Also, when you can find every single compound on the label, you can be sure that you won't take something that can cause allergies, and this is a very important point. This is the only way you will have access to a controlled, clean product, which lets you know beforehand, all its ingredients.

### 9.2.5 FDA

The Food and Drug Administration was formed in 1906, and ever since, its task has been to protect the public by regulating and supervising food, dietary supplements, over-the-counter and prescription drugs, and also an entire range of biopharmaceuticals.

These registered facilities are highly monitored and inspected regularly. This prevents them from fraudulent actions. Those facilities are often allowed to produce over-the-counter drugs, which fall under very strict regulations. However, to get even more security that you have the best product, look for the OTC qualification label.

In order to obtain an FDA drug facility registration, a company must respect a very strict set of rules, because this certificate means that it is also able to produce prescription drugs, which fall under different laws. When you choose a supplement made in a facility verified and approved by the FDA, you can be sure that you are going to receive top quality.

### 9.2.6    GMO Free

GMO Stands for Genetically Modified Organism, and a company that has even one ingredient that has been tampered with at this level, won't be able to obtain this certificate.

Using genetically modified organisms in a supplement will change the nutritional value of the entire product, and it can affect the health of the consumer in the long term.

You probably are aware of the controversy behind the use of GMO, and you know that certain studies have linked them to cancer. This is why it is extremely important to only use supplements that have this certificate, ensuring that none of the ingredients inside have been genetically modified.

### 9.2.7    BSCG

The Banned Substances Control Group gives certificates to those companies producing dietary supplements that do not contain any prohibited substances. This means that if you buy supplements with this particular certificate on the label, you will receive a product that won't interfere with your athletic performance, and you will be able to pass any anti-doping test.

This aspect doesn't just interest athletes, because the banned substances affect health generally, not just performance.

### 9.2.8    EPA

The Environmental Protection Agency certifies companies that have high water quality. If you are going to buy water or water purifiers, you want to make sure that the manufacturer respects EPA standards. This will confirm the fact that the water is, or will be, free of pollutants, bacterial, chemical and viral agents.

### 9.2.9 Your Key Points to Remember

✓ *Supplements are unregulated and there are dangerous products on the market*

✓ *Many labels do not state everything that is inside the product*

✓ *Only go for certified quality to achieve maximum benefit*

✓ *Certificates are given to companies to attest the quality of their products*

✓ *It is of extreme importance to check the label for the certificates, before buying the products*

✓ *You always want to buy products that are treated by the manufacturer as a drug, not as simple food*

✓ *Look for the USP and OTC label to be certain of the cleanest and best quality*

✓ *USP certifies the best absorption*

✓ *Genetically modified organisms can be found in many nutritional supplements. Look on the label for the GMO Free certificate to avoid such dangers*

## 9.3    How you can Choose the Unchoosable

*"When you make a choice, you change the future"*
*~ Deepak Chopra*

*...and the quality of your choice determines the quality of your future.*

But, how do you make a quality decision about this? What makes a supplement good? How can you make a safe choice that will provide you with the right nutrition at no risk? How do you know that you can trust a certain brand?

Those are very good questions, since the market is overwhelmed by new products, and all of them promise the same benefits, but only a few really deliver.

It is important to buy the best there is, because your future and the future of your family depends on it. Even in today's economy, keep in mind that when you are thinking about your health, you always want the best. Don't fall into the trap and choose something cheaper but inferior.

Most people know that whatever you buy in the $1 store is not super high quality, yet some people still buy supplements there. It is a waste of money and probably a danger to your health.

You want the best there is for your health and your family's health, right?

It might be confusing when you first start researching products, but after you read the "rules", you will be able to pick the products that best suit your needs.

The most important aspects to look for in the products:

✓ *Ingredients: The best clean toxin-free ingredients from the best sources*

✓ *Combination: Ingredients that for a synergistic effect and amplify each other*

✓ *Delivery: Bio-availability to promote absorption and use and packaging that supports it*

Let's go over a few traps or warnings that are relatively easy to check so you can get an idea of the quality of any product. Go over the following warning items in sequence. This will allow you to check the label quickly and effectively.

For example you first need to be able to trust what is on the label (warning 5) before it makes sense to look at the ingredients. If it is sold very cheap (warning 1) it is probably not even worth looking any closer, they cannot provide high quality for a cheap price.

### 9.3.1   Stay SHARP about your choices

In order to remember how to select the best supplements that will actually help you restore or improve your vitality levels you can use the following system.

The system is called SHARP. You should stay SHARP when investing in your health. All items in the SHARP system will make the difference enabling you to distinguish between a mediocre nutritional product and exceptional product.

**Select
S.H.A.R.P.**

# Synergy

All the ingredients should work synergistically. Meaning they should enhance each other. Like curcumin for example, when combining that with bioperine it becomes about 200 times stronger, remember? These synergistically effects should be carefully designed within the actual product. If the product is not carefully designed the ingredients could counteract each other and you will have a useless product.

# Holistic

You need to supplement your entire system. It makes no sense to have a strong heart and weak lungs. So whenever selecting your products, make sure that all of your organs and systems will be supported. This is why claims like "just one a day", and "everything you need is inside" are just not true. Make sure you select a balanced set of supplements to support your whole body

# Activators

The actual ingredients need to be of the purest and highest quality available. There are many forms of fish oils, many forms of vitamin C etc. There are only a few forms that are really effective, the other forms are usually cheap fillers. This is important to know. Check the individual chapters for more in depth knowledge.

Part of the activation program is of course how the nutrients are being stored and delivered to your cells. Remember the tablet vs capsule discussion? Choose capsules.

# Reliable

How reliable is the company and product? Have they been sued in the past for fraudulent labeling, or did they create products that were harmful to people?

Always ask the company about their external certifications (OTC, FDA, NSF, GMP, GMO FREE). If they do not carry these certifications you have no guarantee that their products are safe. They will mention that they have tested it themselves in the best way possible. Yeah, right... Go and check the external certifications mentioned above.

### *P*romise

Does the packaging promise you a cure or an improvement? Maybe they guarantee results. This is not allowed by law, so if the company breaks this law, how many others did they break that you do not know of?

Stay: **S**ynergy **H**olistic **A**ctivators **R**eliable **P**romise

Unleash Your Vitality .com

Help for Health

A useful, quick memory device; stay SHARP about your supplement choices.

### Note:

When looking for the best supplement in stores, please consider that many big brands available in different 'health' stores are actually owned by big pharmaceutical companies, your health is not their primary concern.

### 9.3.2    Warning 1 – Cheap product

Price does reflect quality. Take a look at the store, what else are they selling? When you become aware of the value of nutritional supplementation you will start noticing this.

Some stores sell high priced supplements and some sell cheap supplements. Would you expect a high quality item to be sold in a 99 Cent store, where everything else is only 99 cents?

Even though price does not tell you everything, one thing is for sure. If the supplement is cheap then you are wasting your money on it. It is far better to use only one high quality supplement than 10 different cheap ones.

## Warning

✓ *It is sold in a' cheap' or ' affordable' store*

✓ *If it is sold 'cheap'*

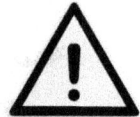

### 9.3.3    Warning 2 - Do they promise to cure you?

This is the first thing you should notice, and it is really easy to spot.

To change your health there are no quick fixes or guaranteed results. There is no such thing. You probably heard the saying "If it's too good to be true, it probably is". So, stay away from anything promising you a quick fix, cure or relief.

Nutrition is a long-term commitment, but it is one of those things that makes your life better, constantly. So, be patient and give the supplements time to work. Rome wasn't built in a day, and in the same way, you won't be able to improve your overall health status in just a few weeks, even though some people will note improvements within a few days.

Taking one multivitamin will not spontaneously cure you of everything. Not even taking one every day. You need a balanced combination of healthy diet and exceptional supplementation to unleash your vitality and maintain your maximized health.

## Warnings:

✓ *Promise a cure*

✓ *Guarantee results or relief*

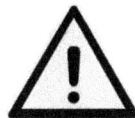

### 9.3.4    Warning 3 – Transparent or light Capsules or Bottles?

This might sound snobbish, but it isn't, in fact the way a supplement is packed can affect its efficiency.

How can that be possible? Well, let's see.

Just by looking at the type of packaging you can tell a bit about the care and quality that a manufacturer has put into their product. If the packaging is not optimal, you can bet that the products inside are not even close to optimal.

For example, Omega-3 fish oil needs to stay in a cool, dark place in order for it not to lose its properties. So, always look for a non-transparent container that contains dark capsules. When the capsules are of a dark color, they have been created specifically to protect the precious cargo inside, so you know that the manufacturer actually cares about what you are receiving.

If the capsules are clear or the bottle is clear it allows the fatty acids to oxidize when they encounter light, rendering them useless. This is a clear sign that the manufacturer does not care about your health.

## Warnings:

✓ *Transparent bottle used*

✓ *Transparent capsules used*

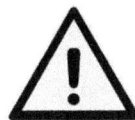

### 9.3.5  Warning 4 – Tablets instead of capsules?

You probably didn't think about the fact that you will also need to choose between capsules and tablets. In fact most people don't give this a second thought, and simply choose whatever seems more convenient at that time.

Let's see the differences between the two, so that you can choose based on evidence about what is best for your health.

#### Tablets

Tablets contain compressed nutrients, the downside is that in order to make the nutrients stick together, chemicals are added. This is some kind of glue, which is ingested along with the nutrients, and it isn't exactly healthy.

The way the nutrients are compressed is not natural either, and most of the time they are compressed with high pressure and heat. The heat can damage the nutrients, causing oxidation. So, you might be swallowing "dead" nutrients held together by… glue.

Moreover, the way tablets are tested for the dissolution properties, isn't similar to what actually happens inside your stomach. They are tested in acid and then pierced with a sharp object.

The truth is that stomach acidity is different for everyone, and piercing, surely doesn't happen inside the stomach. Even if they dissolve well in the test, that test does not mimic your stomach activity.

So with tablets you have 3 main problems:

- ✓ *You take in additional glues*
- ✓ *Absorption is much lower*
- ✓ *Ingredients are heat treated (reducing their effectiveness)*

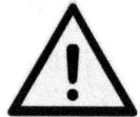

### Capsules

The best part about choosing a capsule over a tablet is the fact that you won't be swallowing any glue. Capsules don't need any binders to hold them together, and they are not thermally processed.

The other important aspect is the fact that the way they are tested for dissolvability really resembles what happens inside your body. They are tested in water, and the capsule is never pierced. So, you can be sure that the moment it enters your body, it starts providing you with nutrients. This ensures that you actually benefit from the nutrients you bought.

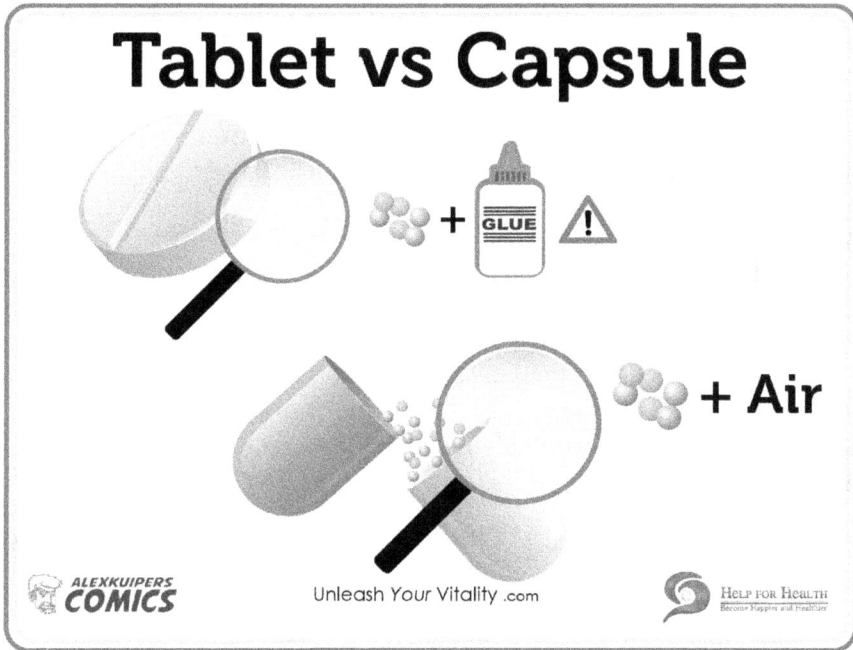

When comparing a tablet with a capsule and how much of the ingested supplement will be actually absorbed by your body, the capsule is far better. So, select a capsule over a tablet whenever you can.

Why are there any tablets on the market, since capsules are so efficient? The answer is simple. It is much cheaper to produce tablets than capsules.

## Warning:

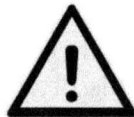

✓ *Tablets used instead of capsules*

### 9.3.6    Warning 5 – No trustworthy certifications?

Is the product you are looking at really certified by qualifying bodies? In the chapter about quality and certification you learned how important this is.

The certifications we discussed are given to the manufacturer to attest various levels of quality, and they give you important information about the product.

There are certificates dedicated to the quality and purity of the product, manufacturing process, and certifications for the ingredients used.

A lack of trustworthy certifications mean that you simply cannot know what is inside the product. The list of ingredients can be amazing, but you never know if it is really inside the product you bought: a waste of money.

## Warning

✓ *Missing OTC certification*

✓ *Missing USP certification*

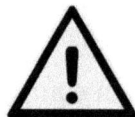

✓ *Missing NSF certification*

✓ *Missing GMP certification*

### 9.3.7   Warning 6 – Missing GMO Free indication

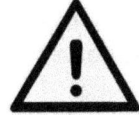

When a product is really GMO free it is mentioned on the packaging. If it is not mentioned, then you can almost be sure that it is genetically modified. That is something you do not want.

## Warning

✓ *Missing GMO Free indication*

### 9.3.8   Warning 7 – Missing 100% natural and toxin free indications?

Always choose supplements that are 100% natural and toxin free. Your body needs to absorb every precious ingredient without chemical additions or pollutants.

You probably agree that it is ridiculous to buy supplements made out of chemicals. Yet many buy purely chemical supplements and hope they work.

Your body absorbs and uses natural supplements in a much more effective way than it would anything else.

Besides natural, look for toxin free products, especially when you are looking for the right Omega-3 fish oils. Why? You may ask. Well, Omega-3 fish supplements are made from fish oil, which comes from…fish. Our oceans aren't by far, as clean as they should be. Think of the numerous oil spills, illegal chemical dumping that is happening. This reflects directly in the fish's health, and by extension in the Omega-3 supplement.

Omega-3 supplements are usually made from big fish, because they have more blubber. The problem is that the bigger the fish, the higher the accumulation of toxins. That is why some people prefer krill oil (very small fish). Whatever the source of the oil, the product needs to be cleaned from all toxins and this process is very expensive, so the more the manufacturer invests in cleaning the oil, the more expensive the supplement will be.

Whether you take your Omega-3 Fish oil from big or small (or even super tiny) fish is irrelevant, the most important part is the cleansing process. It is better to buy very pure fish oil from a large fish than partly contaminated from a small fish. Although it makes sense, many people do not look at it this way.

So, if you intend to choose a less expensive version, you can be sure that you are at risk of ingesting toxins like mercury and dioxin.

A very good way of making sure that you are getting a clean, healthy and most important, safe Omega-3 fish supplement is by checking to see if it is certified by the United States Pharmacopoeial Convention (more on this in the section on quality labels).

## Warning

✓ *Missing toxin free indication*

✓ *Missing 100% natural indication*

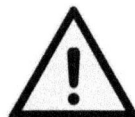

### 9.3.9    Warning 8 – Fillers or harmful substances used?

In order to mislead the consumer or to reduce the nutrients in the product, some manufacturers use fillers. These ingredients will be useless at best, but you are still paying for them.

Omega-3 is often combined with Omega-6 or Omega-9. Yes it is true you need all three, but that does not mean you need to supplement all 3. You already get an overdose of the other Omega in your normal diet. The value of supplementing is to restore the 3-6-9 balance. So only use Omega-3 fish oil.

If Omega-6 or 9 is used (and put on the label) you are sure that the manufacturer is trying to deceive you with useless and even slightly harmful ingredients.

In other cases harmful substances are used to make the product easier to swallow or more tasty. Look out for these ingredients.

You are taking the supplement to become healthier, not because they taste great, right?

## Warning

✓ *Titanium Dioxide used (filler)*

✓ *Magnesium Stearate used (filler)*

✓ *Omega-6 used (filler)*

✓ *Omega-9 used (filler)*

✓ *Artificial sweeteners used (harmful)*

✓ *Aspartame or maltodextrin used (harmful)*

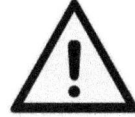

### 9.3.10 Warning 9 – Cheaper ingredients used?

Health is or should always be your number one priority. This is why you should never settle for less than you deserve. Supplements are your way of rebuilding your system, and making sure that you will stay healthy for a long time. This means that you should always choose the highest quality available.

This might mean that you will have to spend more on supplements, but look at it as an investment in your long-term health. Even if it doesn't look attractive now, it is definitely a better deal than investing thousands in the hope of regaining your lost health.

High quality nutritional supplements are your health insurance. It ensures your optimal health (instead of the health insurance that pays for the hospital bills, it does not insure your health at all)

If you choose a low quality supplement, you won't be able to notice the small improvements in your health that you read about.

There are many forms in which a particular nutrient can be found, you must make sure that you choose the one that is most efficiently absorbed by your body. This can sometimes be a daunting task.

You need to realize that this task will pay off, as there is a huge difference in how the body can absorb different forms of nutrients.

Take magnesium for example, you can buy it as "magnesium oxide" (for oxide, think of rusting iron). This only has an absorption rate of 4%. You can also buy the more expensive magnesium in the form of "magnesium taurinate" but this one has a much higher absorption rate, and is therefore much more effective.

Looking at Vitamin K and its two main forms K1 and K2 you will notice that K2 is much stronger and more potent than K1. So, when you choose your supplement, make sure that it will be one with the best forms of nutrients.

## Warning

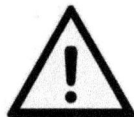

✓ *Calcium citrate used*

✓ *Calcium maleate used*

✓ *Magnesium-oxide used*

✓ *Vitamin K1 used*

✓ *Vitamin K used (missing the 'K2' specification)*

✓ *Vitamin D used (missing the 'D3' specification)*

✓ *Ubiquinone used (none = do not use)*

✓ *Coenzyme Q10 used (missing the Ubiquinol or Ubiquinone specification)*

✓ *Omega-3 used (missing the EPA/DHA specification)*

✓ *ALA used as Omega-3*

### 9.3.11 Warning 10 – Just about the right amounts

A one-a-day multivitamin is not going to be sufficient for vibrant vitality. You need a balanced combination to get the most out of it. Most vitamins and minerals work best in synergy with specific others.

As we previously discussed, the RDA levels are just defining the amount of a certain vitamin that you need to prevent a severe form of deficiency. This is why a balanced supplement needs to contain more than the Recommended Daily Dose. Such a supplement is aimed at enhancing the quality of life, and keeping free radicals at bay.

When the supplement contains about 100% of the RDA, you know that this is not enough, you need more.

## Warning
✓ *One a day is sufficient*

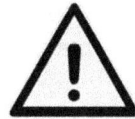

### 9.3.12 Warning 11 – Non effective combinations

Each part of your body is important, even the parts that we neglect. Each gene on the DNA has a purpose, even if we are not aware of it yet.

The same way, each nutrient has a function. Even if each vitamin and mineral can be targeted to treat a particular deficiency, or to improve a condition, you need to have the optimal combination to achieve perfect health.

Think of all the nutrients as being musicians that play in an orchestra. Every individual is uniquely talented and they play magnificently. The flute player is the best in the world, the violinist just won a prize for the best performance. The pianist is sought-after for his concerts all over the planet and so on.

But in order to make the orchestra work, they need to be working with each other, in perfect harmony. Only then the audience can enjoy the beautiful melody. If each of them played what they liked, it would sound like chaos and noise.

Nutrients act the same way, they need to be able to complete each other, and in the case of this spectacular orchestra, the leader is the manufacturer of the supplements.

Scientists of the U.S. National library of Medicine have discovered that the right combinations of vitamins reinforce each other and create enormous synergetic effects[391].

You can take as much calcium as you want, but without the proper amount of vitamin D, it will be useless. Taking the calcium without the proper levels of magnesium can even lead to a heart attack.

In the same way, you need vitamin C to process iron, and you need calcium to improve B12 absorption[392]. These are just a few examples. This is why you need to choose a high quality supplement that balances all the nutrients the right way.

Also keep in mind that Bioperine helps in the absorption of nutrients, so it's always a good idea to take your supplements with it, or to look for a supplement that already contains it.

## Warning:

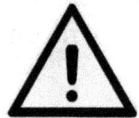

✓ *Missing Bioperine*

✓ *Calcium without magnesium*

✓ *Calcium-magnesium not 1:1*

### 9.3.13 Summary Checklist

When you are searching for a supplement brand look for the following warning signs listed in the table below. The more of the following items you can find on their packaging, the faster you should put it back and select a different brand.

When you can find even one product that does not qualify, then you can safely assume that other products from that company are not to your standards either. Go look for a different brand.

This list is not extensive but it gives some pointers what to look out for. Start from the top and work your way down the list. This is the fastest and easiest way to check the products.

# Warning Signs

**Cheap store warning**
- ☐ Sold in cheap store
- ☐ If it is sold 'cheap'

**Cure promise warning**
- ☐ Promise a cure
- ☐ Guarantee results or relieve

**Transparent packaging warning**
- ☐ Transparent bottle used
- ☐ Transparent capsules used

**Tablets warning**
- ☐ Tablets used

**No trustworthy certifications warning**
- ☐ Missing OTC certification
- ☐ Missing USP certification
- ☐ Missing NSF certification
- ☐ Missing GMP certification

**Missing GMO free warning**
- ☐ Missing GMO Free indication

**Missing toxic free and natural warning**
- ☐ Missing toxic free indication
- ☐ Missing 100% natural indication

**Just the right amounts warnings**
- ☐ One a day is sufficient

**Fillers or harmful substances warnings**
- ☐ Titanium Dioxide used (filler)
- ☐ Magnesium Stearate used (filler)
- ☐ Omega-6 used (filler)
- ☐ Omega-9 used (filler)
- ☐ Artificial sweeteners used (harmful)
- ☐ Aspartame or maltodextrin used (harmful)

**Cheaper Ingredients Warnings**
- ☐ Calcium citrate used
- ☐ Calcium maleate used
- ☐ Magnesium-oxide used
- ☐ Vitamin K1 used
- ☐ Vitamin K used (no 'K2' specification)
- ☐ Vitamin D used (no 'D3' specification)
- ☐ Ubiquinone used (none = do not use)
- ☐ Coenzyme Q10 used (no Ubiquinol or Ubiquinone specification)
- ☐ Omega-3 used (no EPA/DHA specification)
- ☐ ALA used as Omega-3

**Non effective combinations warnings**
- ☐ Missing Bioperine
- ☐ Calcium without magnesium
- ☐ Calcium-magnesium not 1:1

*Unleash Your Vitality* .com

HELP FOR HEALTH
Become Happier and Healthier

This checklist is also in the resource pack so you can print it and keep it in your wallet for when you go shopping.

# Select your products S.H.A.R.P.

# *Your Amazing Insights and Actions*

Date: __ / __ / _____

## What are your insights and learnings from this section?

Now we have come to the conclusion of this chapter. Write down your main insights about what you learned and about yourself.

## What are you going to do differently starting today?

Insights alone will not unleash your vitality. You need to take actions. What are the actions you are going to do in order to implement these insights in your life?

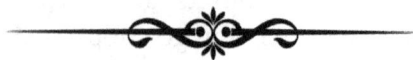

# Nutritional Plan
## Changing Your Nutritional plan is a Cinch!

### 10.1   What can you do?

Health is the first issue anyone should consider when thinking about the future. Without it, everything we do won't be as efficient or beautiful as it could be. Sadly, nutrients are no longer widely available. We can't just eat the right foods, and stay healthy, because nature has been compromised, and it can no longer sustain us the way it should. Besides that many people have a diet that is less than ideal for vibrant vitality.

> *"Healing in a matter of time,*
> *but it is sometimes also a matter of opportunity."*
> *~ Hippocrates*

So, what can you actually do to change the odds in your favor?

Thankfully, the power to influence this particular side of the future is found in your hands. You are the only one who can do something about it, and once you engage on this path, you will only benefit from the changes.

One of the most important aspects concerning nutrition is related to what you eat and the choices you make in food and supplementation. This means that you need to pay attention to your nutritional patterns. Stop indulging in junk food and other health-depriving foods, and start supplementing your nutrients with high quality vitamin and mineral supplements.

There are two main things you need to do to optimize your health:

1. *Eat the right foods*

2. *Use supplements*

## 10.2   Fabulous Food choices

Which are the rules that one must follow, nutrition wise, in order to stay healthy or become healthier?

Although this book is not a diet plan, or an authoritative book on what to eat and what not to eat, I will share some of the basics that you can implement immediately.

The first thing that you must do is to take advantage of what nature preserved for us. Therefore, use the superfoods that you can find to make a smoothie for yourself every morning. This will boost your energy levels right away and it will also keep your glucose levels steady.

> *"The more you eat, the less flavor;*
> *the less you eat, the more flavor."*
> ~*Chinese Proverb*

Super fruits have additional benefits, and you already know this. It might be difficult and time consuming to find all the fruits you need at your local grocery store. So, if you don't have the time, or the energy to go "fruit-hunting", you can find a pre-juiced version and use that one.

As long as you get a 100% natural and toxic free juice, and it comes from a trustworthy source, that has the certificates to prove its authenticity, you can be sure that you are making a great choice, and your body will thank you for it.

*Finish all the vegetables from the plate.*

Did your mother insist that you needed to finish the veggies if you wanted any dessert? Well, she had a point, and you might want to consider listening to her.

Vegetables are rich in chlorophyll and nutrients, well… richer than most other foods. They are also packed with fiber that improves your digestion.

This might not seem important, but having a healthy digestive system will improve your entire life. You will feel less tired, you will absorb important nutrients better, you won't feel bloated, you will sleep better, and even your mind will be clearer.

So, now that we've established the fact that mom was right, let's move on to the part of the program that is not so friendly, but equally important.

### Remove what is harming you.

Many of the foods we eat torture our bodies. Every individual is unique, and everyone should learn what doesn't work for them. This is the purpose of the chart, but there are a few items that stand out, and cause problems for the vast majority of people.

### Restrict sugar intake.

You already know that refined sugar is bad for you; we all know it and we all love it.

Sugar isn't just represented by the beautiful and tasty white crystals. Your body also transforms other foods into glucose. One of the other glucose sources is fructose, which is found in a wide variety of foods, such as beverages and processed foods.

You need to pay attention to what you eat, and make sure that you keep your fructose intake smaller than 25 grams a day.

There are countless diseases that affect people, and many of these are caused by simply eating too much sugar. When you expose your body to too much sugar, you can develop insulin and leptin resistance. Leptin is the hormone that suppresses the appetite. This means that your body will be forced to produce more of these hormones, in order to function properly. This, in turn will cause a general imbalance, which translates into you becoming sick.

Moreover, fructose is able to further affect your balance by increasing uric acid levels. This will influence blood pressure and kidney function.

The worst part is that if your uric acid levels keep increasing, you can develop a disease called Gout, which causes your joints to swell and horrible pain.

The way to stay healthy is to avoid sugar and fructose. This doesn't mean that you can't eat fruit. Fruit contains a balanced amount of fructose that won't harm you. Actually, if your diet was based on fruits and vegetables, you would be much healthier.

### *If sugar is bad, artificial sugar is worse.*

Nowadays, we have everything in the "sugar-free" version. If someone tells you something that sounds too good to be true, it probably is. Artificial sweeteners are chemicals that, not only interact with digestion, growth and metabolism, but they also are able to create mutations.

Aspartame, for example is one of the most controversial artificial sweeteners. It can cause headaches, dizziness and even cancer. So, be aware of these hidden dangers.

If you need to use a sweetener for your coffee, tea or lemonade, use Stevia, which is 100% natural and it has 0 calories.

### *Drink Water*

Water is one of the most vital elements in health. Without water you will not only dehydrate, nutrients will not be absorbed and transported to your cells and waste products cannot be eliminated. We need to drink about 2 liters of water each day to stay hydrated. If you are on a weight-loss program, you need even more water per day to detoxify.

Watch the color of your urine. When it is colorless or has a very light color, then you are properly hydrated. When it is dark (and smelly), then there is a high concentration of waste products. This means you need to drink more to excrete the waste products more gradual.

## *However, make sure the water is clean and purified.*

### *Keep it simple*

Yes we can easily create a 1,000 step program to increase your vitality. But seriously, would you follow all the steps? Maybe you would, however most people will not.

If you want to extend these steps, also look into the positives and negatives of different types of cooking (steaming, boiling, microwave, or not cooking at all). Look into what kind of oils/fats you use for preparing food. Or even how you eat (rushing or mindfully). There are many great books out there that give you more insights into these topics.

## Let's keep it simple for now.

When you start this nutrition plan, you will change many bad behaviors. You will eat less processed sugar, less fructose and fewer carbohydrates. Your body has adapted to your excesses by producing more insulin. When you stop eating bad foods, it will take a while until your insulin levels normalize. This means that you must make sure that you have a steady glucose level and you won't encounter hypoglycemia.

The way to do it is by eating smaller, healthier meals more often. Eat 4, 5 or 6 times a day, according to your needs. By doing this your insulin, leptin and cortisol levels will achieve balance.

## 10.3   Superior Supplements

Even though you will be eating a healthy and balanced diet, you still need to obtain all nutrients. Scientists have looked for a way to achieve this for decades. The good news is that they managed to come up with the best way to do this, in the form of nutritional supplements.

You might think that buying the raw superfoods gives you what you need, however there is no guarantee about the quality of those products, or that they are free of toxins either.

Science has developed ingenious methods to extract valuable nutrients from food sources and to turn them into supplements, keeping their properties unaltered, while not adding any nasty chemicals. This makes it much easier to benefit from all the properties of the superfoods.

Supplements are designed to give the body the right ingredients to create healthy cells and to have a strong immune system.

### Supplements as food or drugs?

People see supplements in one of two ways. They either view them as food or as drugs.

Supplements are not food, they are the part that food is missing! They are developed precisely to address individual needs on a cellular level.

**Supplements provide what food is missing**

Supplements are not drugs either, as we are led to believe. The right supplements should be considered as highly concentrated and balanced foods. You can view them as regular food if you like, but food that is not depleted. Good supplements contain a balanced combination of nutrients that address your needs directly.

### *Food is not enough*

In today's world, we cannot just depend on food alone. As you read in previous chapters there are many problems with soil depletion and food not containing the nutrients we need anymore.

We need to provide for our family, and ourselves. The only available option is to use supplements to correct our imbalances and provide our body with the essential ingredients needed for vibrant vitality.

### *We need supplementation*

Many health experts and scientists agree: vitamin supplementing plays a vital role in your overall health and wellbeing[393].

Much research has already been conducted on how supplements influence health in the long term. One of the first completed studies dates back to 1992. This research showed that subjects, who consumed extra vitamin C, lived an average of 5 years more than then those who didn't. The same study concluded that a vitamin C supplement dramatically helps in the reduction of the number of times that people contract colds[394,395]

The U.S. Food and Drug Administration (FDA) stated in a consumer report on their website that supplementing vitamins and minerals may help meet nutritional needs for:

✓ *elderly*

✓ *young children*

✓ *women who may become pregnant*

✓ *people with various illnesses*

✓ *people with a medical conditions*

✓ *people dealing with stress*

✓ *people who are taking certain medications*

So if you do not belong to this group, you must be someone from out of this earth I think. In other words, nearly everyone should be taking quality natural health supplements[396]

## 10.4   Your next question: "What do I need?"

Now that you understand the extent of the situation, the most difficult task begins. What to take, how much to take and most important which brands to trust?

That is the most daunting task, and really knowing that is a real science. This orthomolecular science focuses to correct the imbalances or nutritional deficiencies.

When considering supplementing your diet, it is important to combine the right elements in the right dosages. Taking just a single vitamin for a prolonged time might result in an imbalance of other important nutrients.

Taking nutritional supplements is a two-pronged approach. The first step is to start using a so-called base package and the second step is to fine-tune it based on your personal needs.

> **Step 1: Basic supplementation**

When establishing the details of your Personal Nutritional Plan make sure that the supplements that you chose are of an advanced quality, providing you with support for your: brain health, bone health, cardiovascular health, eye health, immune system health, while still packing an impressive quantity of antioxidants.

### 10.4.1   Foundation Nutrients

Your vitality plan needs to include a few supplements that every person on earth should take, and besides those basics include your specific needs.

Use a high-quality multivitamin, which will repair your deficiencies and restore your health. Even if you feel better in a couple of weeks, don't forget that you need to take a supplement for at least six months, in order to create a strong reserve.

Remember to get a supplement that sustains your bones, your immunity and also offers protection against cancer. For this look for a supplement that contains calcium, magnesium, vitamin K2 and especially vitamin D, since 90% of the population has some level of vitamin D3 deficiency.

### 10.4.2   Personal Needs

One thing that you can do to determine your deficiencies would be to test your blood for particular minerals and vitamins.

This is not as easy as it seems. Why? First of all, tests like these are truly expensive. Second of all, and more importantly, the body doesn't work like that.

Let's take calcium for example. Testing just the calcium level in your blood wouldn't cost you a fortune, but the test would be completely irrelevant. The human body is so beautifully engineered that if you have a calcium deficiency, it wouldn't show on the test. This is due to the fact that when the blood loses calcium, it extracts it from where it can to keep the levels balanced in the blood. Otherwise, you'd die in just a few minutes. Because if your calcium levels drop below a certain point, your heart would be so stressed that it would stop.

**Step 2: Specific supplementation for your needs**

The problem is that calcium is extracted from places it is also needed, like bones.

So, you see, taking tests wouldn't reflect reality, they would just show you that your body knows what it's doing.

To know where your deficiencies are, you can also go to an orthomolecular specialist and request a full body diagnosis, which includes blood, feces and urine samples and complete physical examination. That is a pretty complex procedure… and it even changes from one day to another. When you had a great party yesterday evening your urine samples will show differences. If you had Chinese 2 days ago, your feces will have different elements.

However, there is a more practical way to address your needs.

If you are prone to cardiovascular disease, or if you have a family history that raises such concerns, take a supplement rich in Coenzyme Q-10 and Omega-3 fatty acids. If you have issues with your weight, look for a natural and safe supplement to help you correct this issue.

If you are exposed to an excess of free radicals, like smokers are, find a supplement that offers a natural combination of powerful antioxidants.

Remember our action plan? We will use that exercise in the next chapter to find the proper supplementation for you. Maybe you need more vitamin D, maybe more Ubiquinol, or maybe something else.

### 10.4.3    I have X, What do I need?

Many people ask me what specific supplements they need for their current symptom. They have read the book or seen my presentation somewhere and they started to realize that certain symptoms can clear when the body receives the proper nutrients. Although that is a good question, because certain nutrients have very specific usages and benefits, it is actually the wrong question to ask.

Let me put it this way:

✓ *Would you rather be blind or deaf?*

✓ *Would you rather have no arms or no legs?*

✓ *Would you rather lose your right arm or your left arm?*

**I hope you answer these questions with…**
**NEITHER !! I want both !!**

✓ *I want to see and hear*

✓ *I want to have both arms AND both legs*

With supplementation, this is the real question to answer:

Do you want to get rid of that specific symptom only – or - Do you want to gain vibrant vitality?

Your answer will probably be that you want to gain vibrant vitality and not just solve one specific symptom. That is very important to realize when you continue your path towards ultimate health.

You do not want to have healthy lungs and a weak heart. You do not want to have strong bones and a malfunctioning liver. You do not want to have plenty of energy and failing kidneys.

Do you remember this example: "Your body needs all the nutrients to form healthy cells. When you want to build a house, but you are missing the roof tiles, your house will leak. Or if you want to build a car, but you are missing the wheels, the car won't move. You need all the pieces to have the right result. "

When increasing your health, all your vitamin and mineral levels should be optimized. It is a whole person approach to health and wellness. Instead of focusing on only one specific symptom we would rather help you towards true vitality in all aspects of your life.

The kind of supplementation you need is a very solid base package that covers all aspects of your body. This supplementation will give you all the basic nutrients for your body to maintain optimal functioning. When you are troubled with symptoms you could take another (or double doses) of specific supplements to give an extra boost to resolve those symptoms.

But first, make sure you have a solid base pack of supplementation suitable for you.

Our coach can help you with that. Just go to the consultation in the resource pack. Fill in the information and our coach will contact you. http://www.UnleashYourVitality.com/resource

## Make Use of Your Assigned Coach ! (it is free)

# *Your Amazing Insights and Actions*

Date: __ / __ / _____

## What are your insights and learnings from this section?

Now we have come to the conclusion of this chapter. Write down your main insights about what you learned and about yourself.

## What are you going to do differently starting today?

Insights alone will not unleash your vitality. You need to take actions. What are the actions you are going to do in order to implement these insights in your life?

**NOTES**

# Action Plan :

## 8 steps to Maximize your health and vitality

*Without action you cannot create change*

After all this bombardment of information, you might feel overwhelmed. Most diseases can be prevented when your body is well nourished. This book contains many useful notions for you to prevent or reverse disease, and you probably wrote down a few.

What should you do right now, to start improving your life immediately?

You are almost at the finish line of THIS part of your journey. You've learned a lot of information that many people are still unaware of. But knowledge alone is not enough; it is time to take some action.

So, what should you do right now to work towards vibrant vitality?

To begin with, take a moment to congratulate yourself for having the will to learn something that will improve your future.

There aren't many people in the world who are responsible enough, and mature enough, to make this choice.

# Ready... Set ... Go !

Unleash Your Vitality .com

Help for Health

Furthermore, appreciate the fact that you had the patience to sit down and read through this, instead of doing something that would have benefited you less. This is a huge accomplishment.

Now, you have all the knowledge you need to improve your health and to unleash your vitality levels. Now you know that by using good quality nutrients, in perfect balance, you can maximize your health.

We have developed a step by step process for you to help yourself towards vibrant vitality.

Before we can start you must have completed reading the entire book and performed all the exercises. Please go over this book again to double check that you filled in all the exercises. If not, do so now, otherwise you will miss part of the effects of the following steps.

Now that we've established the importance of vitamins and minerals, and we have looked at what you want and need. Now the next step is to actually start implementing that in your life.

## Let's start.

## 11.1  Step 1 – Your Extensive Health Check

Before we are going to take the journey together we need to know where you are. Without knowing where you are you will never see progression, right?

---

*"The doctor of the future will no longer treat the human frame with drugs,*
*but rather will cure and prevent disease with nutrition."*
*~ Thomas Edison*

---

We created a special online questionnaire that you can fill out to give you an overview of your health status right now.

This will be your benchmark, so you can check in the future how much you improved. Part of the personal benchmark is that you have a clear before and after image.

Whenever you take this health check, also take some photographs of yourself from the front and left and right side. Make sure the pictures have the dates stamped on them. We have seen some amazing results and it is such a pleasure seeing those before and after pictures.

You will notice it when you have reached the next level. Even though taking a picture now might not be an attractive proposition, after you reach the next level, you will wish you were be able to compare the results. So take that photograph with a date on it.

### *Tracking*

To make your changes visible it is good to track them over time. Our suggestion is to complete this extensive health check (including pictures) again in:

✓ *1 month*

✓ *3 months*

✓ *6 months*

✓ *12 months*

Doing it multiple times gives you a nice overview of your progression and helps your motivation to continue on the program.

### *Set Reminders*

To help you remember there is a special website that sends out reminders. Just go to http://www.futureme.org/, type in the reminder to yourself to fill in the extensive health check again. This website will automatically send you an email when that date comes. It is best to include the link to the health check, so you do not have to search for it in a few months from now.

This link is: http://www.UnleashYourVitality.com/healthcheck

Go online now and set the reminders so you will know when it is time to fill in the questionnaire again.

### *Fill in the questionnaire*

When you have set the reminder, do the questionnaire and fill in the score.

Go online to: http://www.UnleashYourVitality.com/healthcheck

And complete the questionnaire.

Copy your scores to the drawing below in this book. This way your book is your personal workbook and you can see easily how much you improved.

# *Exercise: 6 – Extensive Health Check*

Complete the questionnaire at:
http://www.UnleashYourVitality.com/healthcheck/

When it is done, you will get a score. Fill in the score in the diagram below.

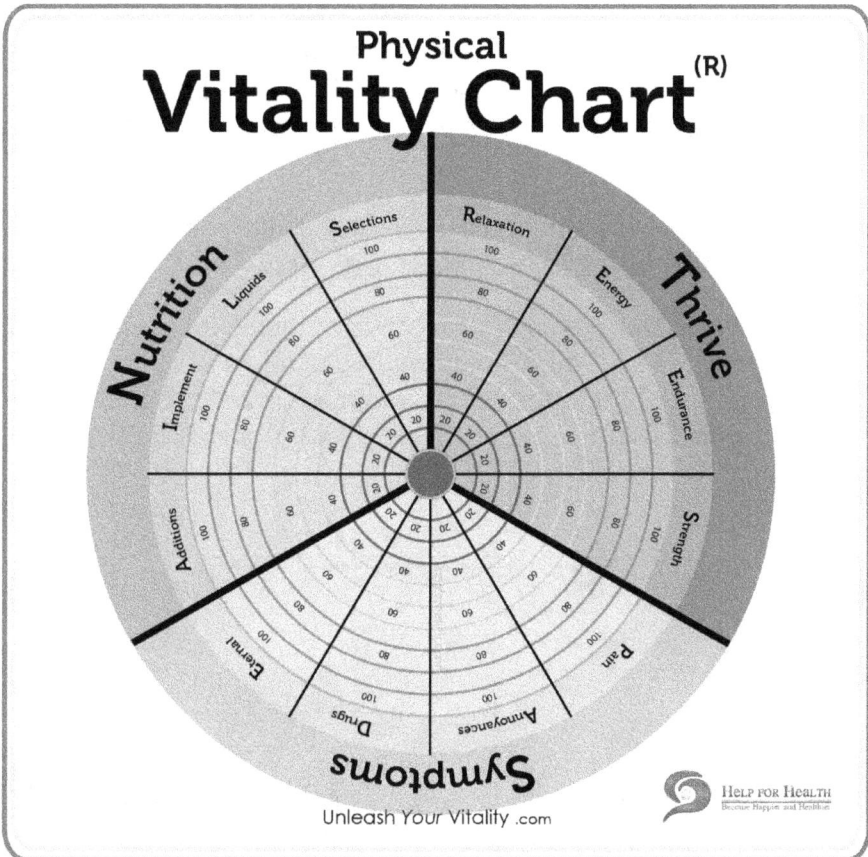

When you have filled in your score, you immediately see where you need to focus your attention on. This is where the wheel is off balance.

### *Strive to make everything a 100.*

Take some pictures of yourself, form the front and from both sides and write the date on them (or rename the picture file with the date in the filename). This is another great benchmark for future reference.

When taking subsequent tests, you can fill them in here on this same chart, just use a different color. Then you have a great overview of your progression: it becomes your wheel of progression.

Get the downloadable version of this chart from:
http://www.UnleashYourVitality.com/resource

This physical wellness wheel is part of our more extensive AMPERE model. The AMPERE model is composed of all areas of life with questionnaire and methods we use in our advanced programs to help people towards complete mental and physical health and wellbeing.

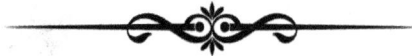

## 11.2 Step 2 – Managing Your Cravings

We all have cravings. We start craving particular foods before we are even born. Inside the wombs of our mothers, we send signals that we need a particular nutrient to develop properly. When we start craving, at first it can be a good thing, but later on in life, we change our behavior and we start wanting foods based on our education.

Now you need to know the fact that cravings have two main causes. One is the purely physical craving and the other is mental-emotional craving.

### *Physical craving*

There is biological craving instinct that kicks in when you are deficient in a certain nutrient. When hormone levels change, people also get suddenly a desire for certain foods. Some people even get cravings for inedible objects, purely on the basis of a nutritional deficiency. The body finds an extreme way to try to reduce that lack of nutrition a little by eating those inedible objects.

The physical element of the craving is dealt with in the nutritional plan. Once you begin that program, your body will come into balance. Your body will then start to emit signals, which translate into good cravings. This will happen because you are "rebooting" your system, and it will become effective again.

So, make sure to pay attention to what your body really needs, and what it is telling you. When you start your Personal Nutritional Plan, you will notice that the frequency and intensity of your cravings will go down.

### *Emotional craving*

Besides the physical aspects of cravings, there are emotional aspects. When people are sad, confused or stressed, some do feel the need to eat something sweet or foods that contain grains. This happens because these foods help the serotonin levels go up, therefore making them feel better.

The trick is to learn to solve problems at the point of origin. So, whenever you have a problem that is more likely to be related to the psychological state, deal with it then and there. This works far better than the temporary 'cure' of eating comforting foods.

What you need to learn is when you have an actual need for a nutrient, instead of an emotional craving.

Although having a better nutrient status will also reduce these emotional cravings, some emotional aspects need to be covered. There are many ways to manage these emotional aspects. But especially for you we created a method for you to start working to reduce your cravings. It also includes a nice poster that you can stick on your fridge to help you remind of your most important goals.

This method is included in the add-on pack at: http://www.unleashyourvitality.com/addon/

### 11.2.1   Step A – Craving List
For this purpose, you can use the exercise below.

Write down any cravings you have. This could be anything… chocolate, chips, fried goods, candy etc. Be as specific as you can.

Take a note every time you crave something, and when that craving goes away or reduces. Especially if it goes away after you feel different or eat something different. If a craving disappears or reduces in a short amount of time after taking a supplement or after having a healthy meal, you will be able to relate it to a particular deficiency.

This will also help you differentiate "physical cravings" from "emotional cravings". In time, you will see a pattern emerging, so you will know yourself better, and you will make better choices.

# *Exercise: 7 – Craving Scale*

Date: __ / __ / _____

Fill in your cravings and how severe they are for you (0-5). So if you have a very heavy craving for chocolate every day, then this might be a 5. If you only have a craving for chips once every 3 months, this might be a 2.

## My main craving for ............... is at a level ...

## This craving starts when:

## It reduces to a level ...... or goes away when:

## My other craving for ............... is at a level ...

## This craving starts when:

## It reduces to a level ..... or goes away when:

11.2.2   Step B – Craving Solution

Now work through the craving solution from the resource pack. Follow the steps exactly and do the exercise as soon as you notice a slight hint of that craving and you will notice the craving reducing or even disappearing.

## 11.3   Step 3 – Your Nutritional Foundation

Respecting a nutrition plan is the second step you must take towards creating the perfect environment in which your body will prosper. Day to day life can be complicated, and you might find it easier to eat whatever you have around.

Keep in mind, however, the fact that most things are only as complicated as you allow them to be, your health, should always be the number one priority.

### *Get in line, stay in line*

The next obvious step is to look for the supplements you need.

You should know that Rome wasn't built in a day, so you will have to give the supplements at least six months to reinforce your body. Even if you feel more energetic in a couple of weeks, you need to give your body time to rebuild reserves and to heal cells and tissues.

> **Get in line...**
> **Stay in line...**

Buy the supplements and use them for at least 6 months. Just getting one package is just not going to give you the results that you are looking for. Either buy them for 6 months, or even better, have them sent to your home every month. Then you do not have to remember it and the vitality program will become easier for you to complete.

A diary might help. Writing down your improvements in a diary or journal has helped many people. Do this every day, even if there is nothing notable to report, then just write that. This will keep you in the loop of writing and what you have learned and how it influences your life.

Keep yourself motivated and write every day. Remember that your main goal is to live a fully vibrant live rather than barely survive.

Choosing the right supplements might seem difficult and confusing, but with all the knowledge you gained from this book, you are certainly able to make good choices. Nevertheless, there is an ocean of supplement manufacturers out there and you have specific needs. Before you buy any supplement, re-read the chapter "Because You're Worth It - How to select the best of the best" to be aware of what to look out for and what pitfalls to avoid.

Find a product range that is well-balanced and high quality so you can even supplement deficiencies that you are unaware of; because as you might remember, not all deficiencies show up immediately, while they will lead to symptoms. Prevention is better than curing.

As a bare minimum start taking the following:

☐ Multivitamin
☐ Calcium & Magnesium
☐ Omega3 Fish Oil
☐ D3

## 11.4   Step 4 – Your Nutritional Personal Needs

Let's take a look at your "Your Action Plan Workbook" (chapter 12) to give you some ideas of your specific personal needs.

Ok, you've read the book, you've done the exercises, but you still don't know what your exact needs are. You know that you need something to boost your energy levels and to ensure your long-term health, but you can't exactly pinpoint your deficiencies.

When you have that exercise in front of you, go online to the consultation page, complete the survey online and we will contact you with a Personal Nutritional Plan.

Go online now and go to the consultation page. Use your personal access code that you can find on the back of this book to access it. After you have filled in the questions, your coach will contact you to help you further. Find it at: http://www.UnleashYourVitality. com/consult/

*Be proactive. Don't wait until your body is worn out.*

## 11.5 Step 5 – Getting Support

This vitality program is an intense process and changing your lifestyle can be hard sometimes. Therefore, it is good that you have help, someone who can support you. Look out for a friend who is willing to keep you accountable, a colleague who is working with you through these steps, or even a professional that can guide you.

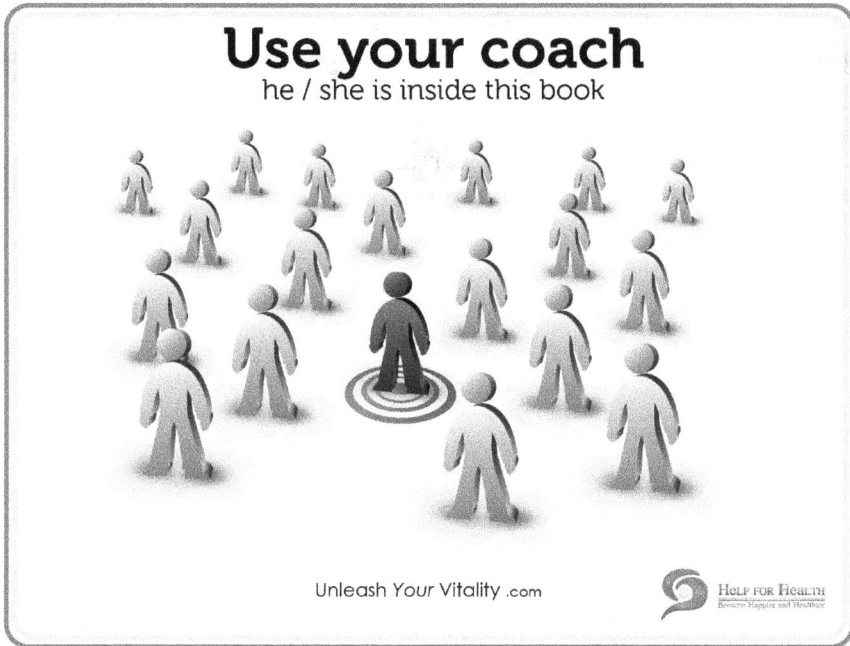

# Use your coach
he / she is inside this book

Unleash *Your* Vitality .com

HELP FOR HEALTH

When you have requested your free consultation (see step 3) then you also have a coach that can help you further. If you have not done so, go to step 3 and do this now, request your free consultation and use your coach. This allows us to help you reach your vitality goals.

If you want even more guidance, look at the special program "Seeking you for The Vitality Challenge". This complete mind-body program will guide you to vibrant vitality.

## 11.6   Step 6 – Your Cell Based Detox

*"By cleansing your body on a regular basis and eliminating as many toxins as possible from your environment, your body can begin to heal itself, prevent disease, and become stronger and more resilient than you ever dreamed possible!"*
*~ Dr. Edward Group III*

When changing your diet and starting to take supplements, it is important that you detox your cells from the amount of toxins they have built up during the last years. There are several detoxing programs available, but one of the really important ones is to detox your fat cells with a combination of pharmaceutical grade optimized zeolite and chlorella. Your fat cells have accumulated a lot of toxins over the years. Now it is time to clean them.

This fat cell detox is especially important when you are working on weight-loss, otherwise the lost weight will be gained back faster than you lost it. These toxins are one of the main causes of a rebound or yoyo effect.

Start with a cellular based fat detoxing program to remove those toxins from your cells.

### Detoxifying your body

This big step forward shouldn't be as difficult as the media presents it. Detoxifying your body shouldn't be about extreme diets and drinking gallons of water. It should be simple and efficient, after all science has developed enough to give us simple solutions.

If you decide to detox your body from all the toxins accumulated, you should:

✓ *Watch your diet. Eat healthy foods as much as you can. Actually, the more you eat the better, as long as you respect the physical nutrition plan (Step 3 – Your Physical Nutrition Plan). Because eating more means accelerating your metabolism.*

✓ *Look for a supplement especially designed restore your body. This is the scientific approach. Instead of eating too little, over-exercising, and drinking gallons of tea, take a supplement that contains pharmaceutical grade optimized zeolite, chlorella, spirulina and activated charcoal2. These elements work great together to attract toxins like a sponge.*

✓ *Drink as much water as you want, but don't overdo it. You just need to drink clean purified water. Watch out from the hidden toxins inside plastic water bottles and for the contaminants inside tap water.*

Detoxification brings many more benefits. It is essential in losing weight; any weight-loss program without a clear emphasis on detoxing is doomed to fail.

It not only makes you look younger, but more importantly, it helps you replace the toxins in your body with nutrients you need.

---

2       Due to the space available in this book, chlorella and some other ingredients are not discussed. Read up on the valuable properties online

## 11.7 Step 7 – Celebrating, Sharing, Feeling Victorious

What else should you do? … Celebrate!

Talk to your friends and loved ones about what you've learned. Most people don't have the patience that you have. They probably will never learn about a better way to live.

Share what you've learned and help others. Personally, I have

**Share and Celebrate you results**

noticed that the more I share my results and experience with my friends, the more I learn from it. Besides that, it really helps them to move towards vibrant vitality. This way you will still have healthy old friends to talk to in your 80's.

Every week, look over your diary and highlight your results and improvements.

Share your results with the world and… share your results with us … We are looking forward hearing how you implemented these steps and the amazing results you booked. Share your results on: http://www.UnleashYourVitality.com/results

### *Special gift*

We love to hear your results and share them with the world to make it a healthier place. Take an after picture with the cover (or printout) of this book. Send the after and before picture to us with your main insights. We will reward you with an exclusive special, $ 250 value, gift for you: a free personal session to help you to the next level of your vibrant vitality just as our way of saying thank you for spreading the word and to make the world a happier and healthier place.

## 11.8 Step 8 – Your Next Level

When you reach this step, you have already made some amazing steps and maybe you have already achieved some wonderful results.

Ultimate vitality is not a do-it-once process. You need to keep working on it. Now it is time to move to the next level of vibrant vitality. This is a constant and never ending personal improvement plan.

Or if you want to see it as a philosophy, adopt the one of CANI meaning Constant And Never-ending Improvement. It is a way of living for continuous openness, learning, improvement and growth.

Are you ready to reach even higher levels?

RE-READ this book from the very first page. No, this is not a joke. Every time you read this book you will find new insights and form new actions. This book was not written for you to absorb it all in one go. The best results are when you read it over and over again and repeat the exercises. Then you will master the material and further develop your vibrant vitality.

Also make sure you read the introduction again, that chapter explains how to get the most out of this book.

✓ *Makes notes*

✓ *Do all the exercises again*

✓ *Make notes*

✓ *Mark your symptoms*

Also when you do the exercises, use the downloaded versions for the 2nd time and store them in a place with the date that you did it. It makes a nice reference for later.

And continue with your 8 steps maximize your health and vitality.

## 11.9 Conclusion

Everything we do, everything we touch, everything we eat, and everything we dream, influences everything else. The fact that humankind has evolved so much is a miracle of nature. There were millions of forces, invisible or not, that created the opportunity which brought us into existence.

Millions of years of evolution have shaped the face of the entire planet. Continents formed, mountains rose, life emerged from a single cell, and today we are the ones who influence life.

Every step we take can change the course of future evolution. Even if you don't see your life as being important, it is. Einstein didn't know who he would become, neither did any of the great personalities who changed science.

Being healthy is not just about living a long and accomplished life, it is about the future. If we want to maintain our position in the food chain, we need to understand that everything is evolving along with us. If we leave any gaps, and allow dangerous life forms to grow inside of us, we could represent the reason for the next great extinction.

> **Proper supplementation provides many health benefits. Are you ready ?**

Nutrition has been extensively researched, but some of the most important information was overlooked. We can no longer depend on food alone for our survival. We need to feed ourselves the right way, before it becomes too late.

What about you? How did you score on the health check? Did you look into your inner mirror?

What have you discovered? Is your life and health as good as it you could be, or are you looking for ways to improve your life and health?

Do you still think that all you need to survive is food, or are you looking for something more?

If you already realized that your body needs a hand, start doing something about it now. Don't fall in the trap of the perpetual tomorrow. Everyone likes to start changing "this Monday", or on the 1st of the month, or on New Year's Eve. The truth is that there is nothing wrong with "today", we just like to postpone important choices, hoping that we'll somehow discover that we don't have to change anything.

Successful people don't wait, they grab every piece of information and they use it to their advantage as fast as possible, because every wasted moment is a chance for failure.

Remember the traffic light metaphor? Will you start driving only when all the lights are green, or will you take action now and get closer to your desires?

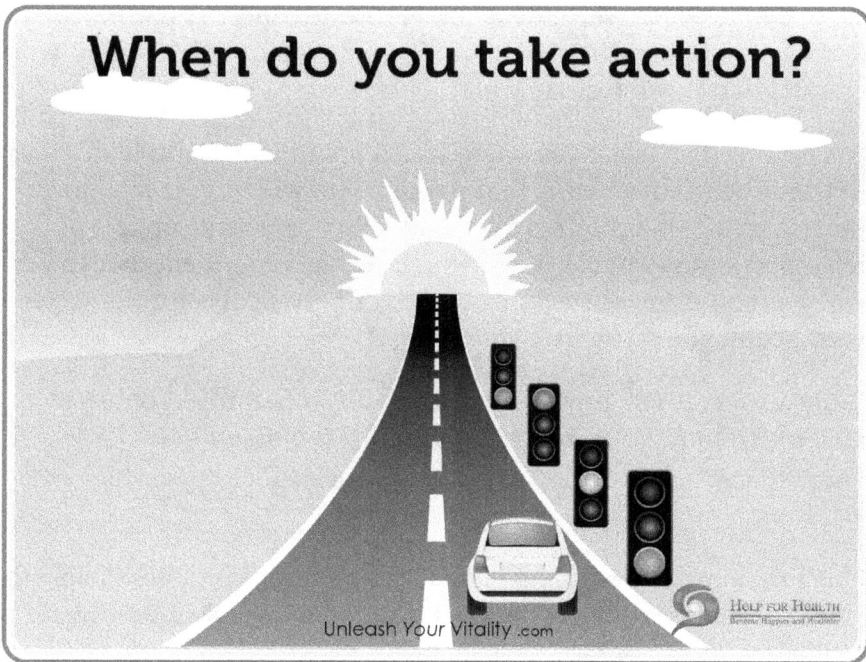

# The choice is yours!

What kind of person do you want to be, and how do you want your health to change?

In a year from now, where will you be, and how will you feel?

Time passes anyway, so why not make it pass with purpose?

Do you have any questions about what you've learned, or do you want to share your newly found knowledge with others? If so, go online and communicate with other people about these important issues.

Even if you are not exactly a sociable person, consider the fact that the more people realize this issue, the more everybody wins.

Maybe, if people started supplementing their diets properly, in a few decades from now, we could eradicate cancer and other terrible conditions. This might not benefit you now, but surely, your grandchildren will feel safer.

Are you ready to start your new life? A life in which you won't have to worry about disease? A life in which you will be able to enjoy the health of your children? A life in which you wake up feeling refreshed and strong? A life in which you feel confident that you will overcome any obstacles because your physical condition and your health allow you to?

If the answer is yes, now is the time to do something about it, to take control over your body and expand its limits.

### Sharing is caring.
Our mission is to "Heal the Planet by Empowering Other People to Heal Themselves". When everyone works on their own health and wellbeing for life, we will be happy.

We aim to touch the hearts of 10 million people inspiring, motivating and encouraging them in a way that means they take action knowing they can do a great deal to improve their personal health. For this we need your help, we cannot do this alone.

Please write your recommendation and publish it on Amazon and other places where people find this book. Your recommendation will help other people to understand the value of this book. Your personal insights will help others to implement this material in their life. We would love to receive and publish your testimonial on our website to, please send it to us.

We hope you consider this mission as important as we do and extend our love and gratitude to you for your support and involvement in this project.

Share your valuable insights and results with the world. With your inspiration and insights other people might take action to improve their vitality.

Teach others this valuable information and you will notice you gain deeper understanding while doing so. At the same time you empower them to improve their lives. Tell people about the book you are reading, and about what it has done for you. They will be grateful for it.

Write down your improvements and share these too. If you didn't catch a cold, even though you were surrounded by sick people, mark it on your chart. It is important to know your successes and failures, because you will learn from them. It doesn't seem likely now, but in a year from now, you will be able to understand how your body responds to certain issues and what effects it will bring.

# Share your results on:

http://www.UnleashYourVitality.com/results

**NOTES**

# Your Action Plan Workbook

## *Exercise: 8 – Action Plan Workbook*

> *"Each patient carries his own doctor inside him."*
> *~ Norman Cousins*

Let's take a look at your current health status.

Start right now. Write down, in this table, the issues that bother you about your health, the period of time in which you intend to resolve them and the steps you are going to take in order to get there. You can fill in the problem you have starting now, and as you read further, you will be able to write down the solutions.

## STEP 1 – Fill in your symptoms

Write your symptoms in the first column. Think of small symptoms, but also include diseases or illnesses. Think of recurring cold, low energy, lack of sleep, and more severe symptoms like diseases and chronic issues.

The more you can write down, the better we will be able to complete the action plan together.

Also fill in the column called SUD (Subjective Unit of Distress). Fill in a number from 0-10. Whereby 0 is that symptom is not really a problem, and 10 is a very severe, maybe life threatening, symptom. The most pressing and serious symptoms have the highest numbers.

So go ahead and fill in all your symptoms, and continue filling them in while you read the rest of the book.

## STEP 2 – Fill in the associated vitamins and minerals

While reading the chapter on vitamins, complete the column with your symptom and the vitamins/minerals associated to it. We are going to use this information later on to create your Personal Nutritional Plan.

Fill in the nutrients while reading the book. If you missed this, then go over the book and find the symptoms and the related nutrients.

| Symptom | SUD | Nutrients |
|---------|-----|-----------|
|         |     |           |
|         |     |           |
|         |     |           |
|         |     |           |
|         |     |           |
|         |     |           |
|         |     |           |
|         |     |           |
|         |     |           |
|         |     |           |
|         |     |           |
|         |     |           |

## STEP 3 – Fill in the superfoods needed

While reading the chapter or superfoods and their benefits, write down the most important benefits for you and the superfood associated with it.

In the Need column, indicate how much you need that benefit on a scale from 0-10. Whereby 10 is the most important benefit in your life, and 0 is not important at all.

| Benefits | Need | Superfood |
|---|---|---|
|  |  |  |
|  |  |  |
|  |  |  |
|  |  |  |
|  |  |  |
|  |  |  |
|  |  |  |
|  |  |  |
|  |  |  |

| Benefits | Need | Superfood |
|----------|------|-----------|
|          |      |           |
|          |      |           |
|          |      |           |
|          |      |           |
|          |      |           |

You will probably need more room than is available in this book. In this case, just download the resource package for this book. It includes a larger form to create your action plan.

This resource pack can be downloaded for free at:
http://www.UnleashYourVitality.com/resource/

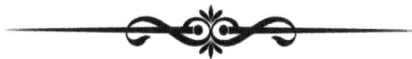

## 12.1 Your VIP Personalized One-One Consultation

Let us help you, contact our office for a more personalized approach and assistance. We can assist you towards more vitality and making the right choises. Just contact our office to make an appointment with one of our certified coaches.

### Contact your coach for free !

**NOTES**

# Appendix

## 13.1 Seeking You for The Vitality Challenge

After reading this book you might want to join our 6 months exclusive mind-body program where we help people unleash their full vitality and maximizing their health.

It is a 6 months program, exclusively for readers of this book, which includes a full mind-body approach to your vitality. When you complete the program we can guarantee you will feel much healthier, have more energy and more fun in life.

Many people have trouble finding the right supplementation for their current diet. We will give you access to our selection of the best products out there, and include all products you need to gain optimal results for this program.

Every month you will have a coaching call with your mentor. This mentor will assist you in overcoming mental blockages or emotional issues around eating and vitality.

Every 2 weeks you receive a new physical 4 min exercise to keep your body in shape. This unique system of a 4 min exercises is easy to follow for all age groups, fitness and exercise experience. Everybody can join in and experience the fitness increase this program will give you.

This program is only for really committed people. If you just want to work a bit towards health, follow all guidance and steps in this book.

However if you want us to help you and really need to make a change in your life, then apply for this program. Contact us, mention "The 6 Months Vitality Challenge" and explain why you think you need this program. Then we will schedule a skype interview with you to explain all the details.

Four times a year we draw a winner of the challenge, a person who changed their health most profound and he or she will get an amazing gift.

## 13.2 Discounts and Special gifts

This book is also an AMAZING gift. Imagine you are invited to a friend's place and you want to bring a gift. What are your taking with you, flowers, chocolate, incense, or even candles? All beautiful gifts but they won't leave the impression of a lifetime. Flowers are easily forgotten, chocolate is easily forgotten. Just for fun, ask yourself what are the gifts you received last time you had a party? Do you remember them?

Here I present you the opportunity to give a life transforming gift, something that actually improves your friend's life. Do you they think they will remember that? I bet you! Your friend will remember that for a lifetime.

About 8 years ago I gave a friend of mine a book. He is still talking about what an amazing life transforming gift that was. Giving this book as a gift is much more than a stack of paper (or bits and bytes). It is an opportunity to increase health and vitality.

We have very a very special opportunity for you to get multiple books for an amazing price. I cannot disclose the price here now, just go to: http://www.UnleashYourVitality.com/gift/

You will find some amazing deals there so that you can present your friends with a life transforming gift, and at the same time spend less money than you would on flowers or chocolate. You will leave an amazing impression.

### 13.2.1   Your GP

Many medical doctors do not know enough about nutrition to give any real solid advice on it.  You might want to give your general practitioner a copy of this book.

He or she will probably first look at the references (if not, point it out to them) and be astounded by the amount of research, next, he or she will probably look at the testimonials and see that other medical doctors endorse this book. Then your doctor will read it, and be thankful for your gift.

You can also give a copy to your local physiotherapist, health practitioner or even to a coach. Share the book with your work colleagues. If you belong to a religious community, sports club, or any other organized group you could even share the book with your peers and and help them to unleash their vitality!

We have special deals for obtaining multiple copies, just check out http://www.UnleashYourVitality.com/gift/

### 13.2.2   Organizations

We have a special offer for corporations, universities, professional organizations, medical facilities, not-for-profit organizations, clubs and other networks of people.

When you want to use this book for increasing the vitality of your organization or network, we have special bulk quantity discounts available. Special books or book excerpts can also be created to fit specific needs. Just contact our office.

## 13.3  Spreading the Word - How to help

We would like to ask you to help us spreading the word. There are many small things you can do to help to make the world a happier and healthier place.

Just to name a few:

* **Tell your friends about this book (or give it as a gift)**
* **Write a review and post it on amazon (even if it is only a line or two**
* **Share your insights and results with people**
* **Write a short (or long) article on your blog or newsletter**
* **Post your insights, actions and progress on social media**
* **Send out an email to your mailing list**

## 13.4  Spreading the Word - Speaking and training

There are speaking and advanced training opportunities available to develop a deeper understanding of this material.

Rob van Overbruggen delivers worldwide different types of keynotes and trainings

His style of presentation is highly dynamic, interactive and fun. It increases the energy of the room and complements the list of presenters, and can be viewed as infotainment; high value content presented in an entertaining way.

If you are interested in booking Dr van Overbruggen for your conference or event, please contact our office.

## 13.5  More in-depth learning

When you want to go even deeper and learn more ways to Unleash your Vitality you can sign up for our:

* **Webinars**
* **Workshops**
* **Home study programs**
* **Advanced one-one coaching**

Check http://www.unleashyourvitality.com for details

## 13.6   Join us ! - Business opportunities

There are business opportunities available if you want to work with us:

✓ *If you are a coach you can join our worldwide network of coaches*

✓ *If you are a trainer you can join our worldwide network of trainers to spread this knowledge*

✓ *If you are representing a corporation or network of people, we can help to increase the vitality of your people*

✓ *Or make your own suggestion how we can work together.*

Many more opportunities for cooperation are available. Just contact us and we will start brainstorming together.

## 13.7   Exclusive Community

We created an exclusive community for you that is free to join. This is where you meet like-minded people, can share your experiences and learn from other people experiences.

**Join now…**

Go to http://www.unleashyourvitality.com/community

## 13.8   Connect with us

If you want to contact us for any reason, just send us an email at: office@helpforhealth.com and we will get back to you.

*Lets Connect on social media too*
\* http://gnoo.net/linkedin_rob
\* facebook.com/helpforhealth

**NOTES**

# Resource Pack

There is a specifically designed resource package for this book. This can be downloaded for free at:
http://www.UnleashYourVitality.com/resource/

During the writing of this book I created many additional documents that just did not make it into the final edit. However, they do cover some very important issues. I decided to include them too in the resource pack.

## Included in this resource pack:

### Health Check

This extensive questionnaire gives you additional insights in how your health is right now. After answering the questions you will receive a beautiful graph that indicates your current health and the areas to improve.

Access this free health check at:
http://www.UnleashYourVitality.com/healthcheck

### *Personal Real Life Coach*

We have a coach for you that helps you obtain the best results. In order for this coach to contact you and provide you with the best advice, you first need to fill in a questionnaire with your goals and what is important to you. Based on this, the coach will contact you on email and/or Skype to help you attain those goals.

Go to: http://www.UnleashYourVitality.com/consult/

Fill in the questions and your information and the coach will contact you.

# Certificate

## Vitality Coaching

The bearer of this certificate is entitled to a vitality coaching session by one of the approved Vitality Coaches

# Price $175

Unleash Your Vitality .com

### *Exercises*

Take them as many times as you want, store them for your reference and to review your progression. By being able to track your progression, you will notice the effects more effectively.

### Checklists

There are many additional checklists available to help you maximize your health in easy ways. New checklists will be added when we develop new materials. These checklists are not for sale, only available as an extra resource to this book.

### Drug Depletion Whitepaper

A full whitepaper of the major pharmaceutical drugs and their influence on vitamin and mineral levels. This will give you additional insights in what extra nutrients to take in if you are on certain medications. This whitepaper will also give you some valuable insights in why certain pharmaceutical drugs have certain side effects and what to do about it.

### Weight-Loss Whitepaper

One bonus chapter is specifically about weight-loss. In this chapter you will learn how to use the information you learned in this book to reduce your weight and keep your ideal weight forever. The clinically proven system described in this chapter is simple yet very effective and supported by many physicians.

You will learn:

- ✓ *Why and how much water you should drink to optimize weight-loss*
- ✓ *How to break through the plateau and reach your desired weight*
- ✓ *Keep the weight off permanently, no more yoyo effect*
- ✓ *How and what sleep does to your weight-loss program*
- ✓ *When to eat and when not to eat*
- ✓ *Food plan for optimal food choices*
- ✓ *Etc.*

### Bone Health Whitepaper

In the bonus chapter on bone health you will learn more about how to obtain the strongest bones and how to maintain them. Calcium is only one part of the equation, there is more to it to build strong and stable bones.

### Reference Illness-Deficiency

This reference list will help you further in your search toward resolution of certain symptoms. Even though you need a solid base pack of nutrients (See: Your next question will be: "What do I need?) you might want to take some additional supplements to aid your body in coping with some specific symptoms.

### Glycemic Index Whitepaper

This document describes many food sources and their glycemic index to give you insights on the effect of their sugar content on your health. You will find some interesting items in here that you would not have thought would have so much negative impact on your health.

### Supplement Selection Checklist

A printable list that you can put in your wallet and take with you to prevent buying poor quality.

### Frige poster

It also includes a nice poster that you can stick on your fridge to help you remind of your most important goals.

# Additional Add-on Pack

### Goal Visualization Audio Program

A specially designed and created audio program to help you focus on your true goals. This program is designed with the help of neuroscientists and cutting edge research into brain waves and neuroformulations.

This program uses neuroripple technology and was designed by http://neuroripple.com/ exclusively for Unleash your Vitality

### Cravings Reduction Method

We created a special method for you to start working to reduce your cravings. This also includes an exclusive audio program to rewire your brain in thinking and eathing healthy. One of the main problems in cravings is emotional craving. In this audio program your brain will be programmed to release those emotions so you can stop when you have enough nutrition.

This program uses neuroripple technology and was designed by http://neuroripple.com/ exclusively for Unleash your Vitality

### Images

The images that are used in this book are provided to you so you can download in full size and full color for your enjoyment. You can even post them online to grab people's attention or to educate people.

Feel free to share these images, but please include a link to: http://www.UnleashYourVitality.com next to your image. Then people know where to get more information.

# Recommended Reading

*"Healing Psyche"*

"Healing Psyche – Successful Psychological Cancer Treatment" by Rob van Overbruggen Ph.D.

This book describes the scientific principles of how the mind influences the cancer process. Learn what and how to implement these strategies in your life or assist your clients.

It has helped thousands of people cope with their personal journey or the journey of their loved ones.

---

*"Healing Psyche is a treasure trove of rigorous research on the mind-body connection for cancer – all presented in practical ways that both doctors and their patients can access and implement easily.*
*This book can save your life"*

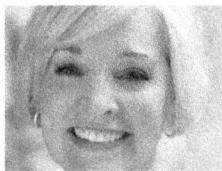

*~ Christiane Northrup MD*

---

*"HEALING PSYCHE is one of the most complete guides to the role of the mind in cancer to appear in years. This practical and authoritative book is a major accomplishment."*
~ **Larry Dossey MD**

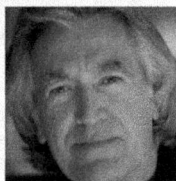

*"Rob van Overbruggen brings us the best review and discussion of theories and research in mind-body influences and interactions with cancer.*
*This book is written clearly, well organized, rich in quotations from the numerous authors cited, replete with case examples, and an excellent resource for anyone interested wholistic healing of cancer."*
~ **Daniel J. Benor MD**

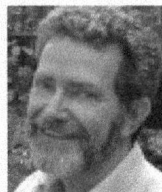

*"I recommend it highly and we will be recommending the book in our next newsletter*

~ **Carl Simonton MD**
*Medical Doctor ~ Carl Simonton is the author of Getting Well Again and The Healing Journey*

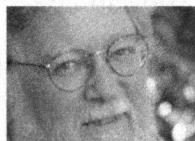

Many more testimonials are available on:
http://www.healingpsyche.com

## Get is now...

Order it now by clicking here

# Commonly Asked Questions

## 16.1  My vitamins are not certified, is that a problem?

YES, The supplement market is a very unregulated market. If your brand or supplement does not have the proper certifications, you have no clue what you are using.

- ✓ *You might end up damaging your health by taking contaminated or toxic products*

- ✓ *You might up wasting your money on products that do not contain any working ingredients*

It would be good to re-read the chapter on certifications and quality labels (chapter 9.2 - Cleaning up your Confusion over Quality Labels) and the chapter on how to select the best supplements (Chapter 9.3 - How you can Choose the Unchoosable)

## 16.2   What do I need for symptom X?

That is a great question to ask, because that means you are already realizing that nutrition can help. The best thing is to re-read the section on this called: Your next question will be: "What do I need?

## 16.3   Some people say that vitamins just make expensive urine, is this true?

NO, When you hear people talk about supplementing their health you have people mentioning that nutritional supplements are not absorbed by the body and are actually only creating expensive urine.

This all depends on the quality of supplement you get. When you get the cheapest product on the shelves, you probably are better to throw it in the toilet straight away than to ingest it. You will not benefit from it.

In the supplement market, is it all about ingredient quality, combinations and absorption of the ingredients. Some products contain weak ingredients, wrong or ineffective combinations and others are not broken down in the stomach, or not absorbed. Those supplements will not help you increase your vitality.

However other supplements (manufactured according to the highest standards) adhere to the US pharmacopeia (USP) standards for absorption of the ingredients. Just make sure you buy the best quality on the market which also have elements to increase absorption. Please reread the chapter on quality selection.

Besides absorption levels there is another side to this story. When you take sufficient high quality vitamins that are optimized for absorption, your body will flourish and unleash your full vitality potential.

When you take more than sufficient, say double the dose, your body takes what it needs and excretes the rest.

Let's paint a picture here.

Assume there is an optimal level for vitamin X at level 60. Below 60 you will have deficiencies. Anything above 60 will help you to maximize your health and vitality.

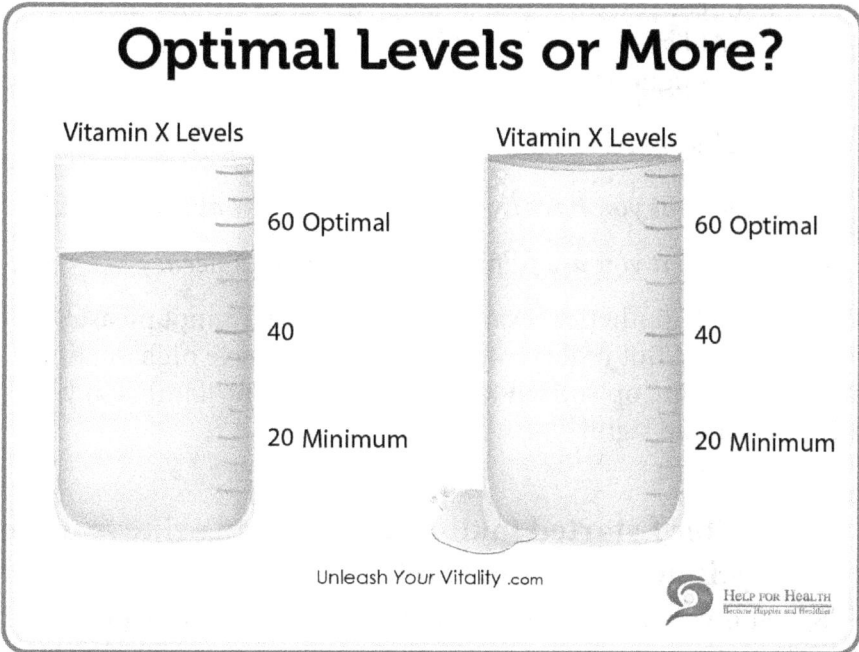

# Optimal Levels or More?

Vitamin X Levels

60 Optimal

40

20 Minimum

Vitamin X Levels

60 Optimal

40

20 Minimum

Unleash Your Vitality .com

Help for Health
Become Happier and Healthier

Now imagine Susan and Rose, both have a level 15 of this vitamin X. Both are seriously deprived and show symptoms. Both women decide to take action and do something about this. They research and find the best source of great absorbable vitamin X.

Susan takes 40 units and reaches level 55, just below the optimal levels. She improves her health tremendously and feels better. Looking at her urine, there is no additional excretion vitamin X.

Rose is really serious and motivated to change her life around, she decides to take 75 units. These additional 75 units will boost her levels to 90. She feels awesome and amazing. Looking at her urine there will be an excretion of the excess vitamin X, and we can find 10units of vitamin X in her urine.

In this case, which one of these ladies will be receiving optimal nourishment? Rose will be, as she filled her entire vitamin X stores until it flooded. Yes, there will be some in her urine, but that is a good sign. At least her body had access to the entire amount of vitamin X it might need.

So when urine levels show increasing vitamin levels it is:

✓ *A sign that you have low quality non absorbable products*

✓ *A sign that you are fulfilling all your bodies needs*

This is just a hypothetical example, because you cannot measure these numbers. But it illustrates that when you have high quality nutrients that are optimized for absorption, extra vitamins in your urine are a good sign!!

## 16.4 After I started taking vitamins my urine is more yellow, is that normal?

YES, that is very normal. Some people say that you have "expensive urine" because you are peeing out the supplements you took. This is not entirely true.

Yes there are lower quality supplements on the market that are very poorly absorbed by your body. If you are taking one of those, then you are indeed wasting your money away. But even worse, lower quality supplements contain contaminants and will hurt your body. You are not spending your money to become sick right? (more on this topic in the quality section)

If you are taking a multivitamin or B-complex it is also normal that your urine will become bright yellow or orange. This is caused by the presence of B2. The body just excretes what it does not need.

## 16.5  How long can I store vitamins?

You might think that they cannot go bad, no matter how old they are. This is not true. You should always observe the expiry date and buy a new bottle if it is past it's time. Vitamins reduce in potency over time. Although it is not dangerous to take slightly date-expired vitamins, it will not benefit you either.

## 16.6  Are supplements safe?

YES very safe, assuming that the supplement is clean, meet safety procedures, are correctly labeled and designed with the appropriate combinations and dosages (see section….).

## 16.7  Thank you, you changed my life and now I want to inspire others, how do I do that?

Excellent, and the credit is all yours. You took the time effort and energy to change your life. We just provided some insights and ways on how to do that.

To inspire others there are a few ways:

1.  *Share your insights and results with everybody who wants to know*

2.  *Post your results on our page:* http://www.UnleashYourVitality.com/results *, this will inspire others to achieve the same results*

3.  *Apply for our coaching program, so you can help people gain the same results. Just send us an email and we will see if this program is for you. We will help you set up your business and change the life of others.*

## 16.8   Why can't they put everything I need in one capsule?

To ensure optimal vitality you need many different nutrients in different combinations. If they put everything into one capsule you would not be able to swallow it!

## 16.9   Why does my doctor not tell me this?

More and more physicians are recognizing the science behind supplementation and how it improves health and vitality. However, not everyone had the time or interest to learn this. In medical school there is just not time to study nutrition and after medical school there is no requirement or incentive to study nutrition any more. This is why most medical doctors are just not aware of the tremendous impact that nutrition has on health, prevention and even on the cure for diseases.

### 16.9.1   Consulting with your physician

Physicians are not trained to understand how nutrition can aid in certain illnesses. When you ask a physician's advice on supplements they will probably say that it will not help. They cannot suggest something they have not studied in detail.

Because they lack the specific study, they tend to react with general remarks as "There is not enough evidence to support that" or "it just creates expensive urine" or something along those lines. Their answer is based on their prior knowledge about the subject and the protection of your safety.

However, you know that nutrition might help you in your situation and you might want to consider taking certain supplementations. When you are using prescription medication it is always a good plan to consult your physician. But what is the best way to ask so you get the best advice possible?

One way to ask is the following:

> **"I want to take these supplements,**
> **I believe they will help me, is that OK?"**

Share your personal ideas, tips, experiences and insights with on our community page. This will help other people to unleash their vitality too.

When the supplement is no good or when it would not be totally safe then they will still let you know. In other cases they agree with your choice. This type of questioning will get you further so you can safely use the supplements to aid your vitality.

## 16.10 How can I help my employees?

Although a bit off-topic, many business owners and human resource specialists have asked me to help with their employees. They already know the tremendous value of good supplementation in their own personal health, and now they want to take it a step further and improve the health of their employees.

There was an economics study done on the effects of disease prevention and the bottom line of a business. They noticed that when a company actively supports their employees in their vitality, the first year they had increased costs. This makes sense because now they have more costs to support the employee. However, in just the second year, while having the same costs, they made more profit - simply because employees were less sick and more productive. So prevention pays off.

> **"Health and happiness of employees will have an impact on**
> **bottom line profits."**
> **~ Professor Vlatka Hlupic Author of "The Management Shift"**

You can easily support your employees by evaluating their health status (or sickness status depending on the person) and then help them make the right choices in supplementing their diet.

If someone is frequently sick then his/ her immune system needs boosting. Support them in changing their lifestyle and it will save you money.

The easiest way to support your employees is to obtain a copy of this book and hand it to them. When you want a more in-depth way to help your employees, contact our office and we will schedule a meeting to discuss how we can help your company.

### 16.11 Other questions?

Do you have other questions that are not addressed in this book? Just connect with us and email your question. We will answer it, and include the answer in the next version of this book. This way you will help others by asking your question.

Feel free to connect to us, we are always happy to help.

http://www.UnleashYourVitality.com

# Unleash Your Vitality™
## 8 Simple Steps to
## Maximize Your Health
# WITH NUTRITION

### by

# ROB VAN OVERBRUGGEN PH.D.

# References

1 - The Center for Health Reform & Modernization 2010

2 - Lee, J. International Journal of Obesity, April 12, 2010; vol 34.

3 - Wu S, Green A. Projection of Chronic Illness Prevalence and Cost Inflation. RAND Corporation, October 2000.

4 - Anderson G, Horvath J The growing burden of chronic disease in America. Public Health Rep. 2004;119:263-70.

5 - Epidemic of chronic disease? BMJ 2009; 339

6 - USDC 1996 werbach, Minerals go down, disease goes up

7 - Ward BW, Schiller JS, Goodman RA. Multiple chronic conditions among US adults: a 2012 update. Prev Chronic Dis. 2014;11

8 - Centers for Disease Control and Prevention. Death and Mortality. NCHS FastStats Web

9 - Centers for Disease Control and Prevention. NCHS Data on Obesity. NCHS Fact Sheet

10 - Hootman JM, Brault MW, Helmick CG, Theis KA, Armour BS. Prevalence and most common causes of disability among adults— United States, 2005. MMWR Morb Mortal Wkly Rep. 2009;

11 - Barbour KE, Helmick CG, Theis KA, et al. Prevalence of doctor-diagnosed arthritis and arthritis-attributable activity limitation—United States, 2010-2012

12 - Melton LJ, 3rd, Atkinson EJ, O'Connor MK, et al. (1998) Bone density and fracture risk in men. J Bone Miner Res 13:1915.

13 - Melton LJ, 3rd, Chrischilles EA, Cooper C, et al. (1992) Perspective. How many women have osteoporosis? J Bone Miner Res 7:1005

14 - Kanis JA, Johnell O, Oden A, et al. (2000) Long-term risk of osteoporotic fracture in Malmo. Osteoporos Int 11:669.

15 - Mark R. Corkins, MD, CNSC, FAAP, Peggi Guenter, PhD, RN, Rose Ann DiMaria-Ghalili, PhD, RN, CNSC et al Malnutrition Diagnoses in Hospitalized Patients United States, 2010 the American Society for Parenteral and Enteral Nutrition

16 - Ferguson M, et al. Nutrition 1999;15:458-464. 2. Banks M, et al. Malnutrition and Pressure Ulcers in Queensland Hospitals. Proceedings of 22nd National DAA Conference,

17 - McWhirter, J.P., Pennington, C.R. (1994) Incidence and recognition of malnutrition in hospital. British Medical Journal; 308: 945-948

18 - Barker LA, Gout BS; Hospital malnutrition: prevalence, identification and impact on patients and the healthcare system.; Int J Environ Res Public Health. 2011 Feb;8(2)

19 - Lisa A. Barker, Belinda S. Gout and Timothy C. Crowe Hospital Malnutrition: Prevalence, Identification and Impact on Patients and the Healthcare System Int J Environ Res Public Health. Feb 2011; 8(2): 514–527.

20 - Lisa A. Barker, Belinda S. Gout and Timothy C. Crowe Hospital Malnutrition: Prevalence, Identification and Impact on Patients and the Healthcare System Int J Environ Res Public Health. Feb 2011; 8(2): 514–527.

21 - Correia MI, Waitzberg DL. The impact of malnutrition on morbidity, mortality, length of hospital stay and costs evaluated through a multivariate model analysis.; Clin Nutr. 2003 Jun;22(3):235-9.

22 - Chima CS1, Barco K, Dewitt ML, Maeda M, Teran JC, Mullen KD., Relationship of nutritional status to length of stay, hospital costs, and discharge status of patients hospitalized in the medicine service., J Am Diet Assoc. 1997 Sep;97(9):975-8;

23 - Kassin MT, Owen RM, Perez SD, et al. Risk factors for 30-day hospital readmission among general surgery patients. J Am Coll Surg. 2012;215:322-330.

24 - R.A. McCance and E.M. Widowson (1940) for the Medical Research Council, UK; 1991: UK Agriculture and Fisheries and Royal Society of Chemistry

25 - Pharmaceutical Company Geigy, Nutrition Laboratory Karlsruhe / Sanatorium Obertal

26 - Michael Via, The Malnutrition of Obesity: Micronutrient Deficiencies That Promote Diabetes, ISRN Endocrinol. 2012; 2012: 103472.

27 - Termanini B, Gibril F, Sutliff VE, et al. Effect of long-term gastric acid suppressive therapy on serum vitamin B12 levels in patients with Zollinger-Ellison syndrome. Am J Med 1998;104:422-30.

28 - Marcuard SP, Albernaz L, Khazaine PG. Omeprazole therapy causes malabsorption of cyanocobalamin. Ann Intern Med 1994;120:211-5.

29 - Saltzman JR, Kemp JA, Golner BB, et al. Effect of hypochlorhydria due to omeprazole treatment or atrophic gastritis on protein-bound vitamin B12 absorption. J Am Coll Nutr 1994;13:584-91.

30 - Recker RR. Calcium absorption and achlorhydria. N Engl J Med 1985;313:70-3.

31 - Bo-Linn GW, Davis GR, Buddrus DJ, et al. An evaluation of the importance of gastric acid secretion in the absorption of dietary calcium. J Clin Invest 1984;73:640-7.

32 - Regolisti G, Cabassi A, Parenti E, et al. Severe hypomagnesemia during long-term treatment with a proton pump inhibitor. Am J Kidney Dis 2010;56:168-74.

33 - Cundy T, Mackay J. Proton pump inhibitors and severe hypomagnesaemia. Curr Opin Gastroenterol 2011;27:180-5.

34 - Doornebal J, Bijlsma R, Brouwer RM. [An unknown but potentially serious side effect of proton pump inhibitors: hypomagnesaemia]. Ned Tijdschr Geneeskd 2009;153:A711.

35 - Kuipers MT, Thang HD, Arntzenius AB. Hypomagnesaemia due to use of proton pump inhibitors--a review. Neth J Med 2009;67:169-72.

36 - Cundy T, Dissanayake A. Severe hypomagnesaemia in long-term users of proton-pump inhibitors. Clin Endocrinol (Oxf) 2008;69:338-41.
37 - Safety Alert. Proton Pump Inhibitor drugs (PPIs): Drug Safety Communication - Low Magnesium Levels Can Be Associated With Long-Term Use. U.S. Food and Drug Administration, March 2, 2011
38 - Laaksonen R, Jokelainen K, Sahi T, et al. Decreases in serum ubiquinone concentrations do not result in reduced levels in muscle tissue during short-term simvastatin treatment in humans. Clin Pharmacol Ther 1995;57:62-6.
39 - Rundek T, Naini A, Sacco R, et al. Atorvastatin decreases the coenzyme Q10 level in the blood of patients at risk for cardiovascular disease and stroke. Arch Neurol 2004;61:889-92.
40 - Caso G, Kelly P, McNurlan MA, Lawson WE. Effect of coenzyme Q10 on myopathic symptoms in patients treated with statins. Am J Cardiol 2007;99:1409-12.
41 - Sattler FR, Weitekamp MR, Ballard JO. Potential for bleeding with the new beta-lactam antibiotics. Ann Intern Med 1986;105:924-31.
42 - Hooper CA, Haney BB, Stone HH. Gastrointestinal bleeding due to vitamin K deficiency in patients on parenteral cefamandole. Lancet 1980;1:39-40.
43 - Goldin BR, Lichtenstein AH, Gorbach SL. Nutritional and metabolic roles of intestinal flora. In: Shils ME, Olson JA, Shike M, eds. Modern Nutrition in Health and Disease, 8th ed. Malvern, PA: Lea & Febiger, 1994.
44 - Conly JM, Stein K, Worobetz L, Rutledge-Harding S. The contribution of vitamin K2 (menaquinones) produced by the intestinal microflora to human nutritional requirements for vitamin K. Am J Gastroenterol 1994;89:915-23.
45 - http://www.webmd.com/hypertension-high-blood-pressure/guide/diuretic-treatment
46 - http://www.nlm.nih.gov/medlineplus/ency/article/000479.htmt
47 - H.H. Mitchell, Journal of Biological Chemistry 158
48 - EWG analysis of water utility test data for 2004-2009 provided to EWG by state drinking water offices
49 - Rebecca Sutton, PhD, Chromium-6 in U.S. Tap Water,

50 - EWG analysis of water utility test data for 2004-2009 provided to EWG by state drinking water offices

51 - Bottled Water - Pure Drink or Pure Hype?, National Resources Defence Council 2013

52 - Summary Findings of NRDC's 1999 Bottled Water Report

53 - Olga Naidenko, PhD, Nneka Leiba, MPH, et al., Bottled water contains disinfection byproducts, fertilizer residue, and pain medication

54 - Olga Naidenko, PhD, Nneka Leiba, MPH, et al., Bottled water contains disinfection byproducts, fertilizer residue, and pain medication – Le 2008

55 - Greifenstein M, White DW, et al Impact of temperature and storage duration on the chemical and odor quality of military packaged water in polyethylene terephthalate bottles. Sci Total Environ. 2013 Jul 1;456-457:376-83

56 - Fan YY, Zheng JL, et al. Effects of storage temperature and duration on release of antimony and bisphenol A from polyethylene terephthalate drinking water bottles of China., Environ Pollut. 2014 Sep;192:113-20

57 - Earth Policy Institute, As You Sow, Container Recycling Institute.

58 - A Systematic Review of Public Water Fluoridation , 2000, Centre for Reviews and Dissemination of the University of York

59 - 'Fluorine and fluorides', Environmental Health Criteria 36, IPCS International Programme on Chemical Safety, WHO 1984.

60 - Jingjing Qian, Dr. A.K. Susheela , Fluoride in water: An overview, UNICEF, Issue 13  December 1999

61 - Jingjing Qian, Dr. A.K. Susheela , Fluoride in water: An overview, UNICEF, Issue 13 • December 1999

62 - Stan C. Frenia ,Exposure to high fluoride concentrations in drinking water is associated with decreased birth rates, Journal of Toxicology and Environmental Health, Volume 42, Issue 1, 1994

63 - San-Xiang Wang, Zheng-Hui Wang, et al., Arsenic and Fluoride Exposure in Drinking Water: Children's IQ and Growth in Shanyin County, Environ Health Perspect. Apr 2007; 115(4): 643–647.

64 - Anna L. Choi, Guifan Sun, Ying Zhang, Philippe Grandjean, Developmental Fluoride Neurotoxicity: A Systematic Review and Meta-Analysis, Environ Health Perspect. 2012 October; 120(10): 1362–1368.

65 - A. K. Susheela1, N. K. Mondal et al. Effective interventional approach to control anaemia in pregnant women , Current Science, vol 98 no 10, 2010

66 - Okada, Haruko C. M.D.; Alleyne, Brendan B.S.; Varghai, Kaveh; Kinder, Kimberly M.D.; Guyuron, Bahman M.D. Facial Changes Caused by Smoking: A Comparison between Smoking and Nonsmoking Identical Twins; Plastic & Reconstructive Surgery: November 2013 - Volume 132 - Issue 5 - p 1085–1092

67 - Li JG, Praticò D. High Levels of Homocysteine Results in Cerebral Amyloid Angiopathy in Mice. J Alzheimers Dis. 2014 Jul 24

68 - Sapolsky R Glucocorticoids, stress and exacerbation of excitotoxic neuron death. Semin Neurosci 1994, 6: 323–331.

69 - 1992 Earth Summit Statistics

70 - Pharmaceutical Company Geigy, Nutrition Laboratory Karlsruhe / Sanatorium Obertal 1985 / 1996 / 2002

71 - R.A. McCance and E.M. Widdowson (1940) for the Medical Research Council, UK; 1991: UK Agriculture and Fisheries and Royal Society of Chemistry

72 - David Thomas, THE MINERAL DEPLETION OF FOODS AVAILABLE TO US AS A NATION (1940–2002) - Nutrition and Health, 2007, Vol. 19, pp. 21–55

73 - Pflipsen MC, Oh RC, Saguil A, Seehusen DA, Seaquist D, Topolski R. The prevalence of vitamin B(12) deficiency in patients with type 2 diabetes: a cross-sectional study. J Am Board Fam Med. 2009 Sep-Oct;22(5):528-34

74 - Murphy AB1, Nyame Y, Martin IK, Catalona WJ, Hollowell CM, Nadler RB, Kozlowski JM, Perry KT, Kajdacsy-Balla A, Kittles R. ; Vitamin D Deficiency Predicts Prostate Biopsy Outcomes.; Clin Cancer Res. 2014 May 1;20(9):2289-2299.

75 - Tang JE, Wang RJ, Zhong H, Yu B, Chen Y.; Vitamin A and risk of bladder cancer: a meta-analysis of epidemiological studies. ;World J Surg Oncol. 2014 Apr 29;12(1):130.

76 - Michel de Lorgeril, Patricia Salen; Helping women to good health: breast cancer, omega-3/omega-6 lipids, and related lifestyle factors ; BMC Med. 2014; 12: 54.

77 - Poulsen HE. ; Oxidative DNA modifications.;Exp Toxicol Pathol. 2005 Jul;57 Suppl 1:161-9.

78 - Poulsen HE1, Prieme H, Loft S.;Role of oxidative DNA damage in cancer initiation and promotion.;Eur J Cancer Prev. 1998 Feb;7(1):9-16.

79 - Valko M1, Rhodes CJ, Moncol J, Izakovic M, Mazur M.; Free radicals, metals and antioxidants in oxidative stress-induced cancer.; Chem Biol Interact. 2006 Mar 10;160(1):1-40. Epub 2006 Jan 23.

80 - Klaunig JE1, Kamendulis LM.;The role of oxidative stress in carcinogenesis.;Annu Rev Pharmacol Toxicol. 2004;44:239-67.

81 - Poulsen HE. ; Oxidative DNA modifications.;Exp Toxicol Pathol. 2005 Jul;57 Suppl 1:161-9.

82 - Poulsen HE1, Prieme H, Loft S.;Role of oxidative DNA damage in cancer initiation and promotion.;Eur J Cancer Prev. 1998 Feb;7(1):9-16.

83 - Valko M1, Rhodes CJ, Moncol J, Izakovic M, Mazur M.; Free radicals, metals and antioxidants in oxidative stress-induced cancer.; Chem Biol Interact. 2006 Mar 10;160(1):1-40. Epub 2006 Jan 23.

84 - Klaunig JE1, Kamendulis LM.;The role of oxidative stress in carcinogenesis.;Annu Rev Pharmacol Toxicol. 2004;44:239-67.

85 - Block, Gladys. The data support a role for antioxidants in reducing cancer risk. Nutrition Reviews, Vol. 50, No. 7, July 1992, pp. 207-13

86 - Block, Gladys. Micronutrients and cancer: time for action? Journal of the National Cancer Institute, Vol. 85, No. 11, June 2, 1993, pp. 846-47

87 - Block, G. Epidemiologic evidence regarding vitamin C and cancer. American Journal of Clinical Nutrition, Vol. 54 (6 suppl.), December 1991, pp. 1310S- 14S

88 - Ames BN. DNA damage from micronutrient deficiencies is likely to be a major cause of cancer. 2001. Mutat Res 475(1-2):7-20.18

89 - Mian Li, Peizhan Chen, Jingquan Li, Ruiai Chu, Dong Xie, and Hui Wang The Impacts of Circulating 25-Hydroxyvitamin D Levels on Cancer Patient Outcomes: A Systematic Review and Meta-Analysis Clin Cancer Res. 2014;20:2289-2299.

90 - Meta-analysis of Vitamin D Sufficiency for Improving Survival of Patients with Breast Cancer, Cedric F. Garland et al., Anti-cancer Research, March 2014.

91 - William B Grant, Cedric F Garland Vitamin D has a greater impact on cancer mortality rates than on cancer incidence rates BMJ 2014; 348

92 - Hertz N1, Lister RE. Improved survival in patients with end-stage cancer treated with coenzyme Q(10) and other antioxidants: a pilot study. J Int Med Res. 2009 Nov-Dec;37(6):1961-71

93 - USDC 1996 werbach, Minerals go down, disease goes up

94 - Rob van Overbruggen Ph.D. "Healing Psyche"

95 - Age-Related Eye Disease Study Research Group. A randomized, placebo-controlled, clinical trial of high-dose supplementation with vitamins C and E, beta carotene, and zinc for age-related macular degeneration and vision loss: AREDS report no. 8. 2001. Arch Ophthalmol 119(10):1417-36.

96 - Tang JE, Wang RJ, Zhong H, Yu B, Chen Y.; Vitamin A and risk of bladder cancer: a meta-analysis of epidemiological studies.; World J Surg Oncol. 2014 Apr 29;12(1):130.

97 - Kim YS, Lee HA, Lim JY et al; B-Carotene inhibits neuroblastoma cell invasion and metastasis in vitro and in vivo by decreasing level of hypoxia-inducible factor-1?J Nutr ;Biochem. 2014 Mar 13. pii: S0955-2863(14)00045-X. doi: 10.1016/j.jnutbio.2014.02.006

98 - Dawson, M.I., The Importance of Vitamin A in Nutrition, Current Pharmaceutical Design, Volume 6, Number 3, 1 February 2000, pp. 311-325(15)

99 - Prof. Paul M. Newberne DVM, PhD, Voranunt Suphakarn SM (2006), Preventive role of vitamin A in colon carcinogenesis in rats, American Cancer Society

100 - H.K. Biesalski, , D. Nohr (2003) 'Importance of vitamin-A for lung function and development', Molecular Aspects of Medicine Volume 24, Issue 6, December 2003, Pages 431–440

101 - Smith AD, Smith SM, de Jager CA, Whitbread P, Johnston C, et al. 2010 Homocysteine-Lowering by B Vitamins Slows the Rate of Accelerated Brain Atrophy in Mild Cognitive Impairment: A Randomized Controlled Trial. PLoS ONE 5(9)

102 - Louwman MW, van Dusseldorp M, van de Vijver FJ, et al. Signs of impaired cognitive function in adolescents with marginal cobalamin status. Am J Clin Nutr. 2000;72(3):762-769.

103 - Smith AD, Smith SM, de Jager CA, Whitbread P, Johnston C, et al. 2010 Homocysteine-Lowering by B Vitamins Slows the Rate of Accelerated Brain Atrophy in Mild Cognitive Impairment: A Randomized Controlled Trial. PLoS ONE 5(9)

104 - Cuskelly GJ, Mooney KM, Young IS. Folate and vitamin B12: friendly or enemy nutrients for the elderly. Proc Nutr Soc. 2007;66(4):548-58.

105 - Wang HX. Vitamin B12 and folate in relation to the development of Alzheimer's disease. Neurology. 2001;56:1188-1194.

106 - Witte KK, Clark AL, Cleland JG. Chronic heart failure and micronutrients. J Am Coll Cardiol. 2001;37(7):1765-1774.

107 - Ambrose, ML, Bowden SC, Whelan G. Thiamin treatment and working memory function of alcohol-dependent people: preliminary findings. Alcohol Clin Exp Res. 2001;25(1):112-116.

108 - Cumming RG, Mitchell P, Smith W. Diet and cataract: the Blue Mountains Eye Study.Ophthalmology. 2000;107(3):450-456.

109 - Gibson GE, Blass JP. Thiamine-dependent processes and treatment strategies in neurodegeneration. Antioxid Redox Signal. 2007 Aug 8;

110 - Lonsdale D. A review of the biochemistry, metabolism and clinical benefits of thiamin(e) and its derivatives. Evid Based Complement Alternat Med. 2006 Mar;3(1):49-59.

111 - Sica DA. Loop diuretic therapy, thiamine balance, and heart failure. Congest Heart Fail. 2007 Jul-Aug;13(4):244-7.

112 - Soukoulis V, Dihu JB, Sole M, Anker SD, Cleland J, Fonarow GC, Metra M, Pasini E, Strzelczyk T, Taegtmeyer H, Gheorghiade M. Micronutrient deficiencies an unmet need in heart failure. J Am Coll Cardiol. 2009 Oct 27;54(18):1660-73. Review.

113 - Rodriquez-Martin JL, Qizilbash N, Lopez-Arrieta JM. Thiamine for Alzheimer's disease (Cochrane Review). Cochrane Database Syst Rev. 2001;2:CD001498.

114 - Steven D. Ehrlich, NMD. "Vitamin B1 (thiamine)". University of Maryland Medical Center (UMMC). Accessed November 5th 2013.

115 - Jane Higdon, Ph.D. "Thiamin". September 2002. Linus Pauling Institute, Oregon State University. Accessed November 5th 2013.

116 - Pantothenic Acid, Biotin, and Choline." Washington (DC): National Academies Press (US); 1998. 4, Thiamin. Accessed November 5th 2013.

117 - Thiamine (Vitamin B1). Natural Medicines Comprehensive Database. National Institutes of Health. Accessed November 5th 2013.

118 - Ba A. Metabolic and structural role of vitamin B1e in nervous tissues. Cell Mol Neurobiol 2008;28:923-31.

119 - Keogh JB, Cleanthous X, Wycherley TP, et al. Increased vitamin B1e intake may be required to maintain vitamin B1e status during weight loss in patients with type 2 diabetes. Diabetes Res Clin Pract 2012;98:40-2.

120 - MacLennan SC, Wade FM, Forrest KM, Ratanayake PD, Fagan E, Antony J. High-dose riboflavin for migraine prophylaxis in children: a double-blind, randomized, placebo-controlled trial. J Child Neurol. 2008 Nov;23(11):1300-4.

121 - Magis D, Ambrosini A, Sandor P, Jacquy J, Laloux P, Schoenen J. A randomized double-blind placebo-controlled trial of thioctic acid in migraine prophylaxis. Headache. 2007 Jan;47(1):52-7.

122 - Mauskop A. Alternative therapies in headache. Is there a role? [Review]. Med Clin North Am. 2001;85(4):1077-1084.

123 - Silberstein SD, Goadsby PJ, Lipton RB. Management of migraine: an algorithmic approach. [Review]. Neurology. 2000;55(9 Suppl 2):S46-52.

124 - Fishman SM, Christian P, West KP. The role of vitamins in the prevention and control of anaemia. [Review]. Public Health Nutr. 2000;3(2):125-150.

125 - Jacques PF, Chylack LT Jr, Hankinson SE, et al. Long-term nutrient intake and early age-related nuclear lens opacities. Arch Ophthalmol. 2001;119(7):1009-1019.

126 - Keligman. Nelson Textbook of Pediatrics, 18th ed. Philadelphia, PA: Saunders Elsevier. 2007.

127 - Head KA. Natural therapies for ocular disorders, part two: cataracts and glaucoma. [Review]. Altern Med Rev. 2001;6(2):141-166.

128 - Maraini G, Williams SL, Sperduto RD, Ferris FL, Milton RC, Clemons TE, Rosmini F, Ferrigno L. Effects of multivitamin/mineral supplementation on plasma levels of nutrients. Report No. 4 of the Italian-American clinical trial of nutritional supplements and age-related cataract. Ann Ist Super Sanita. 2009;45(2):119-27.

129 - Horigan G, McNulty H, Ward M, Strain JJ, Purvis J, Scott JM. Riboflavin lowers blood pressure in cardiovascular disease patients homozygous for the 677C?T polymorphism in MTHFR. J Hypertens. 2010;28(3):478-486.

130 - Wilson CP, Ward M, McNulty H, et al. Riboflavin offers a targeted strategy for manageing hypertension in patients with the MTHFR 677TT genotype: a 4-y follow-up. Am J Clin Nutr. 2012;95(3):766-772.

131 - Prakash R, Gandotra S, Singh LK, Das B, Lakra A. Rapid resolution of delusional parasitosis in pellagra with niacin augmentation therapy. Gen Hosp Psychiatry. 2008;30(6):581-584.

132 - Spronck JC, Nickerson JL, Kirkland JB. Niacin deficiency alters p53 expression and impairs etoposide-induced cell cycle arrest and apoptosis in rat bone marrow cells. Nutr Cancer. 2007;57(1):88-99.

133 - Kostecki LM, Thomas M, Linford G, et al. Niacin deficiency delays DNA excision repair and increases spontaneous and nitrosourea-induced chromosomal instability in rat bone marrow. Mutat Res. 2007;625(1-2):50-61.

134 - Jacobson EL. Niacin deficiency and cancer in women. J Am Coll Nutr. 1993;12(4):412-416.

135 - Canner PL, Berge KG, Wenger NK, et al. Fifteen year mortality in Coronary Drug Project patients: long-term benefit with niacin. J Am Coll Cardiol. 1986;8(6):1245-1255.

136 - Wink J, Giacoppe G, King J. Effect of very-low-dose niacin on high-density lipoprotein in patients undergoing long-term statin therapy. Am Heart J. 2002;143(3):514-518.

137 - Bissett DL, Oblong JE, Berge CA, et al. Niacinamide: A B vitamin that improves ageing facial skin appearance. Dermatol Surg. 2005;31:860-865;

138 - Brown BG, Zhao XQ, Chalt A, et al. Simvastatin and niacin, antioxidant vitamins, or the combination for the prevention of coronary disease. N Engl J Med. 2001;345(22):1583-1592.
139 - Guyton JR. Niacin in cardiovascular prevention: mechanisms, efficacy, and safety. Curr Opin Lipidol. 2007 Aug;18(4):415-20.
140 - de Jager CA, Oulhaj A, Jacoby R, et al. Cognitive and clinical outcomes of homocysteine-lowering B-vitamin treatment in mild cognitive impairment: a randomized controlled trial. Int.J.Geriatr. Psychiatry 2012;27(6):592-600.
141 - Ford AH and Almeida OP. Effect of homocysteine lowering treatment on cognitive function: a systematic review and meta-analysis of randomized controlled trials. J.Alzheimers.Dis. 2012;29(1):133-149.
142 - Marti-Carvajal AJ, Sola I, Lathyris D, et al. Homocysteine-lowering interventions for preventing cardiovascular events. Cochrane.Database.Syst.Rev. 2013;1:CD006612.
143 - Myung SK, Ju W, Cho B, et al. Efficacy of vitamin and antioxidant supplements in prevention of cardiovascular disease: systematic review and meta-analysis of randomised controlled trials. BMJ 2013;346:f10.
144 - Yoshihara K, Kubo C. Overview of medical treatment and management of chronic fatigue syndrome. Nippon Rinsho. 2007 Jun;65(6):1077-81.
145 - Barringer TA, Kirk JK, Santaniello AC, Foley KL, Michielutte R. Effect of a multivitamin and mineral supplement on infection and quality of life. A randomized, double-blind, placebo-controlled trial. 2003. Ann Intern Med 138(5):365
146 - Tveden-Nyborg, Johansen LK; Vitamin C deficiency in early postnatal life impairs spatial memory and reduces the number of hippocampal neurons in guinea pigs.; Am J Clin Nutr. 2009 Sep;90(3):540-6.
147 - Li W, Maeda N; Vitamin C deficiency increases the lung pathology of influenza virus-infected gulo-/- mice. J Nutr. 2006 Oct;136(10):2611-6.
148 - Stone, I; Eight Decades of Scurvy. The Case History of a Misleading Dietary Hypothesis.". AscorbateWeb. Archived from the original on March 18, 2009.

149 - Chatterjee, IB; "Evolution and the Biosynthesis of Ascorbic Acid". 1973 Science 182 (4118): 1271–1272.

150 - Vieth R, et al, Efficacy and safety of vitamin D3 intake exceeding the lowest observed adverse effect level, Am J Clin Nutr 73:288-94, 2003

151 - A. Mithal, D.A. Wahl, J-P. Bonjour et al. on behalf of the IOF Committee of Scientific Advisors (CSA) Nutrition Working Group. Global vitamin D status and determinants of hypovitaminosis D (2009) Osteoporosis International,in press.

152 - Michael F Holick Vitamin D: importance in the prevention of cancers, type 1 diabetes, heart disease, and osteoporosis 2004 American Society for Clinical Nutrition

153 - Michael F Holick Vitamin D: importance in the prevention of cancers, type 1 diabetes, heart disease, and osteoporosis 2004 American Society for Clinical Nutrition

154 - Michael F Holick Vitamin D: importance in the prevention of cancers, type 1 diabetes, heart disease, and osteoporosis 2004 American Society for Clinical Nutrition

155 - William B Grant, Cedric F Garland Vitamin D has a greater impact on cancer mortality rates than on cancer incidence rates BMJ 2014: 348

156 - William B Grant, Cedric F Garland Vitamin D has a greater impact on cancer mortality rates than on cancer incidence rates BMJ 2014; 348

157 - Meta-analysis of Vitamin D Sufficiency for Improving Survival of Patients with Breast Cancer, Cedric F. Garland et al., Anti-cancer Research, March 2014.

158 - Mian Li, Peizhan Chen, Jingquan Li, Ruiai Chu, Dong Xie, and Hui Wang The Impacts of Circulating 25-Hydroxyvitamin D Levels on Cancer Patient Outcomes: A Systematic Review and Meta-Analysis Clin Cancer Res. 2014;20:2289-2299.

159 - Saltman PD, Strause LG. The role of trace minerals in osteoporosis. 1993. J Am Coll Nutr 12(4):384-9.

160 - Age-Related Eye Disease Study Research Group. The Age-Related Eye Disease Study: a clinical trial of zinc and antioxidants--Age-Related Eye Disease Study Report No. 2. 2000. J Nutr 130(5S Suppl):1516S-9S.

161 - Ginde AA1, Scragg R, Schwartz RS, Camargo CA Jr. Prospective study of serum 25-hydroxyvitamin D level, cardiovascular disease mortality, and all-cause mortality in older U.S. adults. J Am Geriatr Soc. 2009 Sep;57(9):1595-603. doi: 10.1111/j.1532-5415.2009.02359.x. Epub 2009 Jun 22.

162 - Meydani SN, Meydani M, Blumberg JB, Leka LS, Siber G, et al Vitamin E supplementation and in vivo immune response in healthy elderly subjects, a randomizedcontrolled trial. 1997. JAMA 277(17):1380-6.

163 - Lloyd, J. K. (1990), The Importance of Vitamin E in Human Nutrition. Acta Paediatrica, 79: 6–11.

164 - Iwamoto,, Ichiro, and Et. Al. "A Longitudinal Study of the Effect of Vitamin K2 on Bone Mineral Density in Postmenopausal Women a Comparative Study with Vitamin D3 and Estrogen–progestin Therapy." The Official Journal of the European Menopause and Andropause Society, 30 Jan. 2009.

165 - Schurgers LJ, Teunissen KJ, Hamulyak K, Knapen MH, Vik H, Vermeer C., Vitamin K-containing dietary supplements: comparison of synthetic vitamin K1 and natto-derived menaquinone-7., Blood. 2007 Apr 15;109(8):3279-83.

166 - Major GC, Alarie FP, Doré J, Tremblay A., Calcium plus vitamin D supplementation and fat mass loss in female very low-calcium consumers: potential link with a calcium-specific appetite control. Br J Nutr. 2009 Mar;101(5):659-63.

167 - Kuanrong Li, Rudolf Kaaks, Jakob Linseisen, Sabine Rohrmann Associations of dietary calcium intake and calciumsupplementation with myocardial infarction and stroke risk and overall cardiovascular mortality in the Heidelberg cohort of the European Prospective Investigation into Cancer and Nutrition study , Heart 2012;98:920e925

168 - Standing Committee on the Scientific Evaluation of Dietary Reference Intakes, Food and Nutrition Board, Institute of Medicine. Dietary Reference Intakes for Calcium, Phosphorus, Magnesium, Vitamin D and Fluoride. Washington DC: The National Academies Press, 1997.

169 - U.S. Department of Agriculture. Results from the United States Department of Agriculture's 1994-96 Continuing Survey of Food Intakes by Individuals/Diet and Health Knowledge Survey. 1994-96. http://www.barc.usda.gov/bhnrc/foodsurvey/ Products9496.html#foodandnutrientintakes.

170 - chauss, A.G. Keynote lecture, Texas Conference on Nutrition and Behavior, University of Texas at Austin, October 28, 1982; and Schauss, A G. Nutrition and Behavior. Journal of Applied Nutrition, 1983; 35:30?43.

171 - Ford ES, Mokdad AH. Dietary magnesium intake in a national sample of U.S. adults. J Nutr. 2003;133:2879-82. Fox C, Ramsoomair D, Carter C. Magnesium: its proven and potential clinical significance. [Review]. South Med J. 2001;94(12):1195-1201.

172 - Schauss, Alexander. Minerals and Human Health: The Rationale for Optimal and Balanced Trace Element Levels. Life Sciences Press: 1995, pp. 1, 5.

173 - Rude RK, et al, Skeletal and hormonal effects of magnesium deficiency, J Am Coll Nutr 28; 2:131-41, 2009

174 - Vieth R, et al, Efficacy and safety of vitamin D3 intake exceeding the lowest observed adverse effect level, Am J Clin Nutr 73:288-94, 2003

175 - Chapuy MC, et al, Prevalence of vitamin D insufficiency in an adult normal population, Osteoporosis International 7:439-43, 1997

176 - Pieczyska J, Grajeta H., The role of selenium in human conception and pregnancy. J Trace Elem Med Biol. 2014 Jul 19.

177 - Hurwitz BE, Klaus JR, Llabre MM, et al. Suppression of human immunodeficiency virus type 1 viral load with selenium supplementation. A randomized controlled trial. Arch Intern Med 167:148-154, 2007.

178 - Margaret P. Rayman, The Importance of Selenium to Human Health , Centre for Nutrition and Food Safety, School of Biological Sciences, University of Surrey,

179 - DR. KATHLEEN CRANDELL Selenium - How Important Is It?

180 - Christopher J. Frederickson, Sang Won Suh, David Silva, et al. 'Importance of Zinc in the Central Nervous System: The Zinc-Containing Neuron1' J. Nutr. May 1, 2000 vol. 130 no. 5 1471S-1483S

181 - Studer M, Briel M, et al. "Effect of different antilipidemic agents and diet on mortality: a systematic review." Archives of Internal Medicine, 2005 April 11;165(7):725-30

182 - S. M. Pilkington, K. A. Massey, S. P. Bennett, N. M. Al-Aasswad, K. Roshdy, N. K. Gibbs, P. S. Friedmann, A. Nicolaou, L. E. Rhodes. Randomized controlled trial of oral omega-3 PUFA in solar-simulated radiation-induced suppression of human cutaneous immune responses. American Journal of Clinical Nutrition, 2013; 97 (3): 646

183 - Farzaneh-Far R1, Lin J, Epel ES, Harris WS, Blackburn EH, Whooley MA. Association of marine omega-3 fatty acid levels with telomeric ageing in patients with coronary heart disease.JAMA. 2010 Jan 20;303(3):250-7. doi: 10.1001/jama.2009.2008.

184 - Dariush Mozaffarian, MD, DrPH; Rozenn N. Lemaitre, PhD, MPH; Irena B. King, PhD; et al. Plasma Phospholipid Long-Chain omega-3 Fatty Acids and Total and Cause-Specific Mortality in Older Adults: A Cohort Study Ann Intern Med. 2013;158(7):515-525.

185 - Jyrki K Virtanen, Jaakko Mursu, Sari Voutilainen, Matti Uusitupa, and Tomi-Pekka Tuomainen Serum Omega-3 Polyunsaturated Fatty Acids and Risk of Incident Type 2 Diabetes in Men: The Kuopio Ischaemic Heart Disease Risk Factor Study Diabetes Care published ahead of print September 11, 2013 1935-5548

186 - American Heart Association Scientific Statement, "Triglycerides and Cardiovascular Disease: A Scientific Statement from the American Heart Association." (April 2011) Circulation 123: 2292-2333

187 - United States Food and Drug Administration (September 8, 2004). "FDA announces qualified heath claims for omega-3 fatty acids". Press release. Retrieved 2006-07-1 0.

188 - The Oxford-Durham study: a randomized controlled trial of dietary supplementation with fatty acids in children with developmental coordination disorder. Richardson AJ, Montgomery P. (2005) Pediatrics 115 (5) 1360-1366.

189 - Simopoulos, Artemis P., MD, FACN. "Omega-3 Fatty Acids in Inflammation and Autoimmune Diseases," Journal of the American College of Nutrition (Dec 2002) Vol. 21 , No. 6, 495-50

190 - James, Andrew M.; Cochemé, Helena M.; Smith, Robin A. J.; Murphy, Michael P. (2005). "Interactions of Mitochondria-targeted and Untargeted Ubiquinones with the Mitochondrial Respiratory Chain and Reactive Oxygen Species: Implications for the use of exogenous ubiquinones as therapies and experimental tools". Journal of Biological Chemistry 280 (22): 21295–312

191 - Hosoe, Kazunori; Kitano, Mitsuaki; Kishida, Hideyuki; Kubo, Hiroshi; Fujii, Kenji; Kitahara, Mikio (2007). "Study on safety and bioavailability of ubiquinol (Kaneka QH™) after single and 4-week multiple oral administration to healthy volunteers". Regulatory Toxicology and Pharmacology 47 (1): 19–28.

192 - Hertz N1, Lister RE. Improved survival in patients with end-stage cancer treated with coenzyme Q(10) and other antioxidants: a pilot study. J Int Med Res. 2009 Nov-Dec;37(6):1961-71.

193 - Canadian government health agency/ Health Canada, COENZYME Q10 (UBIQUINONE-10) Monograph, November 22, 2007. (url: http://www.hcsc.gc.ca/dhp-mps/prodnatur/applications/licen-prod/monograph/mono_coenz-q10-eng.php)

194 - Etsuo Niki, "Biomedical and Clinical Aspects of Coenzyme Q," Molecular Aspects of Medicine, Volume 18, Supplement 1, 1997, Pages 63-70

195 - Ernster, L; Dallner, G (1995). "Biochemical, physiological and medical aspects of ubiquinone function". Biochimica et Biophysica Acta 1271 (1): 195–204. PMID 7599208

196 - Giovanni Ravaglia, Paola Forti, Fabiola Maioli, et al., "Effect of micronutrient status on natural killer cell immune function in healthy free-living subjects aged _90," American Journal of Clinical Nutrition, Vol. 71, No. 2, 590-598, February 2000

197 - Ghirlanda, G; Oradei, A; Manto, A; Lippa, S; Uccioli, L; Caputo, S; Greco, AV; Littarru, GP (1993). "Evidence of plasma CoQ10-lowering effect by HMG-CoA reductase inhibitors: a double-blind, placebocontrolled study". Journal of clinical pharmacology 33 (3): 226–9. PMID 8463436

198 - Family Practice News, May 15, 2013, p. 3.

199 - CoQ10. ConsumerLab.com. ConsumerLab.com LLC, 2013. 13 June 2013.

200 - Coenzyme Q10. Natural Standard –The Authority on Integrative Medicine. Natural Standard, 2013.

201 - Coenzyme Q-10. Natural Medicines Comprehensive Database. Therapeutic Research Faculty, 2013. 8 November 2013.

202 - Suzuki, T. et al. Atrovastatin-Induced Changes in Plasma Coenzyme Q10 and Brain Natriuretic Peptide in Patients With Coronary Artery Disease. Int Heart J (2008) 49, 423-433

203 - Adarsh, K. et al. Coenzyme Q10 (CoQ10) in isolated diastolic heart failure in hypertropic cardiomyopathy (HCM). BioFactors (2008) 32, 145-149

204 - Langsjoen, P.H., Langsjoen, A.M. et al. Supplemental ubiquinol in patients with advanced congestive heart failure. BioFactors (2008) 32, 119-128

205 - Schmelzer, C. et al. Functions of coenzyme Q10 in inflammation and gene expression. BioFactors (2008) 32, 179-183

206 - Wyman, M. et al. Coenzyme Q10: A therapy for hypertension and statin-induced myalgia? Cleveland Clinic Journal of Medicine (2010) 77, 435-442

207 - Molyneux, S.L. et al. Coenzyme Q10, An Independent Predictor of Mortality in Chronic Heart Failure. JACC (2008) 52, 1435-1441

208 - Wada H, Goto H, Hagiwara S, Yamamoto Y. Redox status of coenzyme Q10 is associated with chronological age. J Am Geriatr Soc. 2007 Jul;55(7):1141-2. PubMed PMID: 17608895.

209 - Vladimir Badmaev, M.D., Ph.D., Muhammed Majeed, Ph.D., and Lakshmi Prakash, Ph.D. "Piperine Derived From Black Pepper Increases The Plasma Levels Of Coenzyme Q10 Following Oral Supplementation" J. Nutr. Biochem. (2000) 11: 109-113

210 - Langsjoen PH, Langsjoen AM. Supplemental ubiquinol in patients with advanced congestive heart failure. Biofactors. 2008; 32(1-4):119-28.PubMed PMID: 19096107

211 - Cleren C, Yang L, Lorenzo B, Calingasan NY, Schomer A, Sireci A, Wille EJ, Beal MF. Therapeutic effects of coenzyme Q10 (CoQ10) and reduced CoQ10 in the MPTP model of Parkinsonism. J Neurochem. 2008 Mar;104(6):1613-21. Epub 2007 Oct 31. PubMed PMID: 17973981.

212 - Sandor, P.S. et al. Efficacy of conenzyme Q10 in migraine prophylaxis: A randomized controlled trial. Neurology (2005) 64:713-715

213 - Hershey, A.D. et al. Coenzyme Q10 Deficiency and Response to Supplementation in Pediatric and Adolescent Migraine. Headache (2007) 47:73-80

214 - Mezadri T, Villano M, Fernandez-Pachon M, Garcia-Parrilla M, Troncoso A (2008). "Antioxidant compounds and antioxidant activity in acerola(Malpighia emarginata DC.) fruits and derivatives". Journal of Food Composition and Analysis 21 (4): 282-290.

215 - Leonardo Di Donna , Giuseppina De Luca ; Statin-like Principles of Bergamot Fruit (Citrus bergamia): Isolation of 3-Hydroxymethylglutaryl Flavonoid Glycosides; J. Nat. Prod., 2009, 72 (7), pp 1352–1354

216 - Badmaev, V, Majeed, M. et al. Piperine, An Alkaloid Derived from Black Pepper, Increases Serum Response of Beta-Carotene During 14 Days of Oral Beta-Carotene Supplementation. Nutrition Research, 19(3) 381-388, 1999.

217 - Majeed, M. Use of piperine as a bioavailability enhancer. US Patent 5744161, October 26, 1999

218 - Shoba G, et al. Influence of piperine on the pharmacokinetics of curcumin in animals and human volunteers. Planta Med; 64(4):353-. 1998.

219 - Badmaev, V. and Majeed, M. Skin as a delivery system for nutrients, nutraceutials and drugs. THP a natural compound with the potential to enhance the bioavailability of nutrients and drugs through the skin. Agro-Industry Hi-Tech. 6-10, 2001 (Jan/Feb).

220 - Shoba G, et al. Influence of piperine on the pharmacokinetics of curcumin in animals and human volunteers. Planta Med; 64(4):353-6. 1998.

221 - Ivankovic S1, Stojkovic R; The antitumor activity of thymoquinone and thymohydroquinone in vitro and in vivo;Exp Oncol. 2006 Sep;28(3):220-4.

222 - Alsayed T Salim; Cancer chemopreventive potential of volatile oil from black cumin seeds, Nigella sativa L., in a rat multi-organ carcinogenesis bioassay; Oncol Lett. Sep 2010; 1(5): 913–924.

223 - Woo CC, Kumar AP, Sethi G, , Thymoquinone: potential cure for inflammatory disorders and cancer. Biochem Pharmacol. 2012 Feb 15;83(4):443-51.

224 - Alsayed T Salim; Cancer chemopreventive potential of volatile oil from black cumin seeds, Nigella sativa L., in a rat multi-organ carcinogenesis bioassay; Oncol Lett. Sep 2010; 1(5): 913–924.

225 - Hamed MA1, El-Rigal NS, Ali SA.; Effects of black seed oil on resolution of hepato-renal toxicity induced bybromobenzene in rats.; Eur Rev Med Pharmacol Sci. 2013 Mar;17(5):569-81.

226 - Woo CC, Kumar AP, Sethi G, , Thymoquinone: potential cure for inflammatory disorders and cancer. Biochem Pharmacol. 2012 Feb 15;83(4):443-51.

227 - Abdullah O Bamosa, Huda Kaatabi, Fatma M Lebdaa, Abdul-Muhssen Al Elq, Ali Al-Sultanb. Effect of Nigella sativa seeds on the glycemic control of patients with type 2 diabetes mellitus. Indian J Physiol Pharmacol. 2010 Oct-Dec;54(4):344-54.

228 - Kamal Mahmoud Saleh Mansi, Effects of Oral Administration of Water Extract of Nigella saliva on Serum Concentrations of Insulin and Testosterone in Alloxan-induced Diabetic Rats , Pakistan Jownal of Biological Sciences 8 (8): 1152-1156, 2005

229 - Murli L. Mathura, b, Jyoti Gaura; Antidiabetic Properties of a Spice Plant Nigella sativa; Journal of Endocrinology and Metabolism Volume 1, Number 1, April 2011, pages 1-8

230 - Hasani-Ranjbar S1, Jouyandeh Z; A systematic review of anti-obesity medicinal plants - an update.; J Diabetes Metab Disord. 2013 Jun 19;12(1):28

231 - Dehkordi FR, Kamkhah AF.; Antihypertensive effect of Nigella sativa seed extract in patients with mild hypertension.;Fundam Clin Pharmacol. 2008 Aug;22(4):447-52

232 - Ali BH1, Blunden G. Pharmacological and toxicological properties of Nigella sativa., Phytother Res. 2003 Apr;17(4):299-305.

233 - National Institute of Allergy and Infectious Diseases – March 2014 _ http://www.niaid.nih.gov/topics/antimicrobialResistance/understanding/Pages/quickFacts.aspx

234 - Michael Gilmore , Superbug: An Epidemic Begins – Harvard Magazine

235 - Mohd Tariq Salman, Rahat Ali Khan, In vitro antimicrobial activity of Nigella sativa oil against multi-drug resistant bacteria, Jawaharlal Nehru Medical College, Aligarh Muslim University, Aligarh 202002. India

236 - Hannan A1, Saleem S; Anti bacterial activity of Nigella sativa against clinical isolates of methicillin resistant Staphylococcus aureus;J Ayub Med Coll Abbottabad. 2008 Jul-Sep;20(3):72-4.

237 - Hannan A1, Saleem S; Anti bacterial activity of Nigella sativa against clinical isolates of methicillin resistant Staphylococcus aureus;J Ayub Med Coll Abbottabad. 2008 Jul-Sep;20(3):72-4.

238 - M Al-Somat, A Al-Adhal, Susceptibility of Clinical Bacterial Isolates and Control Strains to Nigella sativa Oil, Britisch biomedical bulletin 2 (1),95-103

239 - Salem EM1, Yar T, Bamosa AO, Al-Quorain, Comparative study of Nigella Sativa and triple therapy in eradication of Helicobacter Pylori in patients with non-ulcer dyspepsia. Saudi J Gastroenterol. 2010 Jul-Sep;16(3):207-14.

240 - W. A. El-Shouny and S. Magaam, "Sensitivity of Multi-drug Resistant Pseudomonas aeruginosa isolated from surgical wound-infections to essential oils and plant Extracts," World Journal of medical Sciences, vol. 4, pp. 104–111, 2009.

241 - Taha, M.; Azeiz, A. Z. Abdel; antifungal effect of thymol, thymoquinone and thymohydroquinone against yeasts, dermatophytes and non-dermatophyte molds isolated from skin and nails fungal infections; December 2010 Egyptian Journal of Biochemistry & Molecular Biology;Dec2010, Vol. 28 Issue 2, p109

242 - M Al-Somat, A Al-Adhal, Susceptibility of Clinical Bacterial Isolates and Control Strains to Nigella sativa Oil, Britisch biomedical bulletin 2 (1),95-103

243 - Gilani AH, Aziz N, Bronchodilator, spasmolytic and calcium antagonist activities of Nigella sativa seeds (Kalonji): a traditional herbal product with multiple medicinal uses. J Pak Med Assoc. 2001 Mar;51(3):115-20.

244 - Gilani AH, Aziz N, Bronchodilator, spasmolytic and calcium antagonist activities of Nigella sativa seeds (Kalonji): a traditional herbal product with multiple medicinal uses. J Pak Med Assoc. 2001 Mar;51(3):115-20.

245 - Abbas AT et al 2005. Effect of dexamethasone and Nigella sativa on peripheral blood eosinophil count, IgG1 and IgG2a, cytokine profiles and lung inflammation in murine model of allergic asthma. Egypt J Immunol. 2005;12(1):95-102

246 - Abbas AT et al 2005. Effect of dexamethasone and Nigella sativa on peripheral blood eosinophil count, IgG1 and IgG2a, cytokine profiles and lung inflammation in murine model of allergic asthma. Egypt J Immunol. 2005;12(1):95-102

247 - Ali BH1, Blunden G. Pharmacological and toxicological properties of Nigella sativa., Phytother Res. 2003 Apr;17(4):299-305.

248 - Taha, M.; Azeiz, A. Z. Abdel; antifungal effect of thymol, thymoquinone and thymohydroquinone against yeasts, dermatophytes and non-dermatophyte molds isolated from skin and nails fungal infections; December 2010 Egyptian Journal of Biochemistry & Molecular Biology;Dec2010, Vol. 28 Issue 2, p109

249 - Al-Ghamdi MS. The anti-inflammatory, analgesic and antipyretic activity of Nigella sativa. J Ethnopharmacol. 2001 Jun;76(1):45-8.

250 - J.A.A. Al-Sa'aidi, A.L.D. Al-Khuzai Effect of alcoholic extract of Nigella sativa on fertility in male rats, Iraqi Journal of Veterinary Sciences, Vol. 23, Supplement II, 2009 (123-128)

251 - El-Abhar HS, Abdallah DM, Gastroprotective activity of Nigella sativa oil and its constituent, thymoquinone, against gastric mucosal injury induced by ischaemia/reperfusion in rats. J Ethnopharmacol. 2003 Feb;84(2-3):251-8.

252 - Al Mofleh IA, Alhaider AA Gastroprotective effect of an aqueous suspension of black cumin Nigella sativa on necrotizing agents-induced gastric injury in experimental animals. Saudi J Gastroenterol. 2008 Jul;14(3):128-34

253 - Kanter M1, Demir H Gastroprotective activity of Nigella sativa L oil and its constituent, thymoquinone against acute alcohol-induced gastric mucosal injury in rats.World J Gastroenterol. 2005 Nov 14;11(42):6662-6.

254 - Mizuno T, Zhuang C, Abe K, Okamoto H, Kiho T, Ukai S, Leclerec S, Meijer L. Antitumor and hypoglycemic activities of polysaccharides from the sclerotia and mycelia of Inonotus obliquus (Per.:Fr.) Pil. Intl J Med Mushrooms. 1999;1:301–316.

255 - N.A. Bisko, N.Y.Mitropolskaya; Melanin Complex from Medicinal Mushroom Inonotus obliquus (Pers.: Fr.) Pilat (Chaga) (Aphyllophoromycetideae); International Journal of Medicinal Mushrooms, Volume 4, 2002 Issue 2

256 - N.A. Bisko, N.Y.Mitropolskaya; Melanin Complex from Medicinal Mushroom Inonotus obliquus (Pers.: Fr.) Pilat (Chaga) (Aphyllophoromycetideae); International Journal of Medicinal Mushrooms, Volume 4, 2002 Issue 2

257 - Rzymowska J.; The effect of aqueous extracts from Inonotus obliquus on the mitotic index and enzyme activities; Boll Chim Farm. 1998 Jan;137(1):13-5.

258 - Kahlos K, Kahlos L, Hiltunen R. Antitumor tests of inotodiol from the fungus Inonotus obliquus. Acta Pharm Fennica. 1986;95:173–177.

259 - Hyun KW, Jeong SC; Isolation and characterization of a novel platelet aggregation inhibitory peptide from the medicinal mushroom. Inonotus obliquus. 2006 Peptides 27: 1173–1178.

260 - Burczyk J, Gawron A; Antimitotic activity of aqueous extracts of Inonotus obliquus.; Boll Chim Farm. 1996 May;135(5):306-9.

261 - Sung Hak Lee, Hee Sun Hwang ; Antitumor Activity of Water Extract of a Mushroom, Inonotus obliquus, against HT-29 Human Colon Cancer Cells; Phytother. Res. (2009)

262 - Lee SH, Hwang HS, Yun JW.; Antitumor activity of water extract of a mushroom, Inonotus obliquus, against HT-29 human colon cancer cells.; Phytother Res. 2009 Dec;23(12):1784-9.

263 - Mizuno T, Zhuang C, Abe K, Okamoto H, Kiho T, Ukai S, Leclerec S, Meijer L. Antitumor and hypoglycemic activities of polysaccharides from the sclerotia and mycelia of Inonotus obliquus (Per.:Fr.) Pil. Intl J Med Mushrooms. 1999;1:301–316.

264 - Lemieszek MK, Langner E, ; Anti-cancer effects of fraction isolated from fruiting bodies of Chaga medicinal mushroom, Inonotus obliquus (Pers.:Fr.) Pilát (Aphyllophoromycetideae); Int J Med Mushrooms. 2011;13(2):131-43.

265 - Mi Ja Chung, Cha-Kwon Chung, Yoonhwa Jeong; Anti-cancer activity of subfractions containing pure compounds of Chaga mushroom (Inonotus obliquus) extract in human cancer cells and in Balbc/c mice bearing Sarcoma-180 cells; Nutr Res Pract. Jun 2010; 4(3): 177–182.

266 - Caifa Chen, Weifa Zheng,; Aqueous Extract of Inonotus bliquus (Fr.) Pilat (Hymenochaetaceae) Significantly Inhibits the Growth of Sarcoma 180 by Inducing Apoptosis; American Journal of Pharmacology and Toxicology Volume 2, Issue 1

267 - Myung-Ja Youn, Jin-Kyung Kim, ; Chaga mushroom (Inonotus obliquus) induces G0/G1 arrest and apoptosis in human hepatoma HepG2 cells; World J Gastroenterol. Jan 28, 2008; 14(4): 511–517.

268 - Kim YO, Park HW, ; Anti-cancer effect and structural characterization of endo-polysaccharide from cultivated mycelia of Inonotus obliquus.; Life Sci. 2006 May 30;79(1):72-80. Epub 2006 Feb 3.

269 - Mi Ja Chung, Cha-Kwon Chung, Yoonhwa Jeong; Anti-cancer activity of subfractions containing pure compounds of Chaga mushroom (Inonotus obliquus) extract in human cancer cells and in Balbc/c mice bearing Sarcoma-180 cells; Nutr Res Pract. Jun 2010; 4(3): 177–182.

270 - Kahlos K, Kangas L, Hiltunen R. Antitumor activity of some compounds and fractions from an n-hexane extract of Inonotus obliquus in vitro Acta Pharm Fennica 1987; 96: 33–40

271 - N.A. Bisko, N.Y.Mitropolskaya; Melanin Complex from Medicinal Mushroom Inonotus obliquus (Pers.: Fr.) Pilat (Chaga) (Aphyllophoromycetideae); International Journal of Medicinal Mushrooms, Volume 4, 2002 Issue 2

272 - Rzymowska J.; The effect of aqueous extracts from Inonotus obliquus on the mitotic index and enzyme activities; Boll Chim Farm. 1998 Jan;137(1):13-5.

273 - Cui Y, Kim DS, Park KC.; Antioxidant effect of Inonotus obliquus.; J Ethnopharmacol. 2005 Jan 4;96(1-2):79-85.

274 - Rzymowska J.; The effect of aqueous extracts from Inonotus obliquus on the mitotic index and enzyme activities. ; Boll Chim Farm. 1998 Jan;137(1):13-5.

275 - Park YK, Lee HB; Chaga mushroom extract inhibits oxidative DNA damage in human lymphocytes as assessed by comet assay.;Biofactors. 2004;21(1-4):109-12.

276 - Babitskaya VG, Scherba VV, Ikonnikova NV, Bisko NA, Mitropolskaya NY. Melanin complex from medicinal mushroom Inonotus obliquus (Pers.:Fr.) Pilat (Chaga) (Aphyllophoromycetidae) Int J Med Mushrooms. 2002;4:139–4

277 - Ham SS, Kim SH, Antimutagenic effects of subfractions of Chaga mushroom (Inonotus obliquus) extract.; Mutat Res. 2009 Jan;672(1):55-9

278 - Sun JE, Ao ZH, ; Antihyperglycemic and antilipidperoxidative effects of dry matter of culture broth of Inonotus obliquus in submerged culture on normal and alloxan-diabetes mice.; J Ethnopharmacol. 2008 Jun 19;118(1):7-13

279 - Joo JI, Kim DH; Extract of Chaga mushroom (Inonotus obliquus) stimulates 3T3-L1 adipocyte differentiation.; Phytother Res. 2010 Nov;24(11):1592-9

280 - Takashi Mizuno , Cun Zhuang; Antitumor and Hypoglycemic Activities of Polysaccharides from the Sclerotia and Mycelia of Inonotus obliquus Int J Medicinal Mushrooms; Volume 1, 1999 Issue 4

281 - Najafzadeh M, Reynolds PD, Baumgartner A, ; Chaga mushroom extract inhibits oxidative DNA damage in lymphocytes of patients with inflammatory bowel disease. ; Biofactors. 2007;31(3-4):191-200.

282 - Ham SS, Kim SH, Antimutagenic effects of subfractions of Chaga mushroom (Inonotus obliquus) extract.; Mutat Res. 2009 Jan;672(1):55-9

283 - Hyun KW, Jeong SC; Isolation and characterization of a novel platelet aggregation inhibitory peptide from the medicinal mushroom. Inonotus obliquus. 2006 Peptides 27: 1173–1178.

284 - Park YM, Won JH, ; In vivo and in vitro anti-inflammatory and anti-nociceptive effects of the methanol extract of Inonotus obliquus.; J Ethnopharmacol. 2005 Oct 3;101(1-3):120-8.

285 - Ko SK, Jin M, Pyo MY.; Inonotus obliquus extracts suppress antigen-specific IgE production through the modulation of Th1/Th2 cytokines in ovalbumin-sensitized mice.;J Ethnopharmacol. 2011 Oct 11;137(3):1077-82.

286 - Kim YO, Han SB, Immuno-stimulating effect of the endo-polysaccharide produced by submerged culture of Inonotus obliquus.; Life Sci. 2005 Sep 23;77(19):2438-56.

287 - Joo JI, Kim DH; Extract of Chaga mushroom (Inonotus obliquus) stimulates 3T3-L1 adipocyte differentiation. Phytother Res. 2010 Nov;24(11):1592-9.

288 - Mizuno T, Zhuang C, Abe K, Okamoto H, Kiho T, Ukai S, Leclerec S, Meijer L. Antitumor and hypoglycemic activities of polysaccharides from the sclerotia and mycelia of Inonotus obliquus (Per.:Fr.) Pil. Intl J Med Mushrooms. 1999;1:301–316.

289 - Gyllenhaal C. Ef_cacy and safety of herbal stimulants and sedatives in sleep disorders. Sleep Med Rev. 2000;4(2).

290 - Sarris, J; Panossian, A; Schweitzer, I; Stough, C; Scholey, A (December 2011). "Herbal medicine for depression, anxiety, and insomnia: a review of psychopharmacology and clinical evidence". European neuropsychopharmacology 21 (12): 841–860. doi:10.1016/j.euroneuro.2011.04.002. PMID 21601431.

291 - Khayyal MT, el-Ghazaly MA, Kenawy SA, et al. Antiulcerogenic effect of some gastrointestinally acting plant extracts and their combination. Arzneimittelforschung 2001;51(7):545-553.

292 - American Chemical Society. "Chamomile Tea: New Evidence Supports Health Benefits." ScienceDaily. ScienceDaily, 4 January 2005.

293 - Atsushi Kato, Yuka Minoshima, et al. Protective Effects of Dietary Chamomile Tea on Diabetic Complication, J. Agric. Food Chem., 2008, 56 (17), pp 8206–8211

294 - Martins MD, Marques MM, Bussadori SK, Martins MA, Pavesi VC, Mesquita-Ferrari RA, Fernandes KP. Comparative analysis between Chamomilla recutita and corticosteroids on wound healing. An in vitro and in vivo study. Phytother Res. 2009 Feb;23(2):274-8.

295 - Atsushi Kato, Yuka Minoshima, Jo Yamamoto et al, Protective Effects of Dietary Chamomile Tea on Diabetic Complications, J. Agric. Food Chem., 2008, 56 (17), pp 8206–8211

296 - Janmejai K Srivastava, Eswar Shankar, and Sanjay Gupta, Chamomile: A herbal medicine of the past with bright future, Mol Med Report. Author manuscript; available in PMC Feb 1, 2011.

297 - Ashok Kumar Panda and Kailash Chandra Swain, Traditional uses and medicinal potential of Cordyceps sinensis of Sikkim, J Ayurveda Integr Med. 2011 Jan-Mar; 2(1): 9–13

298 - Zhu JS, Halpen GM, Jones K. The scientific of an ancient Chinese medicine: Cordyceps sinensis. Part-1. J Altern Complement Med. 1998;4:289–303

299 - Zhu JS, Halpen GM, Jones K. The Scientific study of an ancient Chinese medicine: Cordyceps sinensis. Part-2. J Altern Complement Med. 1998;4:429–57

300 - Wang ZX, Wang XM, Wang TZ. Current status of pharmacological studies on Cordyceps sinensis and Cordyceps hyphae. Chung-Kuo Chung His I Chieh ho Tsa Chih. 1995;15:255–6

301 - de Paiva Gonçalves, Ortega AA; Chemopreventive activity of systemically administered curcumin on oral cancer in the 4-nitroquinoline 1-oxide model; J Cell Biochem. 2014 Dec 16.

302 - Eom DW, Lee JH; Synergistic effect of curcumin on epigallocatechin gallate-induced anti-cancer action in PC3 prostate cancer cells. ; BMB Rep. 2014 Dec 2.

303 - Michal Heger, Zinc phthalocyanine-containing multi-targeting liposomes for the treatment of solid tumors by photodynamic therapy following chemopreventive preconditioning with curcumin, AMC, afdeling AMC-Experimentele chirurgie

304 - S.K. Krishnadath Evaluation of dendritic cell therapy and curcumin as a combinatorial therapy for treating oesophageal cancer, AMC, afdeling; Gastro-enterologie en Hepatologie

305 - Aggarwal, Bharat B.; Shishodia, Shishir (2006). "Molecular targets of dietary agents for prevention and therapy of cancer". Biochemical Pharmacology 71 (10): 1397–421. doi:10.1016/j.bcp.2006.02.009

306 - Choi, H.; Chun, Y.-S.; Kim, S.-W.; Kim, M.-S.; Park, J.-W. (2006). "Curcumin Inhibits Hypoxia-Inducible Factor-1 by Degrading Aryl Hydrocarbon Receptor Nuclear Translocator: A Mechanism of Tumor Growth Inhibition". Molecular Pharmacology 70 (5): 1664–71.

307 - Ströfer, Mareike; Jelkmann, Wolfgang; Depping, Reinhard (2011). "Curcumin Decreases Survival of Hep3B Liver and MCF-7 Breast Cancer Cells". Strahlentherapie und Onkologie 187 (7): 393–400.

308 - Roschek B Jr1, Fink RC, McMichael MD, Li D, Alberte RS. "Elderberry flavonoids bind to and prevent H1N1 infection in vitro."Phytochemistry. 2009 Jul;70(10):1255-61. doi: 10.1016/j. phytochem.2009.06.003

309 - Kinoshita E1, Hayashi K, Katayama H, Hayashi T, Obata A. "Anti-influenza virus effects of elderberry juice and its fractions." Biosci Biotechnol Biochem. 2012;76(9):1633-8.

310 - Rao VS1, de Melo CL, Queiroz MG, Lemos TL, Menezes DB, Melo TS, Santos FA. "Ursolic acid, a pentacyclic triterpene from Sambucus australis, prevents abdominal adiposity in mice fed a high-fat diet." J Med Food. 2011 Nov;14(11):1375-82. doi: 10.1089/ jmf.2010.0267.

311 - Cao GW, Yang WG, Du P, Observation of the effects of LAK/ IL-2 therapy combining with Lycium barbarum polysaccharides in the treatment of 75 cancer patients, Second Military Medical University, Department of Microbiology, Shanghai. Zhonghua Zhong liu za zhi [Chinese Journal of Oncology] [1994, 16(6):428-431]

312 - Drake, Victoria J. Ph.D., Linus Pauling Institute, Oregon State University, Carotenoids & Health Laboratory, 2009, June.

313 - Enginar H, Cemek M, Karaca T, Unak P., Effect of grape seed extract on lipid peroxidation, antioxidant activity and peripheral blood lymphocytes in rats exposed to x-radiation., Phytother Res. 2007 Nov;21(11):1029-35.

314 - Vigna GB, Costantini F, Aldini G, et. al., Effect of a standardized grape seed extract on low-density lipoprotein susceptibility to oxidation in heavy smokers., Metabolism. 2003 Oct;52(10):1250-7.

315 - N. Yahara, I. Tofani, K. Maki, K. Kojima, Y. Kojima, M. Kimura , Mechanical assessment of effects of grape seed proanthocyanidins extract on tibial bone diaphysis in rats, J Musculoskelet Neuronal Interact 2005; 5(2):162-169

316 - Asha Devi S, Sagar Chandrasekar BK, Manjula KR, Ishii N., Grape seed proanthocyanidin lowers brain oxidative stress in adult and middle-aged rats. Exp Gerontol. 2011 Nov;46(11):958-64. doi: 10.1016/j.exger.2011.08.006

317 - Bagchi D, Sen CK, Ray SD, et al. Molecular mechanisms of cardioprotection by a novel grape seed proanthocyanidin extract. Mutat Res. 2003;523- 524:87-97.

318 - Mezadri T, Villan˜o M, Fernandez-Pachon M, Garcia-Parrilla M, Troncoso A (2008). "Antioxidant compounds and antioxidant activity in acerola(Malpighia emarginata DC.) fruits and derivatives". Journal of Food Composition and Analysis 21 (4): 282-290.

319 - Shimoda, Hiroshi, et al. "Inhibitory effect of green coffee bean extract on fat accumulation and body weight gain in mice," Oryza Oil & Fat Chemical Co., Ltd., Research & Development Division, 1 Numata Kitagata-cho, Ichinomiya, Aichi 493-8001, Japan. BMC Complement Altern Med. 2006; 6: 9.

320 - Ochiai R, Chikama A, Kataoka K, et al. Effects of hydroxyhydroquinone-reduced coffee on vasoreactivity and blood pressure. Hypertens Res. 2009 Nov;32(11):969-74.

321 - Setiawan VW, Zhang ZF, Yu GP, et al. Protective effect of green tea on the risks of chronic gastritis and stomach cancer. Int J Cancer. 2001;92(4):600-604.

322 - Shankar S, Ganapathy S, Hingorani SR, Srivastava RK. EGCG inhibits growth, invasion, angiogenesis and metastasis of pancreatic cancer. Front Biosci. 2008;13:440-52.

323 - Yuan JM. Green tea and prevention of esophageal and lung cancers. Mol Nutr Food Res. 2011 Jun;55(6):886-904.

324 - Nakachi K1, Suemasu K, Suga K, Takeo T, Imai K, Higashi Y., Influence of drinking green tea on breast cancer malignancy among Japanese patients. Jpn J Cancer Res. 1998 Mar;89(3):254-61.

325 - Kovacs EM, Lejeune MP, Nijs I, Westerterp-Plantenga MS. Effects of green tea on weight maintenance after body-weight loss. Br J Nutr Mar 1, 2004;91(3):431-437.

326 - Westerterp-Plantenga MS, Lejeune MP, Kovacs EM. Body weight and weight maintenance in relation to habitual caffeine intake and green tea. Obes Res Jul 2005;13(7):1195-1204.

327 - Diepvens K, Westerterp KR, Westerterp-Plantenga MS. Obesity and thermogenesis related to the consumption of caffeine, ephedrine, capsaicin and green tea. Am J Physiol Regul Integr Comp Physiol. 2007;292(1):R77-85

328 - Haskell CF, Kennedy DO, Milne AL, Wesnes KA, Scholey AB (2008). "The effects of l-theanine, caffeine and their combination on cognition and mood". Biol Psychol 77 (2): 113–22.

329 - Juneja LR, Chu D-C, Okubo T, et al. L-theanine a unique amino acid of green tea and its relaxation effect in humans. Trends Food Sci Tech 1999; 10:199-204.

330 - Juneja, LR; Chu, DC; Okubo, T; Nagato, Y; Yokogoshi, H. (1999). "L-Theanine - a unique amino acid of green tea and its relaxation effect in humans". Trends in Food Science & Technology 10 (2): 199–204.

331 - Yokozawa T, Dong E. In_uence of green tea and its three major components upon low-density lipoprotein oxidation. Exp Toxicol Pathol 1997; 49(5):329-335.

332 - Kakuda T, Nozawa A, Unno T, et al. Inhibiting effects of theanine on caffeine stimulation evaluated by EEG in the rat. Biosci Biotechno Biochem 2000; 64:287-293.

333 - Mason R. 200 mg of Zen; L-theanine boosts alpha waves, promotes alert relaxation. Alternative & Complementary Therapies 2001,April; 7:91-95

334 - Degenring FH, Suter A, Weber M, et al. A randomised double blind placebo controlled clinical trial of a standardised extract of fresh Crataegus berries (Crataegisan) in the treatment of patients with congestive heart failure NYHA II. Phytomedicine 2003;10(5):363-369.

335 - Fugh-Berman A. Herbs and dietary supplements in the prevention and treatment of cardiovascular disease. Prev Cardiol. 2000;3(1):24-32.

336 - Pittler MH, Schmidt K, Ernst E. Hawthorn extract for treating chronic heart failure: meta-analysis of randomized trials. Am J Med 2003;114(8):665-674.

337 - Tadic VM, Dobric S, Markovic GM, Dordevic SM, Arsic IA, Menkovic NR, Stevic T. Anti-in_ammatory, gastroprotective, free-radical-scavenging, and antimicrobial activities of hawthorn berries ethanol extract. J Agric Food Chem. 2008 Sep 10;56(17):7700-9.
338 - Schandry R, Duschek S. The effect of Camphor-Crataegus berry extract combination on blood pressure and mental functions in chronic hypotension - a randomized placebo controlled double blind design. Phytomedicine. 2008 Oct 15.
339 - Fugh-Berman A. Herbs and dietary supplements in the prevention and treatment of cardiovascular disease. Prev Cardiol. 2000;3(1):24-32.
340 - Nanba H, Kubo K. Effect of maitake D-fraction on cancer prevention. Ann NY Acad Sci. 1997;833:204-207
341 - Nanba H. Activity of maitake D-fraction to inhibit carcinogenesis and metastasis. Ann NY Acad Sci. 1995;768:243-245.
342 - Lin H, de Stanchina E, Zhou XK, et al. Maitake beta-glucan promotes recovery of leukocytes and myeloid cell function in peripheral blood from paclitaxel hematotoxicity. Cancer Immunol Immunother. 2010 Jun;59(6):885-897.
343 - Kubo K, Nanba H, The effect of maitake mushrooms on liver and serum lipids. Alternative Therapies in Health and Medicine [1996, 2(5):62-66] Department of Microbial Chemistry, Kobe Pharmaceutical University, Japan.
344 - Nanba H, Kubo K. Effect of maitake D-fraction on cancer prevention. Ann NY Acad Sci. 1997;833:204-207.
345 - Jung HA, Su BN, Keller WJ, Mehta RG, Kinghorn AD (March 2006). "Antioxidant xanthones from the pericarp of Garcinia mangostana (Mangosteen)". Journal of Agricultural and Food Chemistry 54 (6): 2077–82.
346 - Escribano-Bailón MT, Alcalde-Eon C, Muñoz O, Rivas-Gonzalo JC, Santos-Buelga C (2006). "Anthocyanins in berries of Maqui (Aristotelia chilensis (Mol.) Stuntz)". Phytochem Anal 17 (1: Jan-Feb): 8–14
347 - Suwalsky, M, et al; "Human erythrocytes are affected in vitro by _avonoids of Aristotelia chilensis (Maqui) leaves;" Int J Pharm. 2008 Nov 3; 363(1-2):85-90.

348 - Miranda-Rottmann S, Aspillaga AA, Pérez DD, Vasquez L, Martinez AL, Leighton F. "Juice and phenolic fractions of the berry Aristotelia chilensis inhibit LDL oxidation in vitro and protect human endothelial cells against oxidative stress." J Agric Food Chem. 2002 Dec 18;50(26):7542-7.

349 - Muñoz O, Christen P, Cretton S, Backhouse N, Torres V, Correa O, Costa E, Miranda H, Delporte C. "Chemical study and anti-inflammatory, analgesic and antioxidant activities of the leaves of Aristotelia chilensis (Mol.) Stuntz, Elaeocarpaceae." J Pharm Pharmacol. 2011 Jun;63(6):849-59.

350 - Heinicke R. The pharmacologically active ingredient of Noni. Bulletin of the National Tropical Botanical Garden, 1985

351 - Heinicke R. The Xeronine system: a new cellular mechanism that explains the health promoting action of NONI and Bromelian. DirectSource Publishing; 2001

352 - Wang, Mian-Ying; et al (2009). "Antioxidant activity of noni juice in heavy smokers". Chemistry Central Journal 3: 13.

353 - Duncan SH, Flint HJ, Stewart CS. Inhibitory activity of gut bacteria against Es cherichia coli 0157 mediated by dietary plant metabolites. FEMS Microbiol Lett 1998; 164: 283-58

354 - Solomon N. The Noni phenomenon. Discover the powerful tropical healer that fights cancer, lowers high blood pres sure and relieves chronic pain. Direct Source Publishing; 1999.

355 - Wang MY1, West BJ, Jensen CJ, Nowicki D, Su C, Palu AK, Anderson G. "Morinda citrifolia (Noni): a literature review and recent advances in Noni research." Acta Pharmacol Sin. 2002 Dec;23(12):1127-41.

356 - American Chemical Society: Noni plant may yield new drugs to fight tuberculosis. Press release the 2000 International Chemical Congress of Pacific Basin Societies. 2000.

357 - Locher CP, Burch MT, Mower HF, Beres tecky J , Davis H, Van Poel B, et al. Anti-microbiol activity and anti-complement activity of extract obtained from s elected Hawaiian medicinal plants. J Ethnopharm 1995; 49: 23-32.

358 - American Chemical Society: Noni plant may yield new drugs to fight tuberculosis. Press releas e the 2000 International

359 - Bushnell OA, Fukuda M, Makinodian T. The antibacterial properties of some plants found in Hawaii. Pacific Science 1950; 4: 167-83.

360 - Schubert SY, Lansky EP, Neeman I (July, 1999). "Antioxidant and eicosanoid enzyme inhibition properties of pomegranate seed oil and fermented juice flavonoids". J Ethnopharmacol 66 (1): 11–17.

361 - L. Mengoni E.S., Vichera G., Rigano L.A., et.al "Suppression of COX-2, IL-1_ and TNF-_ expression and leukocyte infiltration in inflamed skin by bioactive compounds from Rosmarinus officinalis" Fitoterapia 2011 82:3 (414-421)

362 - Paller CJ, et al. A randomized phase II study of pomegranate extract for men with rising PSA following initial therapy for localized prostate cancer. Prostate Cancer and Prostatic Diseases. 2013;16:50.

363 - Pantuck AJ, et al. Phase II study of pomegranate juice for men with rising prostate-specific antigen following surgery or radiation for prostate cancer. Clinical Cancer Research. 2006;12:4018.

364 - Koyama S, et al. Pomegranate extract induces apoptosis in human prostate cancer cells by modulation of the IGF-IGFBP axis. Growth Hormone and IGF Research. 2010;20:55.

365 - Chan WK, Lam DT, Law HK, et al. Ganoderma lucidum mycelium and spore extracts as natural adjuvants for immunotherapy. J Altern Complement Med. 2005 Dec;11(6):1047-57.

366 - G.Q. Qiu, X. Qiao; Hippophaë 10 (4) 39-41 (1997)

367 - Dharmananda S. Sea buckthorn, Institute of Traditional Medicine Online, 2004

368 - Jong SC. and Birmingham JM. Medicinal and therapeutic value of the shiitake mushroom. Advances in applied microbiology 39, 153-184 (1993)

369 - Chihara G, Hamuro J, Maeda Y, Shiio T, Suga T, Takasuka N, Sasaki T. Antitumor and metastasis-inhibitory activities of lentinan as an immunomodulator: an overview. Cancer Detect Prev Suppl. 1987;1:423-443

370 - Ikekawa T, 1969. Antitumor activity of aqueous extracts of edible mushrooms. Cancer Res 29(3), 734-735

371 - Mori, H.1987. Effect of immunostimulants and antitumor agents on tumor necrosis factor (TNF) production. Int. J. Immunopharmacol. 9: 881-882.

372 - Borchers AT, Stern JS, Hackman RM, Keen CL, Gershwin ME. Mushrooms, tumors, and immunity. Proc Soc Exp Biol Med. 1999;221:281-293.

373 - Fang N, Li Q, Yu S, Zhang J, He L, Ronis MJ, Badger TM. Inhibition of growth and induction of apoptosis in human cancer cell lines by an ethyl acetate fraction from shiitake mushrooms. J Altern Complement Med. 2006;12:125-132.

374 - Laraine C. Abbey, R.N., M.S. Functional Nutrient Deficiency in Chronically Multi-symptomatic People — A Pilot Study, Journal of Orthomolecular Medicine Vol. 4, No. 2, 1989

375 - Steven G Newmaster, Meghan Grguric, Dhivya Shanmughanandhan, et al. DNA barcoding detects contamination and substitution in North American herbal products BMC Medicine 2013, 11:222

376 - Geyer H, Parr MK, Mareck U, Reinhart U, Schrader Y, Schanzer W. Analysis of non-hormonal nutritiional supplements dor anabolicandrogenic steroids – results of an international study. Int J Sports Med. 2004; 25, 124-129

377 - Geyer H1, Parr MK, Koehler K, Mareck U, Schänzer W, Thevis M., Nutritional supplements cross-contaminated and faked with doping substances., J Mass Spectrom. 2008 Jul;43(7):892-902.

378 - Green GA, Catlin DH, Starcevic B, "Analysis of over-the-counter dietary supplements.", Clin J Sport Med. 2001 Oct;11(4):254-9.

379 - Van Thuyne W, Van Eenoo P, Delbeke FT, "Nutritional supplements: prevalence of use and contamination with doping agents.", Nutr Res Rev. 2006 Jun;19(1):147-58.

380 - Geyer H, Parr MK, Koehler K, Mareck U, Schänzer W, Thevis M, "Nutritional supplements cross-contaminated and faked with doping substances.", J Mass Spectrom. 2008 Jul;43(7):892-902.

381 - Hasegawa T, Saijo M, Ishii T, Nagata T, Haishima Y, Kawahara N, Goda Y, "Structural elucidation of a tadalafil analogue found in a dietary supplement.", Shokuhin Eiseigaku Zasshi. 2008 Aug;49(4):311-5.

382 - Judkins CM, Teale P, Hall DJ, "The role of banned substance residue analysis in the control of dietary supplement contamination.", Drug Test Anal. 2010 Sep 1.
383 - Cohen PA, Ernst E, "Safety of herbal supplements: a guide for cardiologists.", Cardiovasc Ther. 2010 Aug;28(4):246-53.
384 - Gebhart F, "Drugs' inactive ingredients drawing government attention", Drug Top.; Vol 141, Nov Suppl, P18S, 20S, 1997
385 - Pifferi G, Restani P, "The safety of pharmaceutical excipients", Farmaco. 2003 Aug;58(8):541-50.
386 - De Smet PA. Herbal remedies. N Engl J Med. 2002;347(25):2046-56.
387 - de Smet PAGM, Wagenaar HWG, Smeets OSNM. Dexamethason in eenniet-geregistreerde creme uit het Verre Oosten. Ned Tijdschr Geneeskd.1997;141(33):1626.
388 - de Smet PAGM, de Visser I, Wagenaar HWG, et al. Westerse geneesmiddelenvrij verkrijgbaar in Chinese winkels. Pharm Weekbl. 1999;134(15):614-8.
389 - de Smet PAGM, Wagenaar HWG. 'Afslankmiddelen' uit Thailand: onverwachtereizigerszorg na terugkeer. Ned Tijdschr Geneeskd. 1998;142(51):2798-800.
390 - Wagenaar HWG, Smeets OSNM. ... het WINAp achterhaalt de componentenwel. Identiteitsonderzoek belicht gevaren niet-reguliere middelen. Pharm Weekbl. 1999;134(29):974-9.
391 - Liu, Rui Hai, "Health bene_ts of fruit and vegetables are from additive and synergistic combinations of phytochemicals," Am J Clin Nutr 2003;78(suppl):517S–20S
392 - Bauman WA, Shaw S, Jayatilleke E, Spungen AM, Herbert V. Increased intake of calcium reverses vitamin B12 malabsorption induced by metformin. Diabetes Care. 2000;13(9):1227-1231.
393 - Willett WC, Stampfer MJ. What vitamins should I be taking, doctor? NEJM 2001; 345:1819-1823
394 - S Sasazuki, S Sasaki, Y Tsubono S Okubo, M Hayashi and S Tsugane "Effect of vitamin C on common cold: randomized controlled trial" European Journal of Clinical Nutrition (2006) 60, 9–17. doi:10.1038/sj.ejcn.1602261; published online 24 August 2005

395 - James E. Enstrom, Linda E. Kanim, and Morton A. Klein "Vitamin C Intake and Mortali ty among a Sample of the United States Population" Epidemiology, Vol. 3, No. 3. (May, 1992), pp. 194-202.

396 - Dietary Supplements Consumer Information: "Tips For The Savvy Supplement User: Making Informed Decisions And Evaluating Information," Jan 2002,

# Index

## A

Abdominal 169, 173, 296
Acid reflux 272
Acne 33, 134, 262
Adrenal fatigue 182, 241
Ageing 84, 89, 94, 98, 106, 170, 179,
    195, 207, 210, 213, 220, 261,
    262, 274
Aggression 173
Alcohol 14, 50, 101, 135, 169, 207,
    219, 229, 276
Allergy 48, 75, 134, 239, 261, 270, 294,
    301
Alzheimer 94, 115, 116, 117, 168, 169,
    251, 256
Anemia 62, 68, 166, 167, 170, 171,
    174, 175, 176, 177, 178, 191,
    197, 198, 266
Anxiety 4, 48, 152, 169, 173, 192, 197,
    208, 238, 239, 258
Apathy 197, 233
Aphrodisiac 248, 249, 268
Arteries 172, 177, 179, 180, 181, 182,
    187, 194, 195, 196, 210, 212,
    241, 250, 257, 258, 261, 267, 268
*Calcification 189*

Arteriosclerosis 116, 134, 255, 263
Arthritis 26, 69, 200, 207, 226, 227,
    245
Asthma 26, 94, 159, 233, 240, 242,
    247, 270, 272
Athletes 187, 235, 302
Attention deficit 36, 65, 137, 169, 174,
    175, 208, 226, 281, 291
Autism 233

# B

Bacterial 7, 40, 43, 46, 51, 53, 56, 57, 63, 64, 65, 108, 110, 123, 130, 147, 149, 166, 201, 203, 224, 229, 230, 231, 232, 238, 245, 246, 256, 265, 292, 302

Bladder 167, 256, 262

*Infection 167, 262*

Bleeding 34, 177, 178, 180, 182, 189

*Nose 189*

Blindness 136, 154, 165, 201, 241, 331

Bloating 169, 245, 324

Blood 4, 17, 43, 49, 50, 51, 53, 82, 94, 108, 109, 115, 117, 134, 135, 136, 137, 140, 166, 170, 171, 172, 174, 179, 180, 181, 182, 184, 185, 186, 187, 188, 189, 190, 191, 194, 195, 196, 197, 198, 199, 200, 201, 206, 210, 212, 213, 219, 220, 222, 223, 226, 230, 233, 236, 237, 238, 239, 246, 247, 250, 251, 253, 256, 257, 258, 260, 262, 263, 264, 266, 267, 268, 269, 270, 282, 297, 325, 330

*Pressure 4, 17, 43, 53, 94, 134, 135, 140, 180, 182, 191, 194, 197, 200, 206, 210, 212, 213, 219, 220, 230, 233, 246, 253, 256, 257, 258, 260, 262, 263, 264, 266, 267, 268, 269, 270, 282, 325*

*Stool 198*

*Sugar 17, 184, 186, 212, 222, 238, 239, 253, 256, 260, 269*

*Urine 189*

Bone 22, 26, 41, 49, 50, 67, 69, 70, 71, 86, 154, 159, 165, 166, 172, 179, 181, 183, 184, 185, 186, 188, 189, 191, 192, 193, 194, 196, 199, 200, 202, 221, 251, 266, 268, 329, 330, 332, 370

*Cancer 69*

*Fractures 67, 69, 149, 196, 199, 251*

*Osteopenia 189*

*Osteoporosis 26, 41, 184, 185, 186, 188, 189, 196, 199, 268*

*Pain 22, 154, 186, 194*

*Skeleton 83*

*Strengthening 268*

Bowel 4, 52, 153, 169, 236, 243

Brain 23, 30, 49, 50, 51, 83, 109, 114, 115, 116, 117, 168, 174, 179, 180, 184, 193, 206, 209, 211, 226, 251, 255, 256, 266, 329

Breast 57, 58, 185, 233, 255

Breathing 91, 149, 242

Bronchial 26, 159, 233, 240, 242, 247, 270

Bruising 177, 178, 182, 189

Burnout 282

# C

Cancer 1, 4, 48, 51, 54, 56, 57, 58, 59, 62, 64, 85, 91, 94, 106, 108, 111, 112, 134, 137, 138, 139, 140, 149, 158, 164, 166, 172, 180, 185, 187, 190, 191, 199, 203, 207, 211, 226, 227, 229, 233, 235, 236, 237, 240, 243, 244, 245, 249, 251, 254, 255, 256, 259, 260, 264, 267, 268, 270, 273, 274, 283, 297, 302, 325, 330, 354, 373

Cardiovascular 185, 187, 188, 189, 193, 206, 207, 213, 220, 223, 242, 261, 262, 271, 274, 329, 331

Carpal Tunnel 174

Children 3, 9, 10, 20, 23, 40, 62, 65, 67, 68, 74, 75, 86, 100, 110, 113, 123, 146, 147, 150, 159, 176, 178, 194, 281, 328, 354

# D

# E

Ear 50
Eczema 43, 175, 239, 262, 281, 282
Elderly 40, 149, 177, 231, 328
Elevates mood 224, 268, 272
Emotions 1, 2, 4, 16, 26, 73, 91, 96,
  103, 114, 138, 152, 174, 190,
  208, 246, 247, 255, 283, 341,
  342, 363
Endurance 241, 242
Energy 3, 4, 10, 22, 23, 32, 33, 46, 48,
  61, 73, 78, 81, 82, 83, 87, 91, 92,
  114, 115, 117, 145, 146, 152,
  161, 168, 170, 190, 195, 197,
  198, 209, 210, 211, 213, 219,
  220, 224, 233, 241, 242, 251,
  258, 264, 270, 273, 285, 292,
  323, 332, 346, 358, 363, 366, 379
Erectile 201, 233, 240, 241, 268
Esophageal 243, 255, 256
Estrogen 53, 58
Excretion 41, 43, 70, 377, 378
Eye 50, 51, 98, 114, 135, 149, 154, 163,
  165, 167, 170, 171, 188, 190,
  197, 203, 223, 249, 282, 329
  *Dry 167*

# F

Fat 32, 33, 48, 82, 165, 168, 170, 204,
  220, 253, 256, 348
Fatigue 4, 21, 28, 33, 34, 37, 38, 40, 44,
  46, 52, 87, 145, 146, 150, 152,
  157, 169, 171, 173, 175, 176,
  177, 178, 186, 192, 194, 197,
  198, 200, 201, 208, 212, 233,
  235, 237, 240, 241, 247, 251,
  260, 264, 270, 282, 324
Fertility 67, 69, 71, 134, 188, 199, 233
Fever 222, 247, 266
Fibromyalgia 212
Fitness 86, 159, 241, 242, 364
Flu 148, 152, 157, 180, 185, 186, 191,

201, 212, 222, 230, 233, 235,
  237, 246, 247, 270
Focus 1, 65, 86, 115, 117, 134, 198,
  256, 283, 286, 340
Fungal 108, 123, 166, 232, 233, 262,
  276
Fungus 222, 232

# G

Gas 33, 61, 87, 201, 209, 245
Gastritis 62
Gastrointestinal 226
Genes 8, 130, 166, 180, 302, 303, 313
Gerd 272
Gingivitis 176, 180
Glands 109
Glucose 82, 83, 136, 168, 197, 230,
  236, 237, 247, 253, 266, 282,
  323, 324, 326
Gonorrhea 230
Gum disease 212

# H

Hair 34, 83, 153, 157, 161, 166, 167,
  176, 180, 182, 188, 191, 200,
  201, 233, 259
  *Greying 233*
  *Loss 188, 200, 201, 233, 259*
Hay fever 247, 260
Heachache
  *Migraine 43, 170, 171, 175, 197, 212,
  266, 282*
Headache 4, 43, 48, 51, 52, 62, 69, 135,
  167, 175, 197, 198, 212, 239,
  247, 266, 282, 325

# M

Malaria 230
Malnourished 27, 28, 29, 30, 32, 33,
    34, 35, 36, 37, 38, 39, 110, 113,
    132, 152, 155, 156, 158
Medication 16, 17, 39, 40, 41, 42, 43,
    44, 45, 46, 53, 63, 64, 81, 96, 97,
    102, 139, 148, 174, 181, 191,
    206, 207, 210, 211, 229, 230,
    232, 252, 257, 272, 277, 281,
    282, 284, 290, 292, 295, 296,
    301, 303, 327, 328, 337, 369, 380
*Contraceptives 53*
*Lipitor 42*
*Methicillin 231*
*Painkillers 53, 283*
*Penicillin 148*
*Statin 206, 210*
*Statins 42, 210, 224*
*Zocor 42*
Memory 14, 20, 114, 115, 116, 117,
    169, 176, 191, 197, 198, 208,
    222, 268, 272, 307
Menopause 220, 268
Menstruation 189, 194, 198, 200, 239,
    262, 266
Metabolism 41, 42, 220, 226, 227, 230,
    253, 256, 260, 325, 349
Metastasis 229, 255
Mindset 26, 48, 91, 96, 114, 117, 138,
    144, 168, 174, 176, 177, 191,
    201, 212, 220, 235, 249, 255,
    262, 340, 341, 363
Miscarriage 176, 199
MRSA 230, 231, 233

Muscle 22, 42, 44, 48, 69, 82, 109, 146,
    154, 169, 174, 175, 176, 185,
    186, 187, 188, 190, 192, 193,
    194, 195, 197, 198, 200, 202,
    203, 210, 222, 239, 241, 242,
    268, 282
*Aches 42, 241, 242*
*Recovery 242*
*Stiffness 48, 69*
*Strenght 69, 169, 175, 186, 197, 210,
    222*

# N

Nails 34, 153, 157, 167, 186, 191, 193,
    194, 200, 208
Nausea 43, 48, 59, 175, 188, 197, 212,
    224, 230, 259, 266, 296
Neurological 68, 266
Neurotransmitters 50, 114, 174
Numbness 175, 178, 188

# O

Obese 26, 27, 28, 32, 38, 184, 193
Obesity 25, 30, 32, 134, 212, 222, 230,
    263
Ovaries 274

# P

Pain 21, 22, 24, 37, 42, 51, 69, 73, 78,
    87, 154, 176, 188, 194, 198, 208,
    224, 245, 250, 251, 258, 259,
    263, 264, 266, 282, 296, 325
Pale 28, 153, 157, 177, 178, 198
Pancreas 172, 187, 190, 229, 230, 255
Parasitizes 62
Parkinson 94, 168, 169
Performance 237, 241, 249, 256, 302,
    317
Periodontal 148, 212
Plaque 180, 182, 195
Poliomyelitis 149

# W

# Heal the World
# by
# empowering
# other people
# to heal
# themselves

### ~Rob van Overbruggen

# Meet the author

Rob believes that healing is always possible. Healing is much more than just curing a symptom or disease. Healing is a holistic approach whereby the quality of your life increases to a level of full vibrancy and vitality. Behind every symptom there is either a stressor or a nutritional deficiency. Solving the emotional turmoil and replenishing the nutritional deficiency will allow the body to restore to full health and vitality.

You deserve a vibrant vitality, and most people do not realize the impact that stress and nutrition has on their total health. By teaching people the possibilities and empowering them to take action, healing is again attainable for everyone.

Rob helps people who want to increase their health and vitality.

* **People who want to take control over their own health.**
* **People with lack of energy**
* **People who want to lose weight**
* **People with emotional problems**
* **People with physical symptoms**
* **People who want to prevent disease from ever happening.**

Rob's passion for health and wellbeing started in 1994. At first he focused on mental health. With the use of hypnosis, neuro-linguistics and energy psychology, he was able to help people to reach their goals quickly and efficiently. After years of misery, clients were able to leave the room happy again.

In 1996, Rob started to study how the mind influences disease processes. He noticed that emotions and beliefs directly influence symptoms and diseases. A change in emotions and beliefs often allows the disease or symptoms to disappear. His first book, "Healing Psyche" (www.healingpsyche.com) was published in 2006. It explains the influence of the mind on the process of cancer from a scientific point of view. Many studies have already proven beyond a shadow of a doubt that the mind influences the cancer process. In this book he reveals the patterns that they all have in common. These patterns are universally applicable in the recovery of any disease or symptom.

His passion for nutrition came from a desire to understand and share about the facts and fiction of nutrition. Good proper nutrition has a tremendous impact on health, yet many people do not know or do not take action on that. Those who do take action often have not researched how to get the best of the best.

His mission is "Heal the World by empowering other people to heal themselves" and this book is in service to that aim.

## *"This book can save your life"*
## *Christiane Northrup MD*

Based on his knowledge and experience he devised several models to help people heal quickly and efficiently. His vision expanded to help people to become happier and healthier across the globe.

Using some of his advanced models he is now able to pinpoint the exact emotional stress that prevents the healing of specific symptoms. By releasing that emotional stress the body can repair itself again.

He makes complex materials simple to understand and to take action upon. Therefore his material is now used and described in at least seven different books, full length documentaries and many online and offline courses.

Rob conducts trainings, lectures and keynotes all over the word. The USA, UK, Australia, India, Egypt, Russia, South America and many other countries have already benefitted from his amazing, dynamic and fun style of teaching.

### *"... a combination of deep meaningful insights and standup comedy..."*

Over the last 20 years Rob has taught more than 4000 people to take more responsibility of their life, health and happiness.

His sought after trainings, both private and public, are considered the best in the industry.

You have a perfectly functioning blueprint inside that allows you to reach and maintain ultimate levels of health and vitality. This blueprint might not be fully expressed due to stress or lack of nutrients. By restoring your nutrient levels you too can become happier and healthier. Allow yourself to experience that.

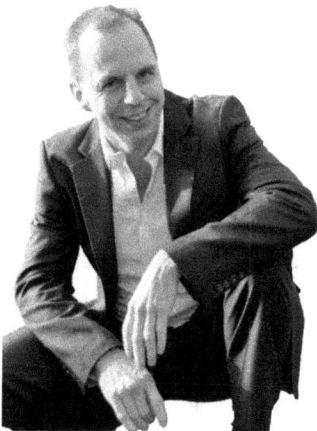

*Join Rob and his team wherever you can...*

*Contact: office@helpforhealth.com*

*Lets Connect:*
* http://gnoo.net/linkedin_rob
* facebook.com/helpforhealth

# Word-of-mouth is CRUCIAL
# for any author to succeed.

If you enjoyed this book then please let us know *WHAT you LIKED and WHY* so we can give you more of that. If you didn't please tell us WHO this book is more suited for.

Leave your review at amazon, even if it's only a line or two. Other people will be grateful for your insights too.

Thank you for this, your review is a **huge help** !"

**Click to review:**
**Amazon USA :** http://gnoo.net/uva_us
**Amazon UK  :** http://gnoo.net/uva_uk

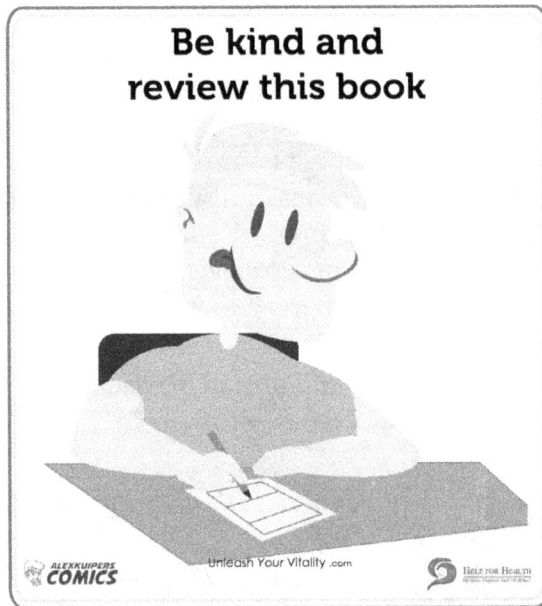

**Be kind and
review this book**

ALEXKUIPERS
COMICS            Unleash Your Vitality .com            HELP FOR HEALTH

**Download the special resource pack with additional chapters, exercises, checklists, whitepapers and other cool stuff.**

Click here to access your resource pack
(http://www.unleashyourvitality.com/resource)

*If reading on e-reader, tablets, phones or computers you need it for the exercises*

www.ingramcontent.com/pod-product-compliance
Lightning Source LLC
Chambersburg PA
CBHW071827270326
41929CB00013B/1916